THE GAME OF BUDGET CONTROL

TAVISTOCK

The International Behavioural and Social Sciences Library

INDUSTRIAL RELATIONS
In 13 Volumes

THE GAME OF BUDGET CONTROL

G H HOFSTEDE

First published in 1968 by
Tavistock Publications Limited

Routledge
2 Park Square, Milton Park, Abingdon, Oxfordshire OX14 4RN
711 Third Avenue, New York, NY 10017

Routledge is an imprint of the Taylor & Francis Group

First issued in paperback 2011

© 1968 Koninklijke Van Gorcum & Comp. N.V.,
Assen, The Netherlands

All rights reserved. No part of this book may be reprinted or reproduced
or utilized in any form or by any electronic, mechanical,
or other means, now known or hereafter invented, including photocopying
and recording, or in any information storage or retrieval system, without
permission in writing from the publishers.

The publishers have made every effort to contact authors/copyright holders
of the works reprinted in the *International Behavioural and Social Sciences
Library*. This has not been possible in every case, however, and we would
welcome correspondence from those individuals/companies we have been
unable to trace.

These reprints are taken from original copies of each book. In many cases
the condition of these originals is not perfect. The publisher has gone to
great lengths to ensure the quality of these reprints, but wishes to point
out that certain characteristics of the original copies will, of necessity, be
apparent in reprints thereof.

British Library Cataloguing in Publication Data
A CIP catalogue record for this book
is available from the British Library

The Game of Budget Control
ISBN 978-0-415-26441-9 (hbk)
ISBN 978-0-415-51388-3 (pbk)
Industrial Relations: 13 Volumes
ISBN 978-0-415-26510-2
The International Behavioural and Social Sciences Library
112 Volumes
ISBN 978-0-415-25670-4

G. H. HOFSTEDE

The Game of Budget Control

LONDON: TAVISTOCK

ASSEN: VAN GORCUM

First published in 1968
By Tavistock Publications Limited
2 Park Square, Milton Park, Abingdon, Oxon, OX14 4RN
In association with Van Gorcum & Comp. N.V.
Reprinted 1969
1. 2
SBN 422 73110 2

© 1968 by Koninklijke Van Gorcum & Comp. N.V., Assen, The Netherland

No parts of this book may be reproduced in any form, by print, photoprint, microfilm or any other means without written permission from the publisher.

Distributed in the U.S.A. by Barnes & Noble, Inc.

PREFACE

The research project upon which this book is based was made possible by a Research Grant from the "Commissie Opvoering Productiviteit van de Sociaal-Economische Raad", the Productivity Committee of the Social Economic Council in the Netherlands. I owe my thanks to the members of this Committee and in particular to its Secretary, Drs. J. E. Hagen, for his aid in obtaining acceptance of the project.

The project was supervised by Dr. H. A. Hutte, Professor of Social Psychology at the University of Groningen, to whom I am deeply indebted for his vision which stimulated me to get the project started, and for his support during the five years we cooperated on it. I also thank the other members of the Supervision Committee representing the c.o.p.: Professor Dr. J. Koekebakker, Mr. H. Luyk, Professor Dr. C. F. Scheffer and Professor Ir. H. K. Volbeda.

I owe my thanks to the Managements of the five Dutch Companies which were farsighted enough to admit a researcher into their plants, and also to the five executives of these companies who joined the Supervision Committee. Finally, within the plants, I am indebted to the one-hundred and-forty nameless interviewees who were willing to go through the stressful experience of a three-hour or even longer interview. I hope that their positive scores on the Attitude Survey item "I enjoyed participating in this c.o.p. Research Project" were not inspired by politeness alone.

Several experts both in the Netherlands and in the u.s.a. have been willing to advise me in various stages of the project. I thank Professor Dr. Chris Argyris, Professor Dr. J. L. Bouma, Professor Ir. W. Monhemius, Drs. H. Philipsen, Professor Dr. F. L. Polak, Mr. H. Reinoud and Professor Dr. Andrew C. Stedry. Mr. P. P. J. de Koning was my partner in all feedback sessions with interviewees. Mr. P. van Leeuwen was my advisor on statistical research techniques. Mr. Palmer B. Hager checked my use and abuse of the American language.

My successive employers, N. J. Menko N.V. and IBM World Trade Europe Corporation, created the opportunity for me to combine the research with my job. I thank them for this unique support.

In spite of all the substantial aid mentioned above, both the project and this book would never have been completed without the highly motivated cooperation of my successive secretaries, Miss Annie de Bruin and Miss Susan Haag, who went beyond the call of duty to make it succeed. Mrs. Hanneke van den Hoek-de Haas assisted me in coding the interview data.

This book is not dedicated to anyone. A dedication would be a poor compensation to the four members of my family who carried the burden of its creation. They suffered under the tightness of their husband's and father's time budget without having participated in setting it. I hope that the completion of this book will restore the scope necessary for the game aspect in our lives.

G. H. Hofstede

CONTENTS

PART IV: THE RESEARCH IMPLICATIONS

APPENDICES:

SUMMARY

The research project

This book is based on a research study carried out by the author in 1964 and 1965. This study covered the budget systems in six manufacturing plants in the Netherlands, belonging to five different industrial companies in different industries: printing, metal products, textiles, electronics and food. The study used both an analysis of company records and extensive interviewing. Altogether about 90 first-, second- and third-line manufacturing managers and about 50 controllers, budget accountants and work study engineers were interviewed: over 400 hours were spent in these interviews, which followed a structured pattern with both open and closed (pre-coded answer) questions. The research method was tried out in the first two plants and thereafter standardized for the remaining four plants. The data collected in the interviews are partly qualitative and partly quantitative. The qualitative data consist of the interviewees' comments, written down as literally as possible. The quantitative data consist of the coding of the interviewees' answers where coding was possible and of data collected from company records. A selected part of the quantitative data was subjected to a statistical analysis (correlation and factor analysis) with the help of a large-scale electronic computer. The results of this statistical analysis were used

I

to test some hypotheses set before or in the beginning of the project. They were also used to explore the data as fully as possible in search for relationships which had not been predicted but which looked meaningful for understanding the functioning of the budget systems in the six plants. Most of the conclusions in this book are based upon this exploration; they are therefore tentative and do not have the value of scientific proof, but they can serve as hypotheses for further studies.

The qualitative data and the statistically treated quantitative data were related to all relevant theoretical concepts available to the author, from the fields of accounting theory, the psychological theory dealing with motivation, and organization theory. The total investigation was guided by a systems conception: the budget system was seen as a part of the larger organizational system and having its own inputs and outputs. The purpose of the study can be interpreted as discovering the relationships between the inputs and the outputs of a budget system and explaining them in terms of different disciplines, mainly accounting, psychology and organization theory. The book is divided for this purpose into four parts:

part I   investigates the existing relevant theory;
part II   describes the research method;
part III applies the theory and the data collected in the research to draw the picture of the input-output relationships of the budget system and to arrive at conclusions;
part IV   translates these conclusions rather freely into practical recommendations for those actually involved in the process of budget control.

The budget system and its outputs

Not everything covered by the term 'budget' is included in the subject of this book. The interest of the project was in budgets as financial plans and in all financial standards and objectives for current operations. It also included technical, non-financial efficiency standards, at least to the extent that these were not primarily set for determining workers' wages but for determining managerial efficiency. The non-financial efficiency standards are the bricks the budget structure is built from. The study did not include investment or capital budgeting: it was limited to budgeting for current operations.

The outputs of the budget system which are considered in this book (see Chapters 1 and 7) are not the outputs in terms of accounting, like profit forecasts or budget variance reports. What is considered an output here is a contribution to the final goals of the organization. The final goals involved are assumed to be profitability in the interest of the stockholders and also the well-being of employees of all ranks. The contributions of budget systems to these goals which were measured in this study are the *motivation of managers to better performance* (as a contribution to profitability) and their *job satisfaction* (as a contribution to their well-being). An implicit issue in the total analysis is the conflict between organizational control and individual autonomy which is present in any management control system and which cannot be seen separated from the democratic ideals of large parts of present-day society. It has its implications for both the motivation and the job satisfaction of the people who were interviewed, but also for the author's attitude towards the total study.

The budget system's contribution to motivation is studied against the background of the psychological theory of job motivation. The motivation of a budgetee (a manager working in a budget system) is split into two components: the *relevance* of budget standards to the budgetee's tasks, and the *attitude* of the budgetee towards the system. Actual motivation to fulfill budgetary standards depends first of all on the relevance component; the attitude component can either reinforce or counteract the relevance component, but it cannot motivate by itself. In the context of job satisfaction of budgetees as an output of a budget system not only their satisfaction with their jobs in a narrower sense but also their feelings of pressure and anxiety in their jobs are considered.

Inputs of a budget system

A number of inputs into a budget system are related to the outputs of relevance, attitude and job satisfaction. Some of these were predicted on the basis of common sense or of research work by others and were found accordingly; other inputs were identified in the exploration of the data in this study. The inputs are classified and the various classes of inputs are described in the chapters 8 through 14 of Part III of the book. The first class of inputs deals with the policy of setting budgetary standards tightly or loosely. The fact that standards are set can have a very real meaning for a budgetee's achievement motivation. Need for achievement is a powerful motivator. In order for a standard to function as a standard for achievement it should be tight, so tight that there is a real risk of its *not* being attained. This means that there should be a difference between such standards and the performance actually expected which is used in coordinating budgets in the accounting system. On the other hand it appears that standards which are so tight that they are seen as impossible destroy motivation. An important role is reserved for the budgetee's superior to judge what level of standards an individual budgetee can tolerate. Interesting results have been obtained by comparing budgetees' evaluations of their departments' performance to the official performance data in the budget variance reports. In some plants the standards appear to be well 'internalized' and to agree with people's personal evaluation standards; in others they are not internalized at all. Besides the level of the standards other factors play a role here as well. These are illustrated in case studies.

Another class of inputs into budget systems deals with the process of participation in the setting of standards by the budgetee. There appears to be a difference in budgetees' reactions to participation in financial and in non-financial standard setting. Budgetees who have no experience in participation in financial standard setting (most of these were first-line managers) generally do not desire it. If they do participate, however, they appear to be much more motivated to fulfill the financial standards that are set. Participation in the setting of non-financial (technical) standards or objectives is considered a prerogative of any manager: they feel dissatisfied if they are not enough involved. The reaction of a budgetee to participation can be shown to be influenced by his personality or culture: authoritarians are less motivated by participation in budget setting than non-authoritarians.

The inputs into a budget system by the controller's department and work study staff consist of a technical contribution and a personal contribution. Both appear to have more negative than positive potential: the staff departments can easily have a negative impact upon the functioning of a budget system, but their possibilities for positively influencing motivation are limited: this depends much more on the superiors of the budgetees in manufacturing management. In the technical part of the staff's task the most important condition is that accounts follow responsibilities. Although this is self-evident and denied by nobody, it is not always done. Assigning responsibilities in accounting terms can even be rather difficult and increasingly so with the development of organizations towards greater interdependence between their parts. The effect of the periodic management information, sucn as budget variance reports, which staff departments produce, appears to depend strongly on its being accompanied by personal two-way communication between staff and line management and even more between the budgetee and his boss. For the staff's contribution to good personal staff-line communication it appears to be most important that the staff man is a competent specialist and that he tries to behave tactfully.

There are some interesting differences in attitude between staff people and line managers in general which undoubtedly play a role in their mutual communication. Staff people tend to assume more of a spectator role, identifying less with what goes on on the shop floor; they also have different satisfactions and frustrations in their jobs than line managers have. From a point of view of personnel management the staff people in this study appear to be somewhat less well managed than the line. The fact that the staff has more scope in spoiling than in improving the functioning of a budget system may be rather frustrating to staff people; the way to overcome this frustration is for the staff to conceive of its role as one of education.

Of all inputs into a budget system the behavior of the budgetee's boss bears the most crucial relationships to its outputs. The boss in his turn depends on his superior, so this type of influence often works plant-wide, however modified by the managerial skills of individual middle-level managers. Superior-subordinate communication can be shown to influence budget motivation through frequent person-to-person contact about budget results and through the use of budget results in performance appraisal. In these cases the increase in motivation will easily be accompanied by an increase in pressure feelings in the budgetee: he will be motivated mainly by outside pressure. This pressure may disrupt teamwork between budgetees and lead to undesirable effects like scapegoating and fighting the system. Superior-subordinate communication has positive effects on motivation without pressure symptoms when it uses group methods of leadership, like the use of department meetings and most important of all, the creation of a game spirit or an atmosphere of sportsmanship around attainment of budgetary goals. The game spirit represents motivation of the budgetee 'from within'. It depends strongly upon the leadership skills of the budgetee's superior, but also upon the way the system is organized: it presupposes a certain amount of free scope and the absence of rigidity, because a game requires a free area to play in. The motivation of adults through games is a neglected area in psychological theory; it could be called a blind spot of psychology, which is surprising because in daily life the motivating forces in game situations can be observed widely. The significance of game situations for our society as a whole has been shown most clearly by the Dutch social historian Huizinga, whose essay 'Homo Lu-lens' has inspired the conclusions in this study about the game aspect of budgeting. Technically the necessary scope in budget control systems to permit the game spirit to operate can be created by the application of statistical techniques similar to those used in quality control, like the use of control limits. The use of statistical techniques in budgeting is still quite rare. None of the five companies which were studied in this project used them, so that this book cannot report on empirical evidence of their effect. Their use is more meaningful for the larger corporation than for the small one.

All inputs into the budget system mentioned so far were *internal* inputs: they could be influenced by management. As budget systems are open systems in interaction with the environment outside the organization, we must also take account of *external* inputs. One group of external inputs consists of the type of people available as budgetees. Their age and generation are important: younger people appear to be more figure-conscious and more independence-oriented. Their length of service in the job will also influence the degree to which they make use of the figures offered to them: budgetees subjected to a system of job-rotation, who are more recent in a job, will automatically have to rely more on the figures for lack of experience as an alternative way of controlling their departments. The personality and the cultural background of the budgetees play a role, for example their 'job involvement': the inner urge to work hard and have tight goals for achievement. Another group

6

of external inputs is given through the technology of the plant, the cost structure of its products and the managerial climate created by its top management, who in their turn are influenced by the market they are operating in. The micro-analysis of management processes within the plants can be made more meaningful when supplemented with an interdisciplinary macro-analysis of forces working on the plant as a whole.

Part I - The Research Subject

CHAPTER 1

CONTROL. AUTONOMY AND THE BUDGET PROCESS

Summary of this Chapter

The budget control process is one of the forms of management control in general. Management control is a necessity for a business. To understand how management controls, I am presenting some interview data, which clearly demonstrate that control is spread over all levels in the hierarchy: it does not only reside at the top.

Management control within an organization can conflict with the individual members' desire for autonomy. The control-autonomy balance is of particular interest to social scientists today. It was of particular interest to me in studying budget control processes.

Two inputs into budget systems dealt with the control-autonomy balance, and both of them appeared meaningful for the way a budget system functions. One input is the amount of participation of lower-level management in the setting of the budgetary standards. The other is the creation of an atmosphere of sportsmanship around budget fulfilment: a game spirit among budgetees which presupposes some free scope for them in budget fulfilment. The importance of this latter input has become the main theme of this book.

Control

To an increasing extent the success of a business depends on its manage-

8

ment. The essence of management is that it gets things done through its relationships with other people. The effectiveness of a manager depends on the impact of these relationships on the others. The fundamental organizational link between the manager and the other people is the control process. In order for an organization to be successful, its control processes must be effective. What has to be done must be done at the right time, in the right way, with the right quantity and quality, and at the right cost.

Control is not limited to one level in an organizational hierarchy, e.g. top management. Control in various ways and to various degrees can be located at all organizational levels. 'Control' in this sense is partly synonymous to the concepts of power[1], 'say', authority and, especially, influence (Tannenbaum, 1962 and Mechanic, 1964)[2]. It is definitely not synonymous with its original meaning in French: inspection. In several European languages, as in the writer's mother tongue, Dutch, the same word exists, but it has kept the original French meaning. This is a source of frequent misunderstandings in translations from the English.[3] The research project described in this book provided an enlightening picture of the various ways in which control can be experienced. In a number of interviews with lower-level line managers and their staff counterparts, I used the 'control graph' as a research tool (Smith and Tannenbaum, 1963; Bowers, 1964). The method itself is described in Appendix A. It implies the question: "In general, how much say or influence do you feel ... (e.g. top management, first-line managers, workers) have on what goes on in ... (in this case I put: this plant)", and the answers were scored on a five-point-scale. After having received some spontaneous comments from interviewees explaining their choice, I decided to add another question: "What kind of influence were you thinking of while answering the previous question?" Altogether 78 persons contributed this time, and I analyzed their answers. Some

---

[1] 'Power' has an unpleasant sound about it. There is still a taboo in management literature to discuss power: "... the power process in management is like sex in the Victorian Age. Everybody knows about it, but nobody ever talks about it" (Dale, 1963). In the Netherlands, Mulder (1963 and 1965) has pointed to the power taboo and conducted research which shows the importance of power as a motivating factor.

[2] A list of '57 varieties' in the connotations of 'control' is given bij Rathe (1960).

[3] There is no exact equivalent of 'control' in the Dutch language. Possible translations are 'beheer', or (in combinations like 'quality control') 'beheersing'.

people gave more than one answer; altogether there were 135 contributions. They could be divided into 6 groups:

1. *Legislative decision-making* (20% of the answers)
   This implied the setting of rules, policies, methods, standards; decisions to invest and to enter a market.
2. *Operational control* (29% of the answers)
   Playing one's role in the organizational process. This implied performing, producing, working up to standards, avoiding mistakes, giving support.
3. *Hierarchical authority* (12% of the answers)
   This was the area of formal leadership and disciplinary action.
4. *Participation in higher management decisions by communication on the shop floor* (13% of the answers)
   This included group decisions, department meetings, being consulted by one's superiors, having a superior who listens to one's suggestions.
5. *Participation in higher management decisions by joint consultation* (7% of the answers)
   In Holland, every enterprise employing over 25 people is obliged by a law, dating from 1950, to maintain a Works Council, in which chosen representatives of the workers and the various levels of management meet with top management; however, this Works Council has no deciding power. The answers in this group dealt with these Works Councils.
6. *Personal, informal influence* (19% of the answers)
   This implied informal contacts, knowing people personally, influencing the atmosphere of the plant or department, enthusiasm, conflict, the strength of one's personality.

Out of this list, 1, 2, and 3 are roughly similar to the 'legislative', 'administrative' and 'sanctions' processes described by Morse, Reimer and Tannenbaum (1951).[4] Recently, Anthony (1965) has devoted a booklet to a classification of 'planning and control systems'. He distinguishes between 'strategic planning', 'management control' and 'operational control'. His strategic planning and management control are both

[4] Other analyses of control processes can be found in Bakke (1950) and Argyris (e.g. 1964).

10

covered by my group 1. His operational control is defined as "the process of assuring that specific tasks are carried out effectively and efficiently" and comes close to my group 2 (my choice of the name 'operational control' for this group, made long before Anthony's work came to my attention, points to an encouraging parallelism in thinking).

The limited percentage in group 3 – answers dealing with hierarchical authority – confirms the thesis of several writers, e.g. McGregor (The Human Side of Enterprise, 1960) about the inappropriateness of hierarchical authority as a means of control in modern industry groups. 4 and 5 are presently a topic of high interest in Holland (e.g. Meynen 1961, Lammers et al. 1965), but also in other European countries (e.g. Kolaja, 1960, Irle, 1963) and in the United States (e.g. Seashore and Bowers, 1962, Patchen, 1965). Category 6, inasfar it applies to the lower levels, is amply discussed by Mechanic (1964). It will be clear that our 6 categories of control were not evenly associated with all organizational levels. Legislative decision-making (1) had its peak for higher management; hierarchical authority (3) for first-line managers; operational control (2) and participation (4, 5) for workers. Informal influence (6) was relatively important for both higher management and workers, less for first-line managers. Staff departments were seen as exercising influence mainly by 2, 4 and 6.

We may now try to formulate a definition of control. Tannenbaum (1962) defines control as follows: " . . . any process in which a person or group of persons determines, i.e. intentionally affects, what another person or group or organization will do". To include more clearly operational control and also impersonal control processes, I will adapt this definition as follows: *"Control within an organizational system is the process by which one element (person, group, machine, institution or norm) intentionally affects the actions of another element"*.[5] Control is defined here as a process. The word 'control' is also used for the condition to which this process leads: a manager can possess control; his business can be 'under control'. This meaning of 'control' is used by Drucker (1964) who also stresses the difference between the singular 'control' and the plural 'controls'. 'Control' with Drucker is an end, 'controls' are the means or tools to achieve this end.

[5] In the case of machines etc., the intention is, of course, given by the designer of the system.

As soon as the actions of *people* are controlled, there arises a controversy between control and individual autonomy. Organizational success asks for effective controls, i.e. a high degree of control in the Drucker sense. It is not this same condition reducing the people controlled to cogwheels in a machine, to yes-men, to 'organization men'? Is it not basically incompatible with the ideals prevailing in a democratic society?

Some people try to deny this conflict, arguing that in business, at least, there is always enough room left for free action and initiative of the controlled. It may be that this is often the case, but again the reason may be that perfectly controlled business organizations are still rare; this fact does not refute the basic character of the conflict. It would be surprising if it did, for the conflict between control and autonomy is as old as organized human group life. Plato dealt with it 2300 years ago ('Politeia'); Rousseau discussed it 200 years ago ('Le Contrat Social'). The conflict has probably become even more acute in recent years. This is because of two opposing tendencies. On the one hand, technological development tends to limit the amount of autonomy left to large groups of workers in their jobs (Boers, 1962; Buiter, 1964), and organizations are developing more sophisticated and more perfect controls. On the other hand, there is a worldwide tendency toward democratization. The masses have reached maturity, social norms are shifting in that absolute dependence is no longer accepted; peoples ask for their share in shaping their own destiny. This development is not confined to business; we see it in world politics, in the family, in the church. (Evan, 1963; Groffen, 1963; Slater & Bennis, 1964).

The sharpening of the control-autonomy conflict in business has aroused modern prophets to defend the individual against organizational control: we can think of W. H. Whyte's 'The Organization Man' (1956), of Argyris' 'Personality and Organization' (1957).

From our previous discussion of the concept of 'control' we should recall that control by people at different levels within an organization is a matter of degree. This is clearly expressed by the six categories of control mentioned before: four out of the six are open at least as much to lower-level participants as to higher levels (the categories 2, 4, 5 and 6). However, their contribution to total control is relatively smaller (see the

Control Graphs in Appendix A). The conflict between control and autonomy is more precisely the conflict between the degree of control available to each member of the organization and the degree of control desirable to him.

In parallel with the definition of control given before, we can define autonomy as "*The degree to which a person within an organizational system is able to affect his own actions and environment*". Autonomy clearly implies to some extent the exercise of control over others.[6] Like control, autonomy has its part synonyms: in this case independence, freedom, self-determination, initiative, self-expression.

Reconciling control and autonomy

Social researchers have tried to reconcile control and autonomy. Using the Control Graph Technique, Tannenbaum (1962) has proved that the total amount of control within a given organization is not limited: control for one level in the hierarchy is not necessarily won at the cost of another level's control. On the contrary, in a number of cases there is a positive relationship between the control of a superior and that of his subordinates. Participation processes (my control category nr. 4) can lead to improved legislation (nr. 1.) and operation (nr. 2). In these cases, the total amount of control in the organization tends to be positively associated with organizational effectiveness.

Researchers have investigated the motivational aspects of autonomy. They have tried to prove that a control process which kills individual initiative is defeating its own ends, as it is frustrating the motivation of the controlled to really perform; and by asking for individual initiative one actually improves organizational performance (Coch & French, 1948; Likert, 1961, van Beinum, 1963; Hutte 1966). To a certain extent they have been successful. On the other hand, situations are known in which initiative-killing controls work very well (Argyris, 1958; Klein, 1965). Also, sometimes increased autonomy does not lead to higher

---

[6] Autonomy and control both are relative concepts. Mulder (1963) puts it: "Interpersonal power is always relative power: A has e.g. more power over B, than B over A" (p 211). We could speak of autonomy to the extent to which A has more power over *A* than B over A. Hutte (1966, p 12) describes relative autonomy as a practical and logical necessity.

motivation and performance (Vroom, 1959; French & Israel & Aas, 1960). The relationship between individual autonomy and organizational performance is by no means a straightforward one.

One might classify 'decentralization', as it is practised by the larger business corporations (by product and geographical area), as another attempt at reconciling control and autonomy. Top-level management defends it on effectiveness grounds: speed of decisions (Bonham-Carter, 1958). But obviously it is also in line with general democratizing tendencies. Within themselves, however, the decentralized units are generally still so large, that for the lower echelons of the organization the increase in autonomy is nonexistent.

In summary, what research and experience can teach us is that control and autonomy are neither fully conflicting, nor fully consonant. In any practical organizational solution we have to deal with both phenomena. One would like to maximize both control and autonomy. It is doubtful if this would ever be feasible, were it only because of the mathematical impossibility of the simultaneous maximization of two functions of the same variables. So the problem becomes one of optimizing: finding a solution giving an optimal balance of control (as a prerequisite for business effectiveness) and autonomy (as a consequence of our democratic ideals). It is well to remember that in the last resort what we call optimal is a matter of ideology. Managers cannot escape from ideological choices, and even social researchers are influenced by them.[7]

The limits of the study: the impact of budgets on lower-level manufacturing management

The research study described in this volume originated from consciousness of the control vs. autonomy polarity. It was designed to investigate management control processes on the one hand, and the possibility of individual autonomy within these processes on the other hand. As the investigation field so defined would be far too wide, three limitations were applied:

[7] In Europe, however, the ideological dilemma of the social researcher is sometimes exaggerated. See e.g. Bolle de Bal, 1965, and Hutte, 1966, p. 84.

14

1. The *budget control process* was selected as the particular part of management control to be studied. The researcher knew the budget process from inside experience; in an existing organization, he had felt and observed both the beneficial and the adverse effects of a tightening of budget controls. Besides, the budget process as a field of investigation was attractive because it has to do with something measurable. Budget levels and budget performance can basically be expressed in figures. Measuring is always a tricky problem in organizational research; it is a rare chance to find such easily available data.

To avoid misunderstanding, let me specify here what I mean by 'budget control' as it was investigated:

a. The interest of the project was in budgets as financial plans, in budgeting as planning translated into monetary terms. Budgeting has another face: that of forecasting. Forecasting is not management control, but just a way of supplying useful (though uncertain) information. As planning, budgeting is control: trying to shape the future. It was planning, not forecasting, which the project focused on.

b. Budgets are used both for investments and for current operations. The project, however, was limited to the study of control through operations budgets, not through investments budgets.

c. Budgets are based on standards, both financial and pre-financial, i.e. technical: quantities, hours, percentages, quality levels. Standards are the bricks the budget structure is built from. So these standards had to be included in the investigation.

2. The study would be limited to manufacturing organizations, the author's own experience being in this field. Within the manufacturing organizations, it would mainly look at "line" departments in which both the input and the output were largely measurable.

3. Interviews would concentrate on first-, second- and third-line managers. Several studies have been devoted to the impact of controls on rank-and-file employees: either tied up with financial incentives (e.g. W. F. Whyte, 1955; Marriott, 1957) or apart from financial incentives (e.g. Morse & Reimer, 1956; Dalziel & Klein, 1960). Studies of the impact of controls on lower-level management are less frequent. On the other hand, the effect of a superior's behavior on his subordinates may be very much dependent upon the way this superior is controlled himself, for example upon his influence with

his own superiors (Pelz, 1951) or upon the decisions he is allowed to make independently (Van Beinum, 1963, partly described in English in Reinoud, 1961/62). The human implications of the conflict between control and autonomy may be all the more severe at the lower and middle management levels (Kahn et al., 1964). I might even have gone higher up in the organizations and concentrated on top management, but I wanted to stay with the controlled rather than with the controllers. So this justified the choice of first-, second- and third-line management as a research field.

The input-output model

Budget control is exercised through definite systems which are part of the larger system which is the organization of the enterprise. Systems like the budget one must be studied on the basis of their *inputs* and their *outputs*. They are set up with certain purposes and the degrees to which they fulfill these purposes are their outputs. Management's contributions to the functioning of the systems as well as the external conditions which influence them are the inputs. The research project can be interpreted as analyzing the relationships between the inputs and the outputs of budget systems.

I chose as the outputs of budget systems:

1. Their contribution to the profitability of the company, at least that part of it which depends on the motivation of those performing against the standards to perform as well as they can.
2. Their impact upon the well-being of the people working in the system, measured by their job satisfaction and their signs of pressure and anxiety. Studies of organizations often consider the well-being of employees only to the extent that it can be proven to contribute to the profitability of the enterprise. In this case I am treating the well-being of the people in the system explicitly as an output in itself, even if it is not related to improved profitability. In this I follow the Charters of several modern corporations, which stress the corporations's responsibility for both the interest of stockholders and of employees (not to mention other interested groups like suppliers and customers).

Participation in standard-setting

As to inputs, the ones I was most interested in were those influencing the balance between individual autonomy and management control. I assumed that this balance would be influenced strongest in the process of the setting of budget standards. This is the 'legislative' element in the budget process. The setting of a standard is a distinct decision in which various levels of management and even non-supervisory employees may participate to various extents. My starting hypothesis was that the amount of participation of lower-level management in standard-setting would be an important input into a budget system leading to higher motivation to perform.

As the study progressed, I developed some doubts as to the importance of participation in budget-setting for motivation. From the interviews I had with lower-level line managers it became clear that many of them did not participate much in budget-setting, were still on the whole well motivated to perform, and seemed not at all eager to have their amount of participation increased. The final statistical analysis of my data showed where I had been led astray. In the first place we must distinguish between the setting of financial and of pre-financial, technical standards. Participation in the setting of financial standards is in general rather alien to those lower-level managers who have never experienced it. Once they participate, however, it does have a strong effect on their motivation to fulfill the budget. Participation in the setting of technical standards is quite normal to all managers and they feel strongly that they should participate here. If they do not, they feel less job satisfaction, but I could not deduce from my data that it influences their motivation.

The game aspect of budgeting

In the course of the study the importance of another input into the budget system became more and more apparent: an input influencing both motivation and job satisfaction and dealing with the control-autonomy balance as well. This was the general atmosphere around budget problems in a department, which was strongly influenced by the way in which the superior of the budgetee (the manager responsible for a budget) handled the feedback on results. This is not the 'legislative', but the 'operational' part of the budget process: what happens in the process of performing against the budgets that are set. I found that both motivation and job satisfaction of a budgetee are positively affected when the atmosphere created around the fulfilment of standards is one of sportsmanship; of seeing budget control as a game. This game atmosphere is related to the control-autonomy balance, because a game presupposes a certain free area to play in, a certain margin or scope or 'play' (the double meaning of the word 'play': 'game' versus 'scope' is significant). Without this freedom, there can be no game spirit. Budgetees need free scope in budget fulfilment.

The game aspect of budget control has become the main theme of this book. We will meet the theoretical background of it in the chapters 3 and 4, the research evidence supporting my conclusions in chapter 12, and the practical implications in chapter 15.

CHAPTER 2
BUDGETS IN ACCOUNTING THEORY

Summary of this Chapter

This chapter shows what I believe to be the major issues in the present accounting theory of budget and standard cost control. It starts with some data from the history of budgeting on both sides of the Atlantic. It analyzes the various functions and the various types of budgets; the relationship of budgets to non-financial efficiency standards and to costing systems. It distinguishes between the 'European' and the 'American' system of budgeting. It deals with variable versus fixed budgets and with a classification of budget variances; with management information systems and cost reduction drives; and with the role of the budget staff and the line departments in a budget system. This chapter also highlights some assumptions in the accounting theory of budgets about human behavior. I am trying to show that although accounting theory is 'neutral' about human behavior and accepts psychological data as fixed constraints, it does, in fact, not escape from making assumptions here. In as far as these may be false, the value of the accounting theory built on it is suffering.

Historical notes

The English word 'budget' stems from the French 'bougette'[1], a leather bag or large-sized purse, which travellers in former centuries hung on the

Footnote on page 20.

saddle of their horse. The treasurer's 'bougette' was the predecessor of the small leather case from which the finance ministers in countries like Britain and Holland still present their yearly financial plan for the state. So the meaning of the word 'budget' shifted to the financial plan itself, but originally only for governments and, metaphorically, for private persons.

The use of budgets as financial control tools for the business enterprise is historically a rather young phenomenon; it seems to date from around 1920.[2] In the United States, early budgetary principles were clearly derived from the budget technique in government (J. O. McKinsey, 'Budgetary Control', 1922, quoted in Reinoud, 1965; Becker & Green, 1962). Paradoxically, this happened in a country where governmental budgets were introduced much later than in Europe (only in 1921), because precisely their novelty got them more attention from the business-men (Limperg, 1965 and A. Mey, 1951). The other source of budgetary principles for business in the United States was the Scientific Management movement, which in the years between 1911 (F. W. Taylor's famous Testimony Before the Special House Committee) and 1935 was conquering the United States' industry. Budget Control Systems can be seen as a logical extension of Taylor's Scientific Management from the shop floor to the total enterprise. Large-scale applications of budget control in U.S. started probably in the depression years after 1930. In 1941, the results of a detailed survey of the organizations of 31 well-established U.S. companies, employing a total of 850.000 people, were published (Holden, Fish and Smith: 'Top-Management Organization

[1] In Mediaeval French 'bolgete', diminutive of 'bolge', vulgar Latin 'bulga', all meaning a leather bag. The English 'bulge' and the verb 'to bulge' stem from the same origin. There is wry humour in this for those having a budget but not feeling exactly 'bulging with money'. There is still an obscure use in the English language of the word 'budget' for the contents of any bag, i.e. 'a collection of things'.

[2] The Concise Oxford Dictionary 1960 still only refers to 'budget' as: the *British* Governmental budget, or a private person's budget. The Petit Larousse 1949 also mentions the use of budgets for Governmental bodies and private persons only, but in the 1961 edition the concept 'contrôle budgétaire' appears, related to the industrial enterprise. The Concise Webster Dictionary 1964 of the American language, however, quite generally describes a budget as "a plan adjusting expenses during a certain period to the expected income for that period", without referring to any particular field of application.

and Control'). Out of these 31, 16 companies used budgetary control in some form, or roughly 50%. In 1958, the results of another survey (Sord and Welsch, 'Business Budgeting') were published. Budgets appeared now to be used for over-all control of company performance by 404 out of 424 companies participating in the study, i.e. about 95%. In Europe, the idea of budget control for business was already formulated by the French organization pioneer Henri Fayol (1841-1925). It found, however, little application. A practical stimulus came from the ideas of the Czech entrepreneur Thomas Bat'a (1876-1932), who introduced the so-called departmental profit-and-loss-control, a kind of artificial free market economy as a tool for decentralizing his international shoe company into a federation of independently run small businesses. The inheritance of Bat'a's ideas can still be traced in Europe (Groot, 1960). The main inducement for the development of budget control in Europe, however, came from across the Atlantic.

In the Netherlands, the pioneer of budget control has been the internationally known Th. Limperg (1879-1961), Professor of Business Administration at Amsterdam University from 1922-1950. His Collected Papers have recently been published (Limperg, 1965). He started teaching Budget Control in 1925. Applications before World War II, however, were limited to a small number of farsighted companies, of which Philips' Lamp is the best known. Only after 1945 did budget control become a common tool in Dutch business, a time lag of around 15 years compared to the U.S. If we assume for a moment that this time lag was maintained, the 1965 situation in the Netherlands with regard to budget application is comparable to the U.S. situation in 1950 – somewhere between 50 and 95% application in 'well-established companies' – an admittedly rough definition. The Dutch writer Scholma (1961) thinks that "the number of really good applications (of budgeting) in our country is still limited" (p.V). In investigating the field for the present study (1963), I found several fair-sized companies where budgets had only recently been introduced or where the system was considered still to be in a pilot phase. In the five companies that finally participated in the study, budget control had been introduced:

1 before 1940, 3 around 1950, 1 about 1958. In some cases it had taken as much as 10 years for the system to reach a state where it could be used as a practical tool for line management.

This chapter will be devoted to the way budget control is seen in current accounting theory. I will do this by raising various issues, which I believe to be the most important ones:
- purposes and functions of budgets
- types of budgets
- budgets and non-financial efficiency standards
- budgeting and costing
- budgeting and decentralization
- fixed and variable budgets, and types of budget and cost variances.
- budgets and management information systems
- budgets and cost reduction drives
- budgets and the budget department
- budgets and the line organization.

Finally, I will try to show what assumptions on human behavior are made in the current accounting theory of budgets.

In all of this, I will draw both on European (mostly Dutch) and on American accounting literature.

Purposes and functions of budgets

Although different writers and practitioners put different stresses, there is common agreement that budgets are a management tool to facilitate the management task of leading the business towards its goals. I shall not enter into the discussion of what *are* the goals of a business here (see Chapter 1); but budgets are primarily intended to achieve the following results, be they considered as goals or as constraints for the business:

1. Higher profitability by coordinating efforts, avoiding waste and improving management decisions.
2. Optimal liquidity and the best way of financing the business because of advance knowledge of cash needs.

Budgets can achieve their purpose in various ways. A Dutch standard textbook on budgeting (A. Mey, 1951, following Limperg) lists the following four basic functions of a budget:

1. Economic forecast for the next period.
2. Authorization for the expenditure of money.

3. Quantified command to management to carry out a certain task for which it is held responsible, wholly or in part.
4. Standard for checking the legality of management's actions and the efficiency of its performance (A. Mey, 1951, p. 285, my translation).

In short (and freely interpreted), the functions of a budget are:
1. Authorizing
2. Forecasting
3. Planning
4. Measuring

The *authorizing* function of a budget is the traditional function of government budgets. In business, investment budgets have primarily an authorizing function. For operating budgets, the authorizing function is mostly subordinate to the other functions. What happens if the authorizing function of an operating budget is taken too literally, is illustrated by the story of a sales office, where at month's end all salesmen used to be sitting at their desks, because their car expense budget was exhausted! The *forecasting* function refers to those influences on performance that are external, i.e. outside control. One forecasts the weather, but one cannot 'control' or 'plan' it! Some parts of a budget are nothing more than forecasts: e.g. inflation percentages. In practice, budgets that could objectively be used for control, are sometimes not communicated to those in a position to exercise this control; and therefore these budgets remain just forecasts.

The main stress in the accounting theory of budgeting, as well as the main interest of this book is concerned with the functions 3 and 4: planning and measuring. Together, they form the *control* aspect of budgeting. The *planning* function is different from the forecasting function in that it is active: it tries to shape the future by coordinating resources (Oxford Dictionary: to forecast = to *estimate* beforehand; to plan = to *arrange* beforehand). As budgeting implies planning, so planning in a business implies budgeting: every plan made must eventually be translated in money, and in this way it becomes a budget. In the German language, the word for 'budgeting' is even derived from 'planning': 'Planungsrechnung' (plan accounting). The *measuring* function implies the use of the budget as a standard for performance. It is important to distinguish sharply between budgets for planning or coordinating and for measuring. This is illustrated by fig. 2-1:

FIG. 2-1. The differences between Standard, Planned and Actual Performance.

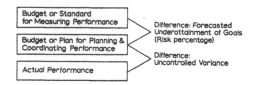

Budgets serving as standards for performance will obviously not always be attained. Not only a lack of effort of the person measured, but also external disturbances may lead to an underattainment of goals. The average risk of such an underattainment can sometimes be forecasted, so that the performance that is actually expected differs from standard performance. Planning, however, must be based on actual expectations. Therefore, when an underattainment of goals can be expected, the same budget cannot be used for measuring and planning purposes. The difference must be resolved by adding a risk percentage to the standard performance. This is technically no problem, but writers about budgeting complain that in practice the difference between the measuring and planning function of a budget is often not understood, leading to confusion (Maris, 1960 and Van Putten, 1960; also Stedry, 1960, who uses the word 'control' where I used 'measuring', Stedry p. 5; 'control' with me implies both measuring *and planning*). The textbook writer who states that "Budget costs ... represent *expected actual costs* under normal operating conditions, assuming a high, yet attainable, efficiency level" (Welsch 1964, p. 404) obviously wants to have the best of two worlds. Fig. 2-1 also draws the attention to the difference between planned and actual performance. If the planning has been good, only a random uncontrollable variance should remain here. In the accounting literature, very little can be found on the size and behavior of this variance. The econometrists Theil and Jochems, writing about 'The Art of Budgeting' (1960) are not able to contribute anything substantial to this subject for lack of data. Only the Holden, Fish & Smith survey report 'Top Management Organization and Control' dating from 1941, stated that "performance against the standards in well-established operations ran within 5%" (p. 160).

When budgets are revised periodically (mostly yearly) and performance improves constantly, the year-to-date (cumulative) difference between actual and average planned performance will follow a curve (fig. 2-2).

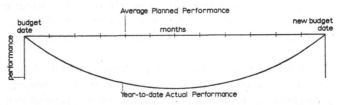

FIG. 2-2. Actual and Average Planned Performance over the Year.

The budget assumes an average performance over the year, which in the first half year is not yet met; therefore, these months show an increasing budget loss, which is compensated in the second half year. In the two companies within the present study where cost reduction was continuous, the fig. 2-2 curve was well known among accountants. In one of these companies even its shape was budgeted.

Types of budgets

In its most complete form, the budget is an extension into the near future of a business' financial reporting system: it culminates in a projected Balance Sheet and Income Statement for the next period (quarter, half-year, year or even longer). At least, a complete budgeting system should include a Profit Plan for the next period.

According to the Dutch textbook by Scholma (1961), the necessary components of a complete budgeting system for an industrial company of some size are:

1. Sales budget
2. Manufacturing budget
3. Inventory budget
4. Purchasing budget
5. Expense budget
6. Capital Investment budget
7. Cash budget
8. Integrated or 'Master' – budget

25

This list could have been extended with:
- Research and Development budget
- Manpower budget, and probably some others

No. 5, the Expense budget, has to be split over the various functions: sales, manufacturing, etc. A recent American textbook (Knight & Weinwurm, 1964) without going into as much detail, gives the same main categories as Scholma.

The study this book is about is only concerned with budgets of current operations (see chapter 1); these are the numbers 1 through 5. More particularly, since the study was carried out in manufacturing organizations, it is concerned especially with manufacturing budgets and manufacturing expense budgets, as well as with the standards these budgets are composed of.

Budgets and non-financial efficiency standards

The word 'budget' is commonly associated with something expressed in money, although for example sales budgets can be made in product units and manpower budgets in numbers of people.

Over-all budgets are composed of a whole structure of more detailed information. Some of this consists of either standard or historical data expressed in money, but much of it is technical, pre-financial information; efficiency standards expressed in weights, numbers, hours, reject percentages, efficiency ratios etc. Accounting textbooks stress that all available technical efficiency standards must be used in composing budgets (In the present study, however, I met a situation where communication between those responsible for setting technical standards and those administering the budget was largely blocked. This probably happens sometimes in practice in other companies outside my sample as well). For this study, I have analyzed the use of non-financial efficiency standards in the five companies along with the use of formal financial budget standards. I considered as a standard everything expressed in numbers which "carries with it the connotation of a 'goal' or 'desired attainment'" (Stedry 1960). I found that, although this has no basis in accounting theory, people in the plants often considered technical and budget standards to be quite different things. The probable reasons for this are:

1. Historically, they have different origines. Technical standards are a direct inheritance from 'Scientific Management', often first designed to set piece rates as financial incentives, and created in the workshop by industrial engineers. Budget standards are a refinement from old fashioned cost accounting practices, created in the office by accountants. In many cases, the responsibility for technical and budget standards still rests with different departments.

2. In Europe at least, financial information still has some status value; it has long been reserved to the owner of the business and his trusted bookkeeper, and has been taboo to other people; this magic is not yet fully removed.

3. It is believed that technical standards can mostly be objectively, 'scientifically' set and that they will generally assume ideal conditions; Financial standards are believed to be less accurate, more often based on historical data and guesses. This, however, is not necessarily true; it depends altogether on the methods of standard-setting in both cases. Recent criticism shows that 'scientifically' set technical standards may not be so accurate after all (e.g. Hesseling, 1963); on the other hand, converting a technical standard into a financial standard does not necessarily mean a loss of accuracy; financial standards need not be less 'ideal' than technical standards.

Budgeting and costing

The word *'costing'* is used for the predetermination of the cost of a product; the actual cost is calculated by *cost accounting*. Predetermination requires some standards; if these standards are at the same time used for comparison with actual cost to obtain product cost control, the system is a *standard cost system*. There are strong ties between the budget system and the standard cost system within a company. If all current costs are charged to products (which is often not the case), the total of standard costs for all products planned to be made during a year must equal the total budget during that year. The difference between the standard cost system and the budget system is, then, that the standard cost systems splits all costs product-wise and the budget system splits all costs department-wise. They are two ways of cutting the pie.

Costs and expenses in an industrial company can generally be divided into four groups:

27

1. Direct product cost, i.e. labor and material cost technically attributable to a certain unit of product.
2. Variable indirect (overhead) product cost, i.e. costs like most production machine maintenance witlich do not belong to 1., but technically still depend on the product volume made.
3. Fixed indirect (overhead) product cost, like production managers' salaries, which do not depend on the number of product units made, but still have some relationship to production.
4. Period costs or operating expenses, like the cost of administrative and personnel departments, for which the relationship with production is very loose.

The limits between the four groups are not absolute and every business has its borderline cases. Now from the above 4 cost elements, 1. is obviously more easily split product-wise and 4. more easily department-wise, while 2. and 3. take in-between-positions. Splitting operating expenses and overhead cost over products is a difficult and always arbitrary and artificial procedure (Riley, 1961). Splitting direct product costs over departments may also be difficult, because, for example, waste in one manufacturing department may be caused by mistakes in another; or total manufacturing unit cost may be influenced by lot sizes, which are imposed by sales.

There are two basic approaches to solving the cost split problem. One originated in the U.S.A. and has also found its way to Europe; the other is more specifically European (Groot, 1960; Blom, 1964). The first, 'U.S.'-system, tries to avoid artificial cost splits as much as possible. Costing in this system is based on variable costs only (group 1 + 2, 'direct costing'), or on variables + fixed overhead (group 1 + 2 + 3) Operating expenses (group 4) are covered from the margin between cost and selling price. Control in the U.S.-system is divided: costs involved in costing are controlled via a standard cost control system, while operating expenses and sometimes overhead costs are controlled via a budget system.

The second, 'European' system, is based on both *integral costing* and *integral budgeting*, the two processes fully interlocking and each involving all four cost groups; furthermore standard indirect and period costs are attributed to direct cost centers, i.e. those departments where the main functions of the business (e.g. manufacturing, selling) occur.

28

For the line manager, the U.S.-system is simpler to understand and to use; it is also more flexible in case of technical changes. The European system, on the contrary, is rather complicated; Van Erp (1965) remarks (and regrets) that at least in Holland budgeting has become more of interest to accountants than to line management. J. L. Mey (1960) rejects any system in which costing and budgeting are combined because standards used for costing should be based on other assumptions than standards used for budgeting. Yet some writers defend the European system on the ground that it will yield a better control of overhead and period cost; this is because the line managers, who get those costs attributed, are supposed to press their indirect department counterparts to keep costs down (Groot, 1960; Scholma, 1961, p. 169). In the present study, I found examples of both the U.S.-system (2 companies) and the European system (3 companies). I included both cost control by standard costs and cost control by budgeting in the survey. In chapter 10 I will show some findings about the operational effects of both systems.

Budgeting and decentralization

An issue which is narrowly related to the one about cost splits is budgetary decentralization.[3] Budgets can be seen as a tool for delegating authority: by making managers at lower levels responsible for a budget, top management delegates a quantified responsibility to them. In the larger corporations, delegation takes the form of decentralization or divisionalization. Decentralized units are generally run on a profit-and-loss base, ultimate control being exercised on the base of divisional profits (Holden, Fish & Smith, 1941, p. 208 ff.; Sord & Welsch, 1958, p. 64, ff.). The trouble, however, is that in many cases divisions are not fully independent, their *inter*dependence being precisely the reason why they belong to the same corporation (Shillinglaw, 1964; Zannetos, 1965). If one division supplies goods and services to another, transfer prices must be set and the divisional profits sometimes depend heavily on the level of

---

[3] A clear definition of decentralization is given by Simon et al. (1954): "An administrative organization is centralized to the extent that decisions are made at relatively high levels in the organization; decentralized to the extent that discretion and authority to make important decisions are delegated by top management to lower levels of executive authority" (p. 1).

these transfer prices. We are running here in the old dilemma of the Bat'a system (p. 21). Bat'a's solution, an artificial internal free market economy where prices were set by bargaining and divisions were free to go to outside suppliers, has rarely proven feasible. The Dutch economist A. Mey reacts sharply to a paper by A. M. Groot, dating from 1942, in which the latter defends the 'free internal market': " . . . the unity of strategy and the consistency of management would disappear. The company would succumb in anarchy and lack of policy" (A. Mey, 1951, p. 354, my translation). In practice, transfer prices in divisionalized companies are mostly set according to rules fixed by higher authority. The internal market is a guided economy.

Now the question arises how far one wants to go in decentralizing from a budgeting point of view. In the European-system of costing and budgeting (p. 28), where all costs are split over direct cost centers, each direct cost center will in fact show its profit or loss: every direct cost center is a 'profit center'. A manufacturing department makes its profit or loss against the standard manufacturing cost price; a sales department makes its profit from the margin between selling price and standard manufacturing cost price, deducting sales expense. The drawback of this system, as I mentioned before, is its complicatedness. In the U.S.-system there is a tendency to run only full units involving manufacturing and selling on the basis of profits and losses; all sub-units of these are only 'expense centers'. In order to maintain control over costs by sub-unit managers, the standard cost control is split over sub-units; each sub-unit gets only control data about those costs and factors affecting cost which he can readily influence. This is called 'responsibility accounting'; it has become particularly popular in U.S. business only in recent years (e.g. Gordon, 1963). In fact, it means a rapprochement between the U.S. and the European cost control systems. It runs into the same problem mentioned before, that it assumes an independence of sub-units which, as we have seen, does not exist. In practice, however, workable compromises are found.[4] The ideal of responsibility accounting is that it should be possible to show on an organization chart the cost variances belonging to the responsibility of each cell (Benard 1963).

---

[4] This is possibly too optimistic. Schleh (1963) thinks 'unique accountability' is simply an erroneous principle and defends a system in which results may be credited or descredited to two or three individuals.

In the present study I was able to compare different solutions to the decentralization issue. In as far as any practical consequences could be traced back to these system differences, they will be further discussed in chapter 10.

Fixed and variable budgets; types of budget and cost variances

One much-discussed issue in the accounting literature is whether a budget should be fixed or variable with regard to volume of sales, or other inputs. Protagonists of the fixed budgets are mostly those companies which can rely on their sales forecasts. When actual sales may vary widely from forecasted sales a variable budget (adaptable to various activity levels) is desired. The necessity for it can be shown from the well-known breakeven charts (e.g. Anthony, 1956, p. 331; Knight & Weinwurm, 1964, p. 45). Its background is the fact that some costs are fixed, and are incurred whatever the sales volume does. Lower activity levels lead to an under-recovery of fixed costs. This is one of the possible causes of budget or cost variances. Altogether, one can distinguish between at least 4 types of budget or standard cost variances:

1. Volume variances: caused by a larger or smaller sales and/or production volume, which leads to an over- or underabsorption of fixed costs.
2. Efficiency variances: due to a larger or smaller technical use of the direct production cost elements: direct labor and direct materials.
3. Expense variances: due to differences in cost per direct labor hour, materials purchasing price, or overhead expense against budget.
4. Accounting system variances: due to changes in the accounting system, for example, in the method of attribution of overhead cost. I am mentioning this fourth group because in practice these 'spurious' variances occur frequently and they can cause much confusion if not recognized properly.

A correct understanding of these 4 types of variances, which have quite different causes, is essential to the use of a budget as a control tool. A further refined analysis of operating variances is described by Mason (1964).

Budget and standard cost systems imply the publishing by the accounting department of budget performance and cost analyses. These are meant to be feedback information to the line manager, for him to base his actions on. They must therefore follow the division of responsibilities (see the previous discussion on 'responsibility accounting'). Henry Fayol is already supposed to have said 'Un budget c'est un monsieur' – 'A budget . . . is a gentleman'. In the U.S. survey of Budgeting Practices by Sord & Welsch (1958) it is reported that for 100% of all (35) companies where they conducted interviews:

– The company's plan of operations is subdivided to indicate the major areas of responsibility.
– The company's system of reporting is designed to pinpoint responsibility for performance.

Yet in the present study I found several cases where reponsibility and performance reporting systems did not coincide, mostly because the rather static reporting system had not followed recent changes in the responsibility organization (see chapter 10).

The responsibility structure delineates what reports must be given to what functions. There still remains to be decided at what level of the hierarchy within the function the information must be aimed: for example department manager, foreman or production operator.

Basically, out of simple logic:

1. the information has to be given to the level where decisions are taken.
2. the decisions have to be taken at the level where the outcome can best be influenced.

In the Dutch literature, there is some suspicion that in practice conditions 1. and 2. are not always fulfilled, that is, that the decision level and even more the information level are traditionally higher than optimal (Zoethout, 1955; Bos, 1955). It is advocated to compensate for the lack of information to the lower levels by quantitative non-financial information, mostly obtained outside the accounting system (Starreveld, 1962). The information to the higher levels gets gradually less detailed and more financial. The total information structure should be pyramidal, like the responsibility structure (Zoethout, 1955). The lower levels should receive the information at least as soon as or sooner than the higher ones.

Budget performance reports, cost analysis reports, and non-financial performance reports are all communication tools. A modern American budgeting textbook (Knight &Weinwurm, 1964) puts it:

"The entire process of developing the budget consists of a series of communications, written and oral, by means of which higher levels of management convey to their subordinates general policies and instructions, and subordinate departments prepare detailed proposals for coordination and approval by their superiors. The control process consists of a similar series of communications, carried out principally by means of budget reports, by which all levels of management are kept informed of the progress of the business and of the extent to which the budget program is actually being carried out" (p. 289).

This quotation mentions oral communication mainly for developing the budget, not for the 'control process'. In general, the accounting literature pays little attention to non-written control reporting. For the purpose of the present study, howerver, I have looked at all extant control reporting systems, whether written or oral (chapter 10, 11 and 12).

On the subject of written reports, there is a lot of literature: about their contents, frequency, timeliness, distribution and shape; whether to use tables, graphs, ratios or percents; whether to give only monthly or also budget-year-to-date figures; whether to use Electronic Data Processing or not (e.g. the appendices to Zoethout, 1955; Scholma, 1961; Starreveld, 1962; Stewart, 1963; Knight & Weinwurm, 1964). Two issues with regard to written reporting are of particular interest for the present study (see also chapter 10):

1. How and by whom is the decision made to publish a periodic report? For many companies that use written reports, managers start to complain of over-information (Stewart, 1963). Basically, written control information to a line manager falls in one of the three categories:

   a. Information required for making decisions.

   b. Information which does not lead to immediate decisions, but which gives useful background data and influences the general attitude and esprit de corps of the reader.

   c. All other information.

   The difference between *a* and *b* information is also noticed by Hall (1965) and Van Russen Groen (1965). All group *c* information is superfluous and acts as 'noise' which may damage the communication of group *a* and *b* messages (Toan, 1965). To avoid group *c* information, the procedure to create a new periodic report should be well studied, and existing reports should be periodically checked; this checking involves consultation between producer and future user about the 'if' and the 'how' (Bos, 1955; Eglin 1965).

2. How much self-help is required from the receiver of the report? Convictions and practices differ widely here. In some cases it is advocated that the budget department should include full explanations of variances (after consulting with the line) in the reports; others maintain that reports should give just the figures and that interpretation is a line task. Sometimes the budget department produces graphs; in other cases the drawing and updating of graphs is deliberately left to the line manager, to stimulate his involvement in the use of the figures (Zoethout, 1955).

Budgets and cost reduction drives

It looks contradictory that in companies using budgets and standard cost control, there should be a need for extra cost reduction drives. Yet one hears of companies where quite apart from the normal budgeting efforts cost reduction teams are set up or even cost reduction departments are installed (OEEC, 1961). Primarily in companies with a relatively stable technology, budget procedures tend to become so much routine that they no longer lead to investigation of all possibilities for cost reduction. As one writer (himself employed by a food company) puts it:

"The control concept is static in the sense that it emphasizes reaching and maintaining a stated level of performance. A standard cost system emphasizing only control can lull supervisors into complacency" (Henrici, 1965, p. 4).

This writer advocates 'superstandards' to measure the effect of long-term cost reduction. Bos (1955) recommends periodic changes in the subjects for control reports; Eglin (1965) thinks "that regular reports ought to be gingered up with shock special investigations . . ." (p. 79). In companies where technology is dynamic, one hears less from special cost reduction drives; here, there is no danger of the kind of blindness to possibilities for improvement described above. Technology dynamics and several other industry differences in the five companies participating in this study are discussed in chaper 14.

Budgets and the budget department

The accounting literature fairly unanimously stresses that the budget department is a staff department, supplying service to management, without formal authority over the line (Knight & Weinwurm, 1964, p. 6). On the other hand, its position within the company is considered a very important (and powerful) one. Ultimate responsibility for the budget department lies in most cases with the controller[5] (Sord & Welsch, 1958, p. 37; Starreveld, 1962, p. 218 ff.). The controller's function is an American creation, which in post-1945 years has been introduced to Europe (Blom, 1965). Of the 5 Dutch companies studied presently, 2 had a formal 'controller' (the same name was used), and in 2 more virtually the same function existed under a different name.

The dilemma between service and power of the controller and his staff is expressed by Anthony (1956):

"... it seems desirable to call attention to the natural, but erroneous, tendency to believe that the controller is the person who is primarily responsible for exercising control... Generally the controller is responsible for the *system* by means of which control figures are collected and reported, but the *use* of these figures in actual control is the responsibility of line management. The controller is something more than an accountant and something less than a chief executive. In addition to his accounting job of collecting historical figures, the controller may also be responsible for analyzing figures, for pointing out their significance to management, and for making recommendations as to what should be done. Moreover, he may police the adherence to limitations on spending laid down by the chief executive. In recent years the controllership function has become increasingly important in companies generally. The controller does *not*, however (unless *de facto* he *is* the chief executive) make or enforce management decisions. The responsibility for control runs from the president down through the line organization, not from the controller, who is a staff officer" (p. 279).

The impact of the budget department, as found in the present study, is discussed in chapter 11.

Budgets and the line organization

What, then, is the task of the line organization? ('line' defined as the hierarchy managing the main functions of the business, like manufacturing and selling). The line is supposed to have a task in

[5] In the Holden, Fish & Smith report (1941) the old name 'Comptroller' is still used (p. 159).

1. Setting objectives
2. Taking action on reported variances.

The setting of objectives is ultimately the responsibility of top management (A. Mey, 1951, p. 357); however, lowel level management takes a part in developing these objectives. Sord & Welsch (1958), in their 35 U.S. companies found amoung others the following common patterns of participation:

1. Lower-level supervisors responsible for a department or for a function participate in planning by actively developing or reviewing plans for the area supervised.
2. Successive screening and coordinating of plans occur at each higher level of management until plans are finally approved by top management (p. 25).

The actual use of participation for lower-level supervisors in the 5 companies is discussed in chapter 9.

Some companies have a *Budget Committee* which prepares the setting and reviewing of standards. The Budget Committee consists at least of some high-level line managers as well as the controller (Sord & Welsch, 1958, p. 302; Scholma, 1961, p. 16). Budget Committees are also known in Holland. Of the 5 companies studied, 1 used a Budget Committee, but only for investment budgeting.

The process by which a manager decides on the basis of periodically reported information is described as 'management by exception' (Anthony, 1956, p. 277; Starreveld, 1962, p. 31); only unfavorable variances are 'red-flagged' so the manager can save the energy of looking at points that are going well. His actions on the red-flagged cases will often be checked by his superiors. In the Sord & Welsch report it is stated that:

"Of the 366 companies indicating (by answering a written questionnaire) the type of action required when significant deviations occur, 52% require a written explanation of causes of significant deviations, 36% require an oral explanation of significant deviations, 49% require an indication of the corrective action taken, and 66% require a discussion of the significant deviation with the immediate superior" (p. 33).

Assumptions about human behavior in the accounting theory of budgeting

The Accounting Theory of Budgeting, as described in the previous pages, takes certain human reactions for granted. If budgets are to function as control devices, the way they control is through the behavior of people; in the first place through the 'budgetees', the managers made responsible for a budget. Therefore, the Accounting Theory of Budgeting is based on the belief that *budgets and cost standards act as incentives for motivating the budgetees*. Taking a closer look at what accountants write about budgets, one can find a number of assumptions about human behavior in it. Some of these are:

1. The only source of control is at the top of the organization; control lines flow from the top downward.
2. The relationship of lower levels to higher levels in the organization can meaningfully be described in terms of accountability.[6]
3. Goal-setting by the organization improves people's performance.
4. Having people participate in this goal-setting improves their performance still more.
5. People will take action when a deviation of an actual situation from a standard is reported to them.
6. The perfect manager manages by exception.
7. People react on control systems as individuals.

The first six of these assumptions can explicitly be illustrated with quotations from the accounting literature. The last one, the assumption that people react on control systems as individuals, is an implicit assumption, proven by negative demonstration: nowhere in the accounting literature I know of, is there any reference made to possible group reactions of people on the budgets they are made responsible for: to the development of informal group norms as to how to live and work with budgets, which standards to take serious and which not, etc. This phenomenon *is* recognized with respect to work standards for rank-and-file employees, but the thought has not been extended to budgets.

Calling the above ideas 'assumptions' does not imply that they are necessarily false. The results of this study in Part III suggest that the assumptions nr. 3, 4, and 5 are true under certain conditions, but that 1, 2, 6 and 7 are only true to such a small extent that in their general formulation they must be considered as misleading. This has, of course,

---

[6] Willemze (1964): "under the influence of accountants the main stress has often been put on accountability and making people responsible ... This means that more attention was paid to the *function* than to the *functioning* (p. 195, my translation).

implications for the practical value of the accounting theory of budgeting built on them.

In the next chapter I will look at budgets from the side of psychological theory and by this correct the above assumptions where necessary.

CHAPTER 3
BUDGETS IN MOTIVATION THEORY: THE GAME SPIRIT

Summary of this Chapter

Chapter 3 consists of two parts. In the first part, a short survey is given of the research done so far into the motivational aspect of budget systems. It culminates in a formulation of the problem for further research against the background of what was already done.

The second part is divided into nine sections. It tries, on the basis of existing psychological theory, to find all sources from which motivational effects of budget systems could be explained and predicted. It uses Vroom's model of motivation and Maslow's hierarchy of basic human needs. For various classes of needs, it investigates where they can be satisfied or frustrated through a budget system: physiological and safety needs, affiliation needs, recognition needs, achievement needs and independence needs. The chapter finally integrates all possibilities for positive motivation into a total picture, which is the picture of a game situation.

Budgeting and the 'human relations' movement

The Accounting Theory of Budgeting, as described in the previous chapter, has its historical roots in traditional organization theory. Just like the 'Scientific Management' movement of the followers of F. W.

Taylor, early budgeting theory started from a mechanistic, materialistic view of human behavior: it believed in the 'one best way' of behaving that could be thought out by specialists, learned by individuals and maintained by appropriate material incentives. The first official acknowledgement of unanticipated consequences of 'scientific management' was made through the Hawthorne experiments (1927-1932); as a result of these, the "Human Relations' movement started to compensate (or rather overcompensate) for scientific management. It was not long before 'human relations' ideas were penetrating into budgeting practice, in the form of 'participation in budget setting':

"By 1930 it was recognized in business circles that imposed budgets resulted in some dissatisfaction and advice was given to prepare them in the departments and have them revised or edited in the central offices"
(quotation from 'Budgetary Control in Manufacturing Industries', National Industrial Conference Board, New York 1931, in Becker & Green 1962, p. 394).

In the Holden, Fish & Smith report about management in 31 leading U.S. corporations (1941) it is stated:

"... it is considered important to secure the maximum possible participation of the organization in both the preparation of the budgets and in following progress ... By this process each person commits himself to a definite accomplishment against which he is checked and can check himself. The results are usually impressive" (p. 206-207).

The same ideas were also found in Europe:

"However, it is out of the question to impose budgets on departments without them having convinced themselves of the feasibility of their realization. Therefore, one ought to obtain the collaboration of those who have to do the carrying out, and to have them participate in the setting of the plans that concern them ... In this way, every manager really feels himself the responsible boss of a cell of the enterprise; he is an associate". (Caussin, 1947, p. 254-255, my translation).

Behavioral studies of budgeting

Both line managers and accountants have a tendency to maintain aprioristic theories about organization even if actual practice does not confirm them. For progress in organization it is necessary that people drop this 'normative' approach and start looking at organization 'empirically'. This means that they try to perceive the reality first, before applying any preconceived notions about how it should be. It implies a behavioral, experimental study of organization. In budgeting, to my knowledge only four attempts have been made to such an experimental study. All four were in the U.S.A.:

1. A study by Argyris (1952[a], 1953)
2. A study by Simon et al. (1954)
3. A study by Stedry (1960)
4. A study by Stedry and Kay (1964[a], 1964[b]).

In Europe, good behavioral analyses of budgeting have been made by Tovey (1963) and Zobrist (1965); both, however, are only based on the available literature and on subjective judgment and experience. The four experimental studies of budgeting mentioned above will now be described in more detail.

1. *The study of Argyris*

The Controllership Foundation of U.S.A. sponsored this study, the results of which have been published in a booklet 'The Impact of Budgetss on People' (Argyris, 1952[a]). From a methodological point of view this was a field study, using open-ended interviews of line and staff supervisors in four middle-sized manufacturing organizations. Its purpose was to explore the socio-psychological implications of budgeting; there were no prior hypotheses, so the study was fully exploratory. The findings of the study were summarized by Argyris as follows:

"... budgets and budgeting can be related to at least four important human relations problems:
– First, budget pressure tends to unite the employees against management, and tends to place the factory supervisor under tension. This tension may lead to inefficiency, aggression and perhaps a complete breakdown on the part of the supervisor.
– Second, the finance staff can obtain feelings of success only by finding fault with factory people. These (the consequent – Hofstede) feelings of failure among factory supervisors lead to many human relations problems.
– Third, the use of budgets as 'needlers' by top management tends to make the factory supervisors see only the problems of their own department. The supervisors are not concerned with other people's problems. They are not 'plant-centered' in outlook.
– Finally, supervisors use budgets as a way of expressing their own patterns of leadership. When these patterns result in people getting hurt, the budget, in itself a neutral thing, often gets blamed[1]". (Argyris, 1952a, p. 25).

[1] In a much later study by Argyris (1962) some similar effects of budgets like those quoted above are described (p. 229-230).

Argyris' study is full of picturesque verbatim comments of interviewees. For example one remark from a supervisor, which is typical for derailed 'human relations' thinking:

"Human factor, that's important. If you treat a human being like a human being, you can use them better and get more out of them" (p. 24).

About 'participation of the line in preparing budgets' as the commonly accepted way of applying 'human relations' thinking to budgeting, Argyris states that all controllers interviewed emphasized the need for participation, but in a somewhat peculiar way:

"We bring them (the supervisors) in, we *tell* them that we want their frank opinion, but most of them just sit there and nod their heads. We know they're not coming out with exactly how they feel. I guess budgets scare them ... some of them don't have too much education ... Then we request the line supervisor to sign the new budget. Then he can't tell us he didn't accept it" (p. 28).

Argyris calls this 'pseudo-participation'. He recommends to move the process of obtaining acceptance of budget changes to small group meetings of supervisors. This, and providing human relations training to finance staff, are his recommendations as a result of the project. Argyris' study, which aroused widespread interest, can be seen as the 'Hawthorne' of budgeting, for two reasons:

1. it gave the first official acknowledgement of its unintended effects
2. its stress on the human side of the problem was so great that it really overcompensated for the traditional budgeting theory. It showed only the negative motivational aspects of budgeting, and failed to show the positive possibilities for motivation inherent in the budget situation. Its influence lasted for many years (e.g. Miller, 1962); probably up to the present day.

2. *The study of Simon et al.*

Like the previous one, this study too was sponsored by the U.S. Controllership Foundation. Its results are published under the title 'Centralization vs. Decentralization in Organizing the Controller's Department' (Simon, Guetzkow, Kozmetsky & Tyndall, 1954). This was again a field study using open-ended interviews of line and staff managers; this time manufacturing, sales and other functions in seven different companies were involved. The research goal was on the one side more limited, as it was mainly aimed at investigating the result of the centralization – decentralization issue mentioned above; on the other side, it was broader, as it tried to weigh all aspects of the problem, human as well as 'technical', in terms of the overall effectiveness of the organization. Like the previous study, this was a qualitative one; it did not use 'counting and measuring' and statistical validations. Also, it did not start from prior hypotheses. What the study produced was a clear picture of the role of the accounting staff in budget and cost control systems, which tended to go far beyond mere 'techniques'. It led to a number of practical recommendations, both about the people and about the system. I will refer back to it in chapters 10 and 11.

A third Controllership Foundation Study, the one by Sord and Welsch (Business Budgeting, a Study of Management Planning and Control Systems, 1958), though it also uses data collected in the field, does not satisfy the conditions of a behavioral, experimental study of organization. It used interviews with 3-7 officials (mostly controllers and top line managers) in each of 35 companies, followed up by a mail survey of 389 other companies. By this approach, it did not escape from the usual stress on what *should* be, rather than on what *is*; its results deal almost exclusively with the formal aspects of budgeting.

3. The study of Stedry

Stedry's results are published in an award-winning doctoral dissertation: 'Budget Control and Cost Behavior' (Stedry, 1960). From a point of view of method, his approach was a laboratory experiment, using university students as subjects, preceded and followed by extensive mathematical model-building. Stedry's main research goal was to investigate the effect of *budget levels* on people's performance: 'the possibility of attaining better performance by the simple means of expecting it' (Stedry, 1960, p. 153). He applied the psychological theory of the 'level of aspiration' to what happens when people get budgets. He found that the performance of his experimental subjects was significantly affected by the budget level, and also by the fact whether or not they had to state explicitly "how much they hoped" to perform, i.e. their aspiration level. The results of his experiment and the additional theory lead Stedry to the conclusion that, in budgeting practice, performances can be improved by choosing budget levels attuned to the motivation structures of the individual managers; he therefore stresses the importance of the difference between budgets for 'planning' and for 'measuring' purposes as discussed in chapter 2 of this book. Stedry's study, to which I will refer again in chapters 4 and 8, is pioneering in its linking of psychological theory and budgeting practices. Of course it is not conclusive: he covers only one small area of the budget process; and the results of his laboratory experiment are not directly valid for the field. The reactions of his student-subjects are not necessarily the same as those of experienced managers. Churchill and Cooper (1964), in a laboratory experiment on the effect of audits, found vastly different reactions between students and industrial employees. Thus, repeating the Stedry experiment with an industrial group might also yield different results. Also, Stedry used a financial incentive in his experiment: whoever made his budget, earned a dollar; whoever missed it, lost a dollar. We do not know to what extent this a valid scale model of the incentives customary in business budget situations; for one thing, these are seldom immediately financial.

4. The study of Stedry and Kay

Recently Stedry was able to test the conclusions of the previous study in a field setting. The results have been published under the title: 'The Effects of Goal Difficulty on Performance' (Stedry & Kay, 1964[a] and 1964[b]). Methodologically, this was a field experiment: the middle way between Stedry's laboratory experiment and the field studies of Argyris and Simon et al., and an extremely difficult, but very promising method. The experiment was carried out among the foremen in a department of a large engineering plant; its purpose was the same as that of Stedry's previous study, to investigate the effects of budget levels on performance.

The results, although not statistically significant because of the small numbers involved, were interesting. Their practical implications are:
1. Over-all job performance is best if an individual is given just one very difficult goal to work on at a time.
2. Difficult goals must be used carefully: a mechanism must be built in

to revise the goal if the individual sees it as impossible; otherwise it will have an adverse effect on performance.

This study will be dealt with in more detail in chapter 8.

Formulating the problem for further research

When the present study was designed, the Stedry and Kay report was not yet published. From the literature then available the following picture could be drawn:

Budgets are intended to motivate managers to perform. There exist psychological processes which make such motivation possible (Stedry). However, in practice a high level of motivation through budgets has been found to be associated with pressure upon employees, inefficiency, aggression towards budgets and conflict between managers (Argyris). Participation of the line managers in setting the budget is advocated to resolve adverse effects, but in practice, there seems to be a lot of pseudo-participation (Argyris); moreover, the beneficial effect of (real) participation in budget setting has not yet been proven experimentally. The budget department plays an important role in the success of a budget system other than by merely using the right 'techniques' (Simon et al.); however, the system itself seems to be a source of conflict between staff and line (Argyris).

All this information came from the U.S. Personally, I had known budget situations in Holland where conflicts were not so noticeable, but where on the other hand nobody seemed to be very involved either; it was doubtful if these budgets motivated anybody.

So the problem was: *how to live with budgets and yet be motivated by them.* In the available information, it looked as if there were two dimensions in budgetee motivation through budgets:

1. The *relevance* of budget standards to the budgetee's tasks, running from low (Holland) to high (Argyris). The word 'relevance' is used here and throughout the book in the sense of the subjective or perceived relevance: as the budgetee sees it.

2. The *attitude* of the budgetee towards the budget or standards system running from negative (Argyris) to positive (Holland).

The challenge now was, *to try to discover the conditions that lead to both high relevance and positive attitude.* The present study was designed to answer this challenge. It had to be a field study (to an outside researcher, field experiments are virtually impossible). Unlike the field studies of Argyris and Simon et al., however, I tried to measure and count, and to apply the modern tool of correlation and factor analysis on an electronic computer to support the exploration. Also I formulated some beforehand ('ex ante') hypotheses.

An application of psychological theory to budgets

The four experimental studies quoted have drawn upon some psychological theory, especially Stedry. The remainder of this chapter will be devoted to a review of these theoretical issues, as well as of other elements of psychological theory that apply to the budget situation.

1. *Performance, Ability, Motivation*

The essence of the psychology of budgeting is, that budgets are designed as control devices, to (compare chapter 1, p. 11) 'intentionally affect the actions of people'. Budgets are intended to act as incentives for people to do a better (more efficient) job. The psychology of budgeting belongs to the field of *job motivation*. Job motivation is a special case of *performance motivation* and this again of *motivation in general*. 'Motivation', according to 'A Dictionary of Psychology' (Drever, 1952) is a 'term employed generally for the phenomena involved in the operation of incentives or drives'.

The study of motivation includes such unbusinesslike areas as the behavior of rats in a maze; it attracts different groups of specialists like depth psychologists, development psychologists and psychological field theorists; it deals with phenomena like sex, power, curiosity, affiliation, achievement and creativity. One recent European reference work, the 13-volume German 'Handbuch der Psychologie' devotes one full 900 page volume to motivation; out of this, 100 pages deal with performance motivation (Heckhausen, 1965). As a main source book on Job Motivation, I have taken the work of Vroom ('Work and Motivation', 1964[a]).[2]

---

[2] Other sources of relevant data I used were Kahn & Morse, 1951; Rotter, 1954; March & Simon, 1958; Cofer & Appley, 1963 and Heckhausen, 1965.

Vroom suggests that:

Performance = f (Ability x Motivation) (Vroom, 1964[a], p. 203)

(f stands for: 'is a function of').

In this, it is assumed that ability and motivation are mutually independent; in fact, 'ability' is defined here so as to include all characteristics relevant to task performance except motivational conditions (Vroom 1964[a], p. 200).[3]

2. Components of motivation

Vroom, in accordance with a number of investigators since K. Lewin, uses a model that can in a simplified form be represented as follows:

Motivation = f (Valence x Expectancy)

in which the concepts are defined as follows:

Motivation: the force to perform a certain act.

Valence: the orientation (preference of attainment above non-attainment) of a person towards a certain outcome of his act.

Expectancy: the degree to which a person believes a certain outcome of his act to be probable.[4]

The above-mentioned relationship has been simplified, in that it considers only one possible outcome of the act. In most cases, many outcomes will be possible. In this case, the relationship is:

Motivation = f [Σ (Valence x Expectancy)] (Vroom 1964[a], p. 18)

i.e. one has to add the valences of all possible outcomes, multiplied by the expectancies of these outcomes.

In the budget situation, the Vroom model must be read as follows:

[3] Heckhausen (1965, p. 669. ff) does not describe the relationship between ability and motivation vs. performance as multiplicative, but the survey of research data he gives fits in quite well with a multiplicative relationship, provided ability is defined so as to exclude motivation. Recently, Lawler (1966) has presented evidence that the multiplicative relationship is justified.

[4] 'Valences' represent the affective, 'expectancies' the cognitive element in motivation (Cofer & Appley, 1963, p. 774).

$$\text{Budget motivation} = f \, [\text{Valence of attaining budget}$$
$$\times \text{ Perceived influence on results}$$
$$+ \, \Sigma \, (\text{Valences of other effects of actions}$$
$$\times \text{ Expectancies of these other effects})].$$

The various concepts mean the following:

Budget motivation: the force to take actions necessary to attain the budget.

Valence of attaining budget: the preference of attaining the budget above not attaining it.

Perceived influence on results: expectancy of the effect of one's actions on budget results.

Valences of other effects of actions: the preferences for these other effects.

Expectancies of other effects: the degree to which the budgetee believes these other effects to be probable.

'Other effects of actions necessary to attain the budget' may be very varied: fatigue, conflict with subordinates, or not meeting other requirements, like quality standards. The 'other effects' are generally unintended and often negative; therefore, the product:

Valence of attaining Budget × Perceived influence on results

must have a sufficiently large value to compensate for them. The 'perceived influence on results' of the budgetee is his perceived '*operational control*' of the particular situation, as described in chapter 1.

The concept of 'valence' needs further clarification. Why does a person prefer the attainment of a certain outcome above non-attainment? Vroom suggests that "*means* acquire valence as a consequence of their expected relationships to *ends*" (Vroom 1964[a], p. 16, italics mine). Many outcomes are just means to other ends, though some outcomes are ends 'per se', for their own sake. The 'ends' involved can be defined as the basic needs, motives or goals of the particular individual ('needs', 'motives' and 'goals' are all used here in the same sense, the first two representing more the point of view of the individual, the third the point of view of the environment; I will in the following use only the word 'needs'). People prefer an outcome because they conceive it to be instrumental to other outcomes, and finally to fulfilment of one or more of their basic needs. In mathematical notation, following Vroom, this means:

Valence of outcome j = f[Valences of other outcomes
         × conceived instrumentality of outcome j to
         these other outcomes]

The 'other outcomes' can all finally be reduced to the fulfilment of basic needs.

Now in the budget situation, we have:

Valence of attaining budget =
         f [Valence of task-fulfilment by the budgetee
         × Conceived instrumentality of budget at-
         tainment to task-fulfilment of the budgetee
         + (Valences of other outcomes possibly re-
         lated to budget attainment
         × Conceived instrumentality of budget at-
         tainment to these other outcomes)]

The first half of the right side of this formula applies to the budgetee's desire to attain the budget just because he thinks this is part of his task. In the second half, the 'other outcomes' mentioned include both those intended and those unintended by the designers of the system. March and Simon remark that a 'stimulus' (like setting a budget) may have unantici-pated consequences because it evokes a *larger* set (= psychological set or frame of reference) than was expected, or because the set evoked is *different* from that expected (March & Simon, 1958, p. 35). This is clearly what happened in the budget situations described by Argyris (p. 41). Several examples of 'other outcomes' will be given in the next pages: expectance of good performance judgment or financial rewards, feelings of fairness or unfairness, feelings of pride or shame. They can lead to both positive and negative attitudes.

Thus, the valence of attaining the budget has been split into a task compo-nent and a non-task component. These components are approximately identical to the two dimensions of manager motivation through budgets introduced on page 45: the *relevance* of budget standards to the budgetee's tasks, and his *attitude* towards the budget system. Both components consist of valences weighted by conceived instrumentalities. The con-ceived instrumentality in the relevance component is the one relating budget attainment to task-fulfilment of the budgetee. It depends among other factors on the availability of alternative ways for the manager to do a good job, apart from budget attainment.[5] The conceived instrumentality in the attitude component depends on the availability of alternative ways to desired other outcomes. For example, to attain a good performance judgment, a budgetee may 'fight the system' and try to show the budget is wrong, instead of spending his energy trying to attain it. All valences in both components can finally be reduced to the basic needs of the budgetee, which will be discussed at length in the next section of this chapter.

Apart from being a component of budget motivation, the factor (budget) *attitude* may also influence the effectiveness of the organization along other lines. This is because the various side-effects of budgeting may generate conflicts within the budgetee, because some needs are fulfilled while simultaneously other needs are frustrated. For example: budget attainment may be expected to bring along a salary increase, but the process of getting it may mean a lot of trouble with subordinates. Now internal conflicts like this will lead to a search for actions that will relieve the conflict.[6] These conflict-relieving actions may have harmful effects upon the organization. One possibility is sickness absence of the budgetee; another one is blaming other departments and damaging interdepartmental cooperation; still another one is lower performance of the budgetee in areas not measured by the budget.

Although negative job attitudes may have no harmful effect on performance of certain routine tasks by non-managerial workers, for the more complicated task of a manager this harmful effect does exist:

"Emotional disturbance has little effect on stereotyped activity, but does have a disrupting effect on nonstereotyped activity" (Schachter et al., 1961, p. 211).

"As tasks become more varied and require greater training and skill, the relationship (between job attitudes and performance) appears to change progressively from the negative to positive" (Likert, 1961, p. 16).

Some of the effects of manager's attitude on the organization's effective-

---

[5] I have assumed (page 45) that relevance will run from zero to very strongly positive. The product of valence and instrumentality on the other hand, can attain negative as well as positive values. In fact, one could imagine cases of negative relevance, but this is unlikely to appear in practice (it would mean that the budgetee would consider himself to do a good job only if he did *not* attain the budget).

[6] A sociologist would describe the conflict in this example as a role conflict. Similar conflicts have extensively been analysed in Kahn et al, 1964.

ness may not be visible on the short term, but only over a couple of years (Likert & Seashore, 1963).
From the above-mentioned factors in budget motivation, I have tried to measure operational control, relevance and attitude. This will be explained at length in chapter 7.

3. Basic needs of the Budgetee

There is no reason to assume that the basic needs of the budgeted manager will be any different from the basic needs of other people. *Classification of needs* is a much-practised art in psychology (Thomae, 1965). Of all possible need classifications I will choose one that seems particularly well adapted to the business situation: the Hierarchy of Basic Needs as developed by Maslow (1954), also used by McGregor (1960).
Maslow's theory states that for most human beings needs can be 'ranked' into a hierarchy. In fig. 3-1 this hierarchy is represented by a pyramid,

FIG. 3-1. Schematic representation of Maslow's Hierarchy of Basic Needs.

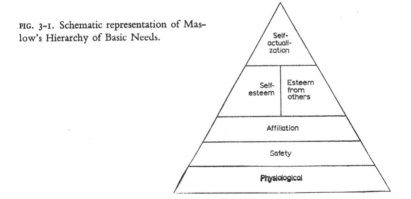

following Buchanan (1961). The hierarchy implies that some needs are more basic than others; these are shown in fig. 3-1 closer to the base of the pyramid. Maslow now states that "man is a wanting animal and rarely reaches a state of complete satisfaction except for a short time. As one desire is satisfied, another pops up to take its place" (Maslow 1954, p. 69). This process follows the hierarchy in such a way, that the needs higher up in the pyramid will emerge as soon as the more basic needs, lower down the pyramid, are satisfied to a reasonable extent; and only *if* the lower needs are thus satisfied. Lowest in the pyramid are the physiological needs, like the desire for food and rest. Until these are reasonably satisfied, they shut out all other needs. Next come the safety needs. In the job situation we may think here of job security, but also of a certain comfortable routine and predictability in the job situation. *Resistance to change* may result from frustration of safety needs. Safety needs are also active in the desire for justice and fair treatment by those in more powerful positions. Above the safety needs are placed the needs for affiliation, social contacts, belongingness, love. Berne (1964) quotes examples where social deprivation gives rise to temporary mental disturbances. The need for social contacts in any sane person is self-evident.

On the next level, Maslow puts the esteem needs. These can be divided into two subsidiary sets:

a. Self-esteem: the desire for strength, achievement, adequacy, mastery, competence, autonomy.

b. Esteem from others: status, recognition, appreciation of one's performances.

Although the word is not used by Maslow[7], the desire for *power* probably also belongs to the esteem group.

Highest in Maslow's hierarchy ranks a need for 'self-actualization'; a rather vague concept which deals with 'doing what one is fitted for': fulfilling the ideas one has about one's own destiny. This may e.g. mean creative activity, though creative activity may serve to satisfy other needs too (Maslow, 1954, p. 92). McCall replaces self-actualization by 'self-expression', which he describes as an 'elan to maximize', to achieve 'the greatest possible self-enrichment psychologically speaking'; he does not put this as a special motive at the head of the hierarchy but as a general principle applicable to all motives generally (McCall, 1963, p. 302). In any case both Maslow's and McCall's conceptions lead to the conclusion that at the top of the pyramid there is an area where need fulfilment can never be complete – there will always be room for striving for more.

[7] See the remark about the power taboo in the footnote on page 9.

The importance of Maslow's hierarchy for motivation is based on two considerations:

a. A satisfied need is no longer active in motivation.

b. Higher placed needs can only be active in motivation if the lower needs are satisfied to a reasonable extent.

One objection against the use of Maslow's theory is, that its total claims have never been proven experimentally, and are very difficult to test anyway. However, the theory accounts very well for some empirical phenomena. It is particularly applicable to the motivation experiments by Herzberg et al. (1959), which have been repeated by Schwartz et al. (1963), Myers (1964), Hofstede (1964b) and others. Most of these experiments have been done with white-collar or managerial employees.

In their most simple form, they consist of asking the subjects to record two situations: one in which they felt *exceptionally good*, and one in which they felt *exceptionally bad* about their job. The situations thus described are classified in a number of categories which Herzberg et al. developed on the basis of the material itself. According to the hedonistic principle that people are motivated towards what makes them feel good, and motivated away from what makes them feel bad, the classification of situations in the Herzberg et al. experiments must distinguish between positively motivating situations (recorded predominantly in the 'good feelings' stories) and negatively motivating situations (recorded predominantly in the 'bad feelings' stories).

Now it appears that the situations recorded predominantly as arousing good feelings have to do with factors like:

> the work itself
> achievement
> recognition
> responsibility
> advancement

These, Herzberg states, are the real *motivators*.

On the other hand, the situations recorded predominantly as arousing bad feelings have to do with factors like

> relationships with superiors
> company policy and administration
> salary
> working conditions.

These factors, mostly concerned not with the job itself – like the first groups – but with the conditions that surround the doing of the job, Herzberg calls factors of *hygiene*, for they can only prevent illness but not bring about good health. The antithesis motivators – hygiene factors is the fundamental conclusion of the Herzberg study (Herzberg et al., 1959, p. 81 and 113 ff). Although some of the hygiene factors, like salary, may be related to several basic needs (e.g. safety, affiliation, and esteem needs), the general tendency of the above list is that the motivators are related to needs considerably higher in the pyramid of fig. 3-1 than the hygiene factors. To understand this in the context of Maslow's Hierarchy of Basic Needs, we must assume that in our culture various occupational groups have developed standards as to to what extent various needs will normally be fulfilled. In the Western countries physiological needs are almost universally satisfied; safety needs to a great extent; on the other hand, the standard for satisfaction of for example achievement needs will be much higher in the case of some occupational groups, for example scientists, than for others, for example assembly line workers.

Now good feelings (leading to positive motivation) will arise when need satisfaction exceeds group standards, but bad feelings (leading to negative motivation) will arise when need satisfaction lags behind the group standards. An interesting implication of this is, that between various occupational groups the difference in factors giving 'good feelings' must be much greater than the difference in factors giving 'bad feelings': the latter have to do with the basis of the pyramid, which is the same for all occupational groups. This is fully confirmed by the findings of Gurin et al. (1960), also recorded in Gurin (1962), for a large sample (n = 2460) of the male, employed American population: The comparison between the two extreme occupational groups: professionals and unskilled workers, is given in fig. 3-2. We see the differences between groups are much greater for 'good' than for 'bad' feelings.

In the case of our budgeted managers, we can expect their group standard of need fulfilment to be fairly high on the fig. 3-1 pyramid. Therefore, attempts on budget motivation by building on the lower level needs for these people will be likely to have either no effect, or possibly a negative one. Positive budget motivation will only be possible by trying to

% of occupational group who mentioned

	professionals technicians	unskilled workers
good feelings only for factors related to satisfaction of "higher" needs	80	29
good feelings only for factors related to satisfaction of "lower" needs	2	29
bad feelings only for factors related to nonsatisfaction of "higher" needs	25	16
bad feelings only for factors related to nonsatisfaction of "lower" needs	31	46

(figures from Americans View Their Mental Health, by G. Gurin, J. Veroff, and S. Feld, Basic Books, Inc., Publishers, New York, 1960, Table 6.8, page 159 and Table 6.9, page 16.1).

FIG. 3-2. Comparison between 2 occupational groups as to type of needs satisfied in job.

fulfil the higher needs: esteem from others, self-esteem and possibly some kind of self-actualization.

In the following pages, I will discuss various ways in which budgets may motivate (positively or negatively) classified by the types of needs involved in the motivation process.

4. *Formal Rewards and Penalties in Budget Motivation, and the Role of Physiological and Safety Needs*

On the basis of Maslow's theory and Herzberg's experiments, we can expect the situations in which physiological and safety needs are involved to be associated with negative attitudes towards budget fulfilment, rather than with positive ones.

It is tempting to consider the total system of formal rewards and penalties connected with budget attainment and non-attainment, as being related to these 'lower' needs. Rewards may take various forms:

a. Budget performance may be one of the indications of overall performance appraisal, for the purpose of granting merit salary increases, status increases and promotions.

b. Budget performance may be the main or even the sole indication for the purpose mentioned under *a.*

c. Direct financial bonuses may be linked to budget performance (a situation similar to that of quota compensation for salesmen and piece rates for workers).

Penalties are the opposite of rewards. Ultimate possibilities are salary cuts, demotions or even dismissal in the case of a severe under-attainment of goals.

There is a rather cynical tendency in some managers to consider salary rewards and penalties as the modern version of the traditional 'carrot and stick' motivation, aiming only at satisfying physiological and safety needs. However, this is a gross oversimplification. As I mentioned before, salary may be related to several basic needs: it may well be mainly a basis for satisfying esteem needs like achievement and recognition, and a tool for obtaining social need gratification. "Like the psychologist's inkblots, money is an essentially neutral object which each man interprets in terms of his own habitual ways of thinking about the world and his relation to it" (Gellerman, 1963, p. 166). In the case of the budget, the effect of financial rewards and penalties will depend on this individual interpretation of each budgetee. This individuality in reactions makes financial rewards and penalties a risky tool, which may have negative effects as well as positive ones. In the Herzberg experiments, salary was referred to in both positive and negative stories; in fact, it was the most ambiguous of all factors found, but still the negative element was predominant.

Status increases and promotions are more clearly related to 'higher' needs, like esteem needs. Yet their use in connection with budget performance also involves some risk. The main risk in both salary and status/promotional incentives is that they will reinforce latent feelings of injustice about the budget. The desire for justice has to be placed with the safety needs. Feelings of injustice or unfairness about a budget are strongly demotivating. In practice it often happens that budget situations are felt as unfairly and arbitrarily handled. Evan (1961) remarks, that the junior or middle manager has 'no protection against arbitrary and capricious authority'; he 'appears to be a member of a new proletariat'. Thus, feelings of injustice can easily arise.

Some other situations within the rewards and penalties system,

where clearly safety needs are frustrated by budget practices, are:
- Management by fear. In some cases, superior managers or controllers use their authority to make subordinates comply with the budget because of fear of what will happen if they don't. This 'what will happen' is seldom openly stated; objectively it may not even exist; fear however, is a subjective and irrational reaction which does not need an objective basis.
- A stress on 'accountability'. If accountability functions at all, it is based on penalties: threatening job security. As one American manager puts it: 'If we don't make a profit, I don't have a job'. (N.I.C.B. 1963, p. 36).

Another way in which the budget can frustrate safety needs, quite apart from the rewards and penalties system, is by breaking the comfortable routine. In a dynamic system of budgeting, budgets may be perceived as 'vehicles of change' (Tovey, 1963); if the budgetee is not well prepared for this change, it may be felt as threatening.

5. The Role of Affiliation Needs in Budget Motivation

The budgeted manager is part of the social network of his organization. He will belong to various small groups in this organization, which to some extent will satisfy his *affiliation* (belongingness) needs. Unlike the lower needs, this group does not mainly induce negative attitudes; actual fulfilment of affiliation needs in the job situation can both exceed and lag behind expectations, so that the attitudes they induce may be both positive and negative.

The social relationships of the budgeted manager in his job in a very simplified scheme look like fig. 3-3.

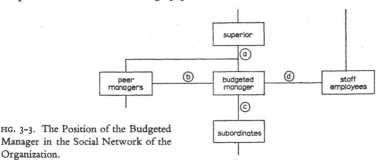

FIG. 3-3. The Position of the Budgeted Manager in the Social Network of the Organization.

The manager is shown in fig. 3-3 as having four main types of social relationships:

a. The relationship with his superior. This is generally a very important one to the budgeted manager. The superior is the direct representative of the organization's formal power over him. Moreover the superior is generally one of the members of the organization with whom he has the most frequent and regular contact about highly relevant matters. The power element in the manager-superior relationship (represented by the possibility of the superior giving financial, status and promotional rewards or penalties) has already been discussed in the context of the safety needs. If it has any motivational implications, there is a strong risk that these are negative.

It is my impression, however, that the meaning of the power element in superior-subordinate relationships in business is often overestimated. In ordinary day-to-day operations, the interpersonal relation and communication between superior and subordinate is of much greater importance for the functioning of the organization than the power relationship. In a sense, superior + subordinate are just a small group together – the smallest possible group, communicating and influencing each other, thereby satisfying partly each other's need for affiliation. Budget motivation may be reinforced by this small group relationship, if the superior himself is sincerely motivated by the budget and communicates this. Vroom (1964ᵇ, p. 78) reports similar effects between first-line managers and workers.

In those cases where superiors and subordinates do *not* have frequent interpersonal contacts, for example when the subordinate is in a geographically different location, the small group relationship between superior and subordinate will be much less tight. In these situations the budget motivation of the subordinate will be less dependent on that of his superior. The whole of chapter 12 is devoted to the superior-subordinate relationship.

b. The relationship between the budgeted manager and his peer managers. While considerable attention has been paid to group processes among rank-and-file employees, studies of group processes among managerial employees have been much more rare. I have already remarked that the accounting theory of budgeting does not show any acknowledgement that people react on control systems other than as individuals (chapter 2). However, there is no doubt that managers are fundamentally not different in their human reactions from any other employees, and therefore will also show group reactions, if the circumstances allow peer group formation. Such peer groups play an important part in satisfying affiliation needs on the job. Group membership means being subject to group pressure toward group norms; the budget motivation problem now becomes a group motivation problem. There are various possibilities:

- There is a closely knit group of peer managers with a group norm against the budget; the effect on the individual's budget motivation will be negative. "There is a fair amount of research evidence indicating that middle and lower management groups tend to develop protective mechanisms which, although more elaborate and considerably more costly to the organization, are psychologically identical to those developed by workers to defeat the administration of individual incentive plans" (McGregor, 1960, p. 150; see also Miles & Vergin, 1966). In the present study, another similarity between manager's group behavior and workers' group behavior towards standards is shown (chapter 8): the development of informal group standards, which may deviate from formal budget standards.
- There is a closely knit group of peer managers with a group norm reinforcing budget motivation; the effect on the individual's budget motivation will be positive. This situation is similar to the one described by Vroom (1964[b], p. 80) for the workers' level:
  "The highest level of performance should occur when the worker strongly desires acceptance by his co-workers, and anticipates that he will receive this acceptance only if he performs effectively".
- There is no strong tie between peer managers for situational reasons. This is a neutral condition with regard to budget motivation.
- Although a group formation of peer managers would be possible and obvious, budget pressure acts in a way that makes the managers department-centered and breaks interdepartmental ties. In this case, budgets themselves are a tool for frustrating affiliation needs; they can be expected to arouse negative attitudes. An illustrative example of this is given in Argyris' book 'Executive Leadership: An Appraisal of a Manager in Action' (1953[b]).

The positive use of group forces to back up budget motivation depends strongly on the formal group leader, most often the common superior of the budgetees.

Group participation in standard-setting will make the standards into group goals and improve performance to reach these goals, as was shown in an experiment by Lawrence and Smith (1950). Likert (1962) reports how the use of *group meetings in discussing results* for groups of salesmen is correlated with higher group productivity.

c. The relationship between the budgeted manager and his subordinates. In many cases the fulfilment of the budget depends on the performance of other people than the budgeted manager himself: his subordinates. Argyris (1960) describes how between manager and subordinates there can exist a 'psychological work contract', to the effect that subordinates will be left alone as long as they do not transgress certain informal rules. If budget pressure breaks this psychological work contract that makes the superior-subordinate contract viable, it will lead to negative feelings for both superior and subordinate.

d. The relationship between the budgeted manager and staff employees, especially those from the controller's department. Generally, the staff people will represent a different sub-culture within the organization from the manager's. Contacts with the staff are not so essential for the manager's affiliation needs. Therefore, the possibilities of positive budget motivation through line-staff contact are limited. Unfortunately, there are many possibilities for negative budget motivation by staff people. Argyris (1952[a]) has reported that the staff can be seen as people who constantly find fault with the line. The staff may represent a certain impersonal bureaucratic power that is resisted. It may be misunderstood, because it speaks another language, and therefore just be seen as a spoil-sport. It may be seen as the personification of disagreeable budget pressure. In the terminology introduced by Herzberg (see p. 54), the line-staff contact is hygienic in its potential, rather than motivating.

The Simon study of controller's departments, described on page 42, has indicated some ways to avoid negative motivation by the staff. The present study also found some clues here, which will be described in chapter 11.

6. The Role of the Need for Esteem from Others in Budget Motivation: Recognition by the Superior

Budget variances are a basis for appraisal of at least three types: self-appraisal of the budgetee, subordinate appraisal by his boss and activity appraisal by higher management (Shillinglaw, 1964, p. 153). Of these three, self-appraisal and subordinate appraisal have motivational implications. Self-appraisal is related to achievement motivation, which will be dealt with in the next section. Subordinate appraisal is related to recognition motivation of the subordinate, which belongs to the 'esteem from others' need group: it can also be related to the immediate attribution of rewards and penalties (see section 4 of this paragraph). Recognition for budget performance does not, of course, need only to come from the boss. Peers or staff may also give such recognition, but as the usual distribution of roles in a hierarchy is such that one looks to his superior for appraisal, I will restrict myself to recognition by the superior. Recognition may take the positive form of praise, or the negative form of criticism. In principle, there is no direct link between budget variances on the one side, and praise or criticism on the other side, because budget variances may be caused by uncontrollable causes through no merit or fault of the budgetee. However, in practice this is often forgotten, especially in the case of negative variances: "the reactions of executives to such situations as unfavorable deviations from standards are probably biased in the direction of 'doing something', of 'taking corrective action'. To some extent this bias probably arises out of the human inclination to pass judgment on others and on situations and to 'improve' things". (Bradshaw & Hull, 1950, p. 192). Therefore a demand for 'explanation' of a negative variance is felt by the subordinate as an implicit criticism or even threat. Unfortunately, the principle of 'management by exception' (the assumption that the perfect manager manages by exception, chapter 2, p. 37), tends to fix the boss' attention precisely on the unfavorable deviations and not on those cases where standards are met. The system is therefore strongly biased towards criticism for insufficient performance, and even unfounded criticism, rather than towards positive recognition. As budget systems are often operated, they are likely to frustrate the need for recognition of good performance by the budgetee, and therefore they are likely to arouse negative feelings here (Stedry, 1964[b], p. 9).

We must not, however, overestimate the effect that the system could have, even if good performance *were* recognized by superiors. Meyer, Kay and French (1965) state on the basis of a study in the General Electric Company, that although "criticism has a negative effect on achievement of goals, praise has little effect one way or another". In the Herzberg experiments, it is shown that the good feelings caused by positive recognition are generally quickly gone and relatively less enduring than good feelings caused by all other factors (the same, incidentally, holds true for the bad feelings because of lack of recognition; Herzberg et al., 1959, p. 72). It looks as if the potential of recognition as a motivator is limited to the short term, at least in our Western culture.

The doubts expressed here as to the adequacy of subordinate appraisal on the basis of budget performance as a motivational tool, actually hold true for performance appraisal in general. Neither subjective performance judgments (McGregor, 1957), nor objective measurements (Ridgway, 1956; Coleman, 1965), seem to be of much use in positively motivating subordinates. Meyer, Kay and French (1965) therefore recommend using appraisal only as a justification for salary action, and to have separate goal-setting interviews for the purpose of motivating subordinates. This takes us to the participation issue, which will be dealt with in section 8 of this chapter. The evidence about the effects of subordinate appraisal in budget motivation collected in this study is presented in chapter 12.

7. *The Role of Achievement Needs in Budget Motivation; Levels of Aspiration*

One of the assumptions about human behavior in the accounting theory of budgets mentioned in chapter 2, was that goal-setting by the organization improves people's performance. Some people, reacting to this, take the position that not goal-setting itself, but only the system of rewards and penalties associated with it has an effect on performance:

"What is not commonly understood is that the budget itself is not intended to act as a motivating force" (Shillinglaw, 1964, p. 154).

Contrary to the opinion quoted, however, there is evidence that the budget can act as a motivating force; what is not commonly understood is, when and why this is the case.

In fact, what we are concerned about here can be defined in terms of the mathematical relationship expressed on page 49, as the *valence of attaining the budget* per se, apart from any other outcomes.

"Succesful performance on a task or job may constitute not only a means or a path to the attainment of other goals, but also may be a goal in itself" (Vroom 1964[b], p. 80).

The basic need that successful budget performance can fulfill, is the need for *achievement*, classified by Maslow as a need for self-esteem. This is one of the higher needs in Maslow's hierarchy, so that it is more likely to be associated with positive motivation than negative. In fact, the Herzberg experiment showed achievement situations to be the single most powerful group of motivating situations for the interviewees (Herzberg, 1959, p. 72).

Now achievement, in order to be felt, must be measured by some standard. By definition budgets are such standards. If the individual sees his budget as a fair and relevant standard, it may be the vehicle for his achievement feelings. 'Fair and relevant' also means that the standard must be sufficiently objective to have meaning to others than himself; achievement implies evaluating himself against others.[8] The presence of objective standards for budgets, be they based on technological data, studies by acknowledged specialists, or comparison with relevant other units, will increase their value as standards for achievement. On the other hand, budgets based on subjective estimates, either by some superior or staff department, or by the employee himself, will have less value as standards for achievement. I will refer back to this when dealing with the participation issue (p. 67).

Actual achievement feelings will arise through self-appraisal, based on *knowledge of results* compared to the standards, i.e. in this case the budget variances. This presupposes that variances are reported regularly, timely

[8] Festinger (1954) in his Theory of Social Comparison Processes, a predecessor and component of his Theory of Cognitive Dissonance, hypothesizes: "There exists, in the human organism, a drive to evaluate his opinions and his abilities". For this evaluation, people use primarily 'objective, non-social means', and secondarily 'the opinions and abilities of others'. Further "In the absence of both a physical and a social comparison, subjective evaluations of opinions and abilities are unstable".

and understandably to those whose performance is reflected in them – a 'technical' condition not always fulfilled in practice.

Knowledge of results, as has been shown in various psychological experiments, leads to improved performance (Maier, 1955, p. 401ff; Gibbs & Brown, 1956; Cofer & Appley, 1964, p. 770-771). This is partly because it conveys information which can be used for acting more effectively on the next trial; but also partly because knowledge of results motivates through satisfying the achievement need. An interesting study in a related field was done some years ago in the Netherlands by Stok (1959). He investigated the effect of control systems using visual presentation of quality on workers' quality performance. He found that visual presentation of quality had both an information and a 'stimulation' (motivation) effect and that both were instrumental in improving performance.

A psychological concept of great importance for the achievement motivation through budgets is the *level of aspiration*, defined as: "The level of future performance in a familiar task which an individual, knowing his level of past performance in that task, explicitly undertakes to reach" (J. D. Frank, 1935, quoted by Lewin et al., 1944). Most psychological literature on level of aspiration goes back on an extensive literature survey by Lewin, Dembo, Festinger & Sears (1944). Recent summaries are given in the Handbooks by Cofer & Appley (1963), and Heckhausen (1965).

Lewin et al. explain the formation of a level of aspiration from a person's different valences and expectations of success and failure at various performance levels, which balance out at a certain level where total weighted valence is maximal (weighted valence = Σ valence × expectation for success + failure). Thus, the level of aspiration is a subjective borderline between performances considered predominantly successful and performances considered predominantly unsuccessful:

"The experiments show that the feeling of success and failure does not depend on an absolute level of achievement. What for one person means success means failure for another person, and even to the same person the same achievement will lead sometimes to the feeling of failure and sometimes to the feeling of success. What counts is the level of achievement relative to certain standards, in particular to the level of aspiration (goal line): if the achievement lies on or above the goal line, the subject will probably have a feeling of success; if it lies below the goal line he will probably feel failure, depending on the size of this difference and the ease with which the achievement has been reached" (Lewin et al., 1944, p. 374-375).

In practice the level of aspiration may be more of a border zone than a border line; also a person may have several levels of aspiration, depending on whether one asks what performance he *hopes* to reach or what he *expects* to reach; Rotter (1954, chapter VI) uses the term 'minimal goal levels' instead of 'levels of aspiration', which again may work out somewhat differently. Important measures introduced in the Level of Aspiration Theory are the

- *goal discrepancy* = level of aspiration
  — past performance
- *attainment discrepancy* = level of actual new performance
  — level of aspiration

Feelings of success and failure tend to be positively associated with attainment discrepancies, but only up to a certain limit; outside that, goals are not taken serious.

Now experiments have shown some indications as to the effects *of* and the effects *on* levels of aspiration. The effect *of* a level of aspiration can be expressed in terms of its goal discrepancy. *Positive goal discrepancies* are generally associated with *high motivation* and *good performance*. Three types of factors are reported to have effects *on* levels of aspiration:

a. Temporary situational factors, i.e. attainment discrepancies in the previous task. Child and Whiting (1954) have proven the following hypotheses:

- Success generally leads to a raising of the level of aspiration, and failure to a lowering.
- The stronger the success, the greater is the probability of a rise in level of aspiration; the stronger the failure, the greater is the probability of a lowering.
- Shifts in level of aspiration are in part a function of changes in the subject's confidence in his ability to attain goals.
- Effects of failure on level of aspiration are more varied than those of success.

They have found some evidence in support of another hypothesis:

- Failure is more likely than success to lead to withdrawal in the form of avoidance of setting a level of aspiration.

b. Cultural and group factors:

"It has been found . . . that nearly all individuals of western culture, when first exposed to a level of aspiration situation, gave initially a level of aspiration which is above the previous performance score, and under most conditions tend to keep the goal discrepancy positive". (Lewin et al., 1944, p. 337).

Ours is an 'achieving society'. McClelland (1961) has, in a book with this title, reported about extensive studies of the cultural element in achievement motivation.

Besides being influenced by the larger culture, the individual may be subject to standards valid for the group he belongs to – what performance is normal for this group – or to standards of other reference groups, which serve as calibration points for his own level of aspiration.

c. Personality factors:

Some people appear to be more motivated by a need to achieve success, while others show more a need to avoid failure. Success-oriented people tend to have positive goal discrepancies, failure-oriented negative ones; some failure-oriented people set quite unrealistic goals, either extremely high or extremely low, without having them affected in any way by actual results. Success-oriented people tend to prefer a calculated risk; failure-oriented people are more the 'gambler' type. The position of an individual between success-and failure-orientation is related to factors like his education, his age and his general experiences of success and failure in his lifetime; these general experiences lead to his *self-concept* and his confidence in his ability to attain other goals.[9]

We see that the level of aspiration both depends on and, in its turn, influences performance. There is a circularity in this process, which makes the good performers perform still better, and the bad performers still worse.

All of the Level of Aspiration Theory dealt with so far is concerned with levels of aspiration set without explicit external standards, like budgets. To test the effect on levels of aspiration of explicit budgets, Stedry (1960) carried out his laboratory experiment mentioned before. The issue was

[9] Vroom (1964b) applics the Theory of Cognitive Dissonance (Festinger, 1957) to explain the degree of consistency between a person's performance and his self-concept.

now to see to what extent external budgets influence aspiration levels and thereby performance – to what extent are the budget levels internalized? "A level of aspiration is fundamentally an operational goal. It is a base for action, stated with perceivable variables and in a simple way". (Starbuck, 1963, p. 58). If, in this quotation, we substitute 'budget' for 'level of aspiration', we get a sentence that would work well in any conventional textbook on budgeting. We see, therefore, that 'level of aspiration' is nothing but an internalized budget; which, however, not necessarily coincides with the formal, external budget.

This is confirmed by the results of Stedry's experiment. I will postpone the discussion of the experiments of Stedry, and of Stedry and Kay to chapter 8, where I can compare them with mine. Thus far we can conclude that a budget in itself can be a standard for achievement for a budgetee and in this way an important contribution to his motivation.

8. *The Role of Autonomy Needs in Budget Motivation; the Issue of Participation in Standard-Setting*

In chapter 1 I have expressed my ideological concern for the possibility of autonomy within the budget control system. The way this autonomy works, is that decisions are taken, or at least prepared, on the lowest hierarchical levels possible. Lower levels participate in decisions that usually have been reserved to higher levels. This is influence group 4 as described in chapter 1. 'Participation in decision-making' is a much used term. To avoid misunderstanding, I will refer to 'participation' only *as perceived by the lower level participant*. This excludes the 'pseudo-participation' described by Argyris (p. 42); my definition of participation is what Vroom (1959) calls 'psychological participation' (the term is also used in French et al., 1960). Participation in decision-making can assume various degrees. In the strongest case, the decision is fully left to the subordinate. In a weaker case, the superior takes the decision after hearing the subordinate. In a very weak case the superior explains his decision to the subordinate after it has been taken, and asks for questions. A full scale for the degree of participation will be given in chapter 9. Participation in decision-making can be exercised both by groups (group decisions) and by individual subordinates; it is useful to keep this difference in mind, for the motivational implications may be quite different.

Many experiments and field studies have proven now that under certain conditions (to be discussed below) participation in decision-making will improve the subsequent performance of the participant. Most experiments have been concerned with group participation. The classic example is the field experiment of Coch and French (1948) in the Harwood Pajama Manufacturing Company, Harwood, Virginia, U.S.A. Having groups of girls participate in the introduction of change in the production programme resulted in an increase in performance without any girls leaving, instead of the performance drop and high labor turnover usual on such occasions.

Another example is a laboratory experiment carried out in the U.S. by Bass and Leavitt (1963). They used business managers and supervisors as their experimental subjects. The subjects, divided into groups of three, performed simple tasks, for which:
– either they had planned in their own group
– or they were given the planning made by another group.

The experiment showed a clear tendency of self-planners to perform better than those operating others' plans.

Further examples can be found in Likert (1961), p. 43 and Vroom (1964ª), p. 220 ff; compare also the discussion of peer group influences in section 5 of this chapter.

Participation in decision-making by *individual* subordinates has, to my knowledge, only been studied in field settings. Recently, two studies in the U.S. have been devoted to joint goal setting by superiors and subordinates as part of appraisal and counseling procedures. One is a field study by Raia (1965) with the Purex Corporation, another a natural field experiment (i.e. a field experiment in which the experimental change occurred unintentionally) with General Electric Corporation (Meyer, Kay & French, 1965; French, Kay & Meyer, 1966). Both studies deal with goal setting for managerial or professional employees. As performance is always difficult to measure in these cases, these studies give only indications of performance improvement, no statistical proofs. Additionally, both report considerable improvements in attitudes. (See also my remarks about "appraisal" in section 6 of this chapter).

Why does participation in decision-making improve performance?

a. One reason is *communication*. Participation by a subordinate in decisions of a superior that affect him, serves to close a feedback cycle between superior and subordinate. This feedback is the essential condition for *learning processes* within the organization; it makes the organization adaptable to change; it guarantees a higher quality of decisions.

b. A second reason is *control.* I have quoted (chapter 1) Tannenbaum's hypothesis that the control of a superior and that of his subordinates can be positively related. This can be explained by a quotation from March and Simon (1958, p. 54) as follows: "The greater the amount of felt participation, the greater the *control of the organization* over the evocation of alternatives, and therefore, the less the evocation of alternatives undesired by the organization".

c. The third reason is *motivation.* Participation in decision-making can satisfy basic needs of the participant. There are several theories as to which basic needs can be satisfied by participation:

- The most obvious supposition is that there is a basic *need for autonomy* and independence at least in our modern, western culture: in line with the tendency towards democratization noted in chapter 1, "There is a widely held cultural norm of independence in decision-making that makes at least *pro forma* participation in decisions a condition for their acceptance without further exploration of alternatives" (March & Simon 1958, p. 54). In the Herzberg experiment, the third most frequently long-term factor mentioned in the 'good' stories (after 'achievement' and 'work itself') was 'responsibility' which included independence (Herzberg et al., 1959, p. 72).
- For group participation, the *need for affiliation* with the group will obviously stimulate performance to comply with group-accepted goals (compare section 5 of this chapter). In a theoretical paper, Patchen (1964) hypothesizes that participation in decision-making in general may lead to *identification* with the organization, which makes the individual more susceptible to *social pressures* from organization members (at various levels in the organization).
- Participation in decision-making can also be related to the *need for achievement.* In the same paper, Patchen hypothesizes that participation may help the individual to get a sense of *personal achievement* from reaching goals in his work. Participation helps to *internalize* the goals

that are set. In the light of section 7 of this chaper, we can interpret this function of participation in that it *stimulates the formation and formulation of a level of aspiration* (this is not to say, of course, that participation is the only way in which levels of aspiration can be formed).

– Argyris (1957[a], p. 191-192), dealing with 'participative' leadership, sees this type of leadership as fulfilling the individual's need 'to obtain optimum self-actualization'. This takes us to the top of the Maslow hierarchy (fig. 3-1). However, as stated before, self-actualization is a rather vague concept; it is difficult to apply it in practice.

It was not long before social researchers discovered that the performance-improving effect of participation in decision-making is conditional upon several other variables. Participation does not always work (Tannenbaum & Schmidt, 1958; Likert, 1958; Davis, 1963). Limitations to the effect of participation on performance can be found in:

a. Personality traits of the participant. Vroom has proven in a field study, that "authoritarians and persons with weak independence needs are apparently unaffected by the opportunity to participate in making decisions. On the other hand, equalitarians and those who have strong independence needs, develop more positive attitudes toward their jobs and increase in performance through participation" (Vroom, 1959, p. 327)

b. Experiences of successful participation in the participant, partly determined by personality traits in the superior. In the goal-setting field experiment with General Electric (French, Kay & Meyer) it was found that a high level of *usual participation* acts as a background factor which promotes the formation of strong personal goals and leads to favorable effects of experimental participation on subsequent performance.

"Under conditions of . . . low usual participation, however, experimental participation has strong *negative* effects on subsequent performance improvement" (French, Kay & Meyer, 1966, p. 18).

c. Cultural influences on the participant, as well as on the superior. I quoted before the Coch and French experiment, which showed the very positive effect of group participation in decision-making in the setting of a U.S. Pajama factory. One of the researchers involved was able to repeat the experiment several years later in a shoe factory in Norway. This time an increase in participation did *not* bring about significant changes in performance. One of the possible reasons for the difference is that:" The Norwegian workers had a stronger tradition of being organized in a union than had the workers in the American factory. This in turn can produce an attitude that the legitimate pattern of participation is through union representatives rather than direct participation" (French, Israel & Aas, 1960, p. 18). Business subculture in itself probably contains some stumbling blocks to participation; it has a strong autocratic tradition. This may be true in U.S.A. as well as in Europe: "... benevolent autocracy, while it is neither idealistic nor inspiring, is practical. It accepts people as they are and recognizes particularly that most people prefer to be led" (McMurry in Harvard Business Review, 1958).

d. The situation. Whether, in a particular case, participation in decision-making will in fact lead to improved performance, depends on a number of situational conditions, e.g.:
- Whether the subordinate possesses information and specialized knowledge that can contribute to the particular performance; or whether only the superior has such information and knowledge.
- To what degree the subordinate's effort is required for the particular performance, so whether his being motivated affects performance or not. Decisions for which the successful implication rests on the subordinate, offer a perspective for participation; the more so, if they may be associated with feelings of fairness and unfairness in the subordinate. Maier (1964) mentions the example of assigning a new typewriter to somebody within a group of typists as an attractive situation for group participation in decision-making.
- To what degree the task can be routinized or even mechanized. Leavitt (1962) stresses that there are many tasks for which an increase in the prescribed structure, so a decrease of individual say in their accomplishment, will lead to improved performance. He refers to the laboratory experiments of Bavelas, Shaw and others with communication nets between small groups of people (circle = decentralized, vs. wheel = centralized). In many cases, the more centralized communication network performs best, although overall satisfaction of the

participants is always higher in the decentralized network. Advanced experiments of this type have been carried out in the Netherlands by Mulder (1963ᵇ). He has shown that for a new and fairly complex task, the decentralized structure generally has the superior performance. If tasks are repeated, however, and thus become routine, the more centralized network soon wins. In the U.S.A., rather similar results were obtained by Carzo (1963). He found also that for complex problems 'loose' communication structures started off with a better performance, but in his case repeating the tasks led to equal performance of all structures.

How much independent decision-making is already present in a subordinate's task. Vroom and Mann (1960) showed in a field study that there were striking differences between two groups of employees in a U.S. delivery company. Truck drivers, who had an independent on-the-road job, had the most favorable job attitudes when working for an *authoritarian* supervisor who permitted little participation in his decision-making. On the other hand, parcel positioners, who worked in a simple routine team job in the plant, reacted most favorably when working for an *equalitarian* supervisor (who permitted more participation).

Which other, and may be more relevant, determinants of performance are present? In the above-quoted Norwegian replication of the Coch and French experiment, another reason given for the lack of correlation between participation and performance is, that with regard to the most relevant determinants of performance: the piece-rates and the group standards for production, there was no difference between the experimental and the control groups (French, Israel & Aas, 1960).

How much time is available for reaching a decision? Obviously, for emergency decisions – like acting in case of fire – there is no possibility for participation.

So far, I have dealt with participation in decision-making in general, without referring to the particular situation of budgeting. Now most of this applies equally to the budget situation. Basically, within a budget system, a subordinate can participate in various types of decisions:

a. Decisions on the structure of the system: e.g. which items will be included, which information will be given to whom, etc. (Bos, 1955, p.23).

b. Decisions on the setting of standards.

c. Decisions about actions on reported variances.

As was illustrated in the beginning of this chapter, the traditional concern is with *b*: 'Participation in the setting of standards' only. In chapter 2, the assumption was noted that "having people participate in goal-setting improves their performance still more" (than goal-setting alone). This sole concern with participation in standard-setting is an oversimplification. On the one hand, there is more in the system to participate in (*a* and *c* above); on the other hand, the use of participation in standard-setting has its limitations, which will be shown in chapter 9. Recently, a polemic about the use of participation in standard-setting has been published between Stedry (1964ᵃ) and Becker and Green (1962, 1964); the latter defend participation.

To my knowledge, previous to the present study there is no empirical, tested evidence of the effects of 'participation in standard-setting' in a budget situation on motivation. The evidence of the present study, which is collected in chapter 9, shows that participation in budget-setting does have a noticeable effect on budget motivation.

9. *An Integrated View of Positive Need Satisfaction through Budgets; The Game Spirit*

The past pages have shown a number of ways in which budgets may motivate positively or negatively, by either satisfying or frustrating basic human needs. It is now time to try to integrate these elements of motivation, to answer our basic problem 'how to live with budgets and yet be motivated by them'. For this reason, I have summarized the main positively and negatively motivating characteristics in budget systems in fig. 3-4. The table in fig. 3-4 is divided according to the types of basic needs mainly involved, going from 'safety needs' to 'autonomy needs'. One sees at a glance that in this sequence the number of negatively motivating characteristics decreases and the number of positively motivating characteristics increases. Many of the negative characteristics have to do with rewards and penalties and other side-effects usually connected to budget performance, but not intrinsically belonging to it; many of the positive characteristics have to do with the challenge of budget performance for its own sake: with the intrinsic aspects of the

Types of basic needs mainly involved	Characteristics in system positively motivating:	Characteristics in system negatively motivating:
Safety Needs (section 4 of this Chapter)		– Heavy stress on salary rewards and penalties, leading to possible feelings of injustice and unfairness. – Heavy stress on status and promotional rewards and penalties – Management by fear – Stress on accountability – Changes for which the budgetee is not prepared.
Affiliation Needs (section 5)	– Frequent communication budgetee-superior, developing in budgetee a positive perception of superior's budget motivation – Formation of coherent peer-groups of budgetees with norms reinforcing budget motivation, by using group methods of supervision.	– Stress on the power element in the budgetee-superior relationship. – Formation of coherent peer-groups of budgetees with group norms against the budget. – Breaking interdepartmental co-operation by budget pressure; making budgetees department-centered; divide and rule. – Breaking 'psychological work contract' between budgetees and their subordinates by budget pressure. – Controller's department exercising bureaucratic power through the system; being misunderstood and seen as spoilsports.
Esteem-from-others Needs (sections 6)	– Moderate use of praise as well as criticism – Separation of appraisal and goal-setting	– Bias towards personal criticism when unfavorable budget variances are shown – Management by unfavorable exceptions only.
Achievement Needs (section 7)	– Knowledge of results – Potential of budgets to be internalized into personal levels of aspiration	

Types of basic needs mainly involved	Characteristics in system positively motivating:	Characteristics in system negatively motivating:
	– Value of budget as a public standard for achievement, having meaning to others than the budgetee only – Balance of success and failure-experiences, adapted to personality, age etc. of the budgetee (see ch. 8) – Budgets seen as challenging (see ch. 8)	– Consistent failure-experiences (see ch. 8) – Budgets seen as easy – Budgets seen as impossible (see ch. 8)
Autonomy Needs (section 8)	– Participation in decisions to structure the budget and variance reporting system – Using external reference points for standards wherever available (see ch. 9) – Participation in finding reference points for standards. (see ch. 9) – Using participation in standard-setting where external reference points are not available, to an extent adapted to the need for autonomy in the particular budgetee. (see ch. 9) – Using standard-setting by higher authority where external reference-points are not available, also to an extent adapted to the need for autonomy in the particular budgetee. (see ch. 9) – Participation in decisions to act on reported variances	 – 'Participation' in standard-setting that is not perceived by the budgetee as such ('pseudo-participation') – Participation in the setting of standards for areas outside operational control. – Using participation in standard-setting indiscriminately (see ch. 9) – Using standard-setting by higher authority indiscriminately (see ch. 9)

FIG. 3-4. Summary of Characteristics in a Budget System Positively and Negatively Motivating Budgetees.

system. This conclusion is identical to that of Herzberg et al. for the total job situation: there is an antithesis between motivators and hygiene factors for the budget situation too.

This is illustrated by one of the side-outcomes of Stedry's budgeting experiment. After participating, the subjects filled out a questionnaire with a number of attitude questions. Three out of the eight questions dealt with the financial rewards Stedry had used: whether the subject enjoyed participating predominantly for the money, or predominantly for the challenge; whether the money rewards had made him try harder; and whether a money reward twice as high would have made him try harder still. For all three questions, those stressing the importance of money had significantly lower performance in the experiment than those not stressing money (Stedry, 1962, table 1-2, *my interpretation of Stedry's data*).

It will also be clear from the analysis in this chapter, that in budget motivation we are dealing with a very complicated phenomenon; we cannot isolate just one characteristic and use it or decide to avoid it; many effects will develop, whether we like it or not. Our problem of designing an optimally motivating budget situation is not solved by a recipe of do's or don't's. What the analysis and fig. 3-4 can do is indicate *the general atmosphere in which budget communication must take place*: it must foster the idea that budget performance is an end in itself, *existing for its own sake*, not primarily leading to some external reward.

Many activities in our society are carried out for their own sake; they are called *play*. Can budgeting be played?

The Dutch social historian J. Huizinga has legalized the 'playing man' with his essay 'Homo Ludens' (1938). In this, he has shown convincingly that to a large extent all human culture *is* play. Huizinga distinguishes between various levels of play: the primitive activity of animals and children, the solo skill exercises of children and adults, and the social games, existing in a regulated activity of a group or community, or of two groups against each other. Especially these latter, higher types of games are historically at the root of many elements of past and present culture: they can be traced in poetry and other arts, philosophy and sciences, law and business.

To avoid misunderstanding, let me stipulate that I use the words 'play'

76

and 'game' in the psychological sense; as defined in Drever, A Dictionary of Psychology (1952):

"Play: activity, physical or mental, existing apparently for its own sake, or having for the individual as its main aim the pleasure which the activity itself yields.

Game: organized play according to definite rules with a definite objective, and usually competitive".

This meaning of 'play' and 'game' is different from that used in the Mathematical Theory of Games, which is a branch of Mathematics dealing with the content of decisions in games, rather than with the process of playing (e.g. Vajda, 1960). It is also different from that used in the 'Transactional Game Analysis' of the psychiatrist Berne (1964), who calls 'games' the recurring sets of transactions people engage upon to gain a mostly irrational, psychological advantage, rather similar to the 'gamesmanship' described by Stephen Potter (1962).

Huizinga analyzes the characteristics that are the essence of 'play'. Amongst these are the following, all very significant to our subject:

a. Play is an activity carried out for its own sake.

b. It has a potential for high motivation and involvement of the players.

c. It entails a challenge for definite achievements.

d. It presupposes a certain free area to play in, a certain margin or scope or 'play', in the sense of chapter 1, p. 18, both in place and in time.

e. It is separated from real life.

f. It follows certain rules, which are voluntarily accepted by the players and conscientiously followed.

g. It has a potential for creating a team spirit. (Huizinga, 1938, chapter I).

I could add to this list, that because play is separated from real life, it is basically safe; a playing dog bites, but it doesn't bite through. Also, that play is something people engage upon out of their own free will: the players maintain their basic autonomy.

Although 'play' is opposite to 'earnestness', this does not mean that players are not earnest when playing. They know they are playing; yet they are fully involved and earnest.

Huizinga points to many play elements in present-day society. He does not, in the first place, include the most obvious element: organized sport life. He notes (p. 204) a paradoxical tendency in organized sport to lose its play characteristic and to become earnestness; contrariwise,

77

economic occupations, which started to be carried out for the sake of interest or need, are acquiring secondarily a play character. They develop an inner culture of their own, in which rules are valid that have no general finality outside their limited 'playground'.

Thus, business is a game. The quotation on the second title page of this book is from the founder of a great business organization. Huizinga quotes another great businessman (A. F. Philips): " . . . both my brother and I have, in fact, never considered our business as a 'task', but as a game . . .". How many managers in business, without stating it so explicitly perhaps, carry out their job as if playing a game? Many and often far-reaching decisions in business are in the last resort taken just because the manager likes taking them. This is not just because rationality in any human organization is limited; it is because these organizations have a rationality of their own, the rules of their game. It is reflected in a well-known slogan: 'There's no reason for it – it's just our policy'. It is one thing to note, philosophically, the game aspects in business, but another to try consciously to use them positively in motivating employees. 'Human Relations' literature seldom refers to play. An exception is a book by Fraser:

"We recognize . . . that sportsmanship is an admirable quality in a person and one which is linked up with emotional maturity, self-control, and the ability to make a strong competitive effort while at the same time keeping it within the framework of a set of rules. In our games environments, . . . we have got the relation between the personal qualities of the individual and the working of the group pretty well sorted out. *We might do well to transfer some of our concepts of sportsmanship to other groupings in life also*, and use them to interpret what is happening in our working life and our familylife. In these groupings the roles have not been so well defined nor do the conventions seem always to have the same kind of authority. If we accepted a similar code of behaviour to that which governs our sportslife in this country at the present day, many of our difficulties might be clarified" (Fraser, 1960, p. 195-196, my italics).

It is probably not by accident that this was written in Great Britain, where games have for centuries had a more important place in culture than probably in any other Western country. Another writer who pays some attention to play is Maier in 'Psychology in Industry' (1955), but he refers mainly to play as a necessity to replace work after retirement (p. 399-400).

One particular area where games have found official acknowledgement in business is as 'business games' for the purpose of educating managers (e.g. Hutte, 1965). The fact that the 'game model' for what happens in real-life business is considered valid, proves at least some openness to the game idea.

The motivation through games and play is a remarkably neglected area, a blind spot in motivation theory, which is all the more surprising in view of its ubiquitous presence in everyday life. There seem to be strong resistances to the idea that play is important; there is, besides, a powerful tradition in psychology to explain phenomena out of their finality to other phenomena, which resists the idea of activities existing for their own sake. Game motivation is discussed as a side issue in psychological textbooks. Play is an acknowledged subject in development psychology (Russel, 1958). However, in one recent motivation handbook (Cofer and Appley, 1964) play and games for adults are not even mentioned (except sex play), in another (Thomae-editor, 1965) on only two out of 900 pages is any reference made to adult play.

Maslow (1954) refers to play as an example of a relatively unmotivated reaction (p. 297-302) together with art, tastes, philosophy etc. This means that these activities are ends in themselves, and that they can all be components of the self-actualization Maslow puts at the highest level of his hierarchy of needs.

White (1959) introduces the concept of competence, of the satisfaction obtained from the ability to control one's environment, a satisfaction sought for its own sake. Gellerman, in interpreting White, gives evidence "that the games and horseplay of seven- and eight-year olds have something to do with events in the executive suite thirty years later" (Gellerman, 1963, p. 114 and 149).

I had been struck by the play element in budget control before entering upon the present study, without realizing its full implications (Hofstede, 1964[a], p. 275). During the interviews with line and staff managers, several of them spontaneously referred to aspects of the budget system in game terms. Tovey (1963, p. 1) quotes a British business executive: 'What is a budget?' 'It's a game – illegal but still a game'. And later (p. 5) 'These people ... begin to look at a budget as something of a game'. Recently in the U.S.A. Fuyuume (1965) has defended the game approach for controllers in working with operating management:

"A metaphorical comparison can be made between the profit and loss statement and a baseball score sheet. Such a comparison can often jolt a manager into realizing his deficiency in understanding the game of management" ... "The psychology of 'game participation' is constructive, while the approach of control for control's sake engenders an attitude of being oppressed" (p. 51). "It is important to gain the foreman's confidence as a participating player by illustrating that every action can materially effect profits" ... The point is, when supervision can think management terms and rules with the same facility and interest as their favorite game, then we have a management body that can begin to play the game as a team, with direction and purpose. That purpose is to make profits as there is no substitute for winning games" (Fuyuume, 1965, p. 52).

In stressing the game element of budgeting, let me make it clear that I do not want to do away with control. Stedry (1964^b, p. 16 ff.) criticizes writers like Argyris (1962), Mc. Gregor (1960) and Likert (1961), in that he feels they negate the need for planning and control. Although I do not necessarily share his interpretation, I have taken the warning not to neglect the formal organization point of view. Now the basic problem is how budgeting can be considered a game, because it is part of a formal, purposeful control system, and it should remain part of it. However, the answer is that this control system has repeatedly proven to be self-destroying when used in a direct, mechanical way. I is so complicated because of all the technological, economic and human elements involved, that in a mathematical sense its operation is 'over-determined' – like five equations with four unknowns. In order to make it viable, a 'play' or margin or tolerance or random element must be introduced into the system, and this is the condition that makes it possible to exercise budget control as a game. This 'play' must therefore be valued positively. March and Simon (1958, p. 126) describe an 'organizational slack' which is unintended play in the control systems of an organization. They relate this to intergroup conflict: if the slack becomes less in crisis periods, there will be more competition between groups for the scarce resources and more intergroup conflict. Their 'organizational slack' has a connotation of wastefulness. My 'play' on the other hand is a condition for reaching a psychological and economic optimum: for avoiding the waste of destroying people's motivation. I also find less intergroup conflict in 'play' situations (chapter 12); March and Simon's explanation can contribute in accounting for this.

The concept of 'play' or 'margin' in the control processes of an organization can be related to several other concepts.[10] The sociologist Merton

[10] These considerations are based on an exchange of views with Mr. H. Wallenburg, soc. drs.

stresses 'the need for privacy' for the individual within social structures. ". . . if the facts of all role behavior and all attitudes were freely available to anyone, social structures could not operate . . . 'Privacy' is not merely a personal predilection; it is an important functional requirement for the effective operation of social structure" (Merton, 1957, p. 375). Thomas, in describing the job situation of German metal workers, stresses the necessity for 'the hidden situation' (Thomas, 1964, p. 85, ff.). Levinson et al. describe in the report of a participative field study in the U.S.A. the element 'distance': "controls were reinforced by the foreman, who did not, however, breathe down their necks. He did permit them to play, still in controlled fashion, when it was appropriate to play" (Levinson et al., 1962, p. 76).

There are strong resistances to be overcome in business culture to officially establish this 'margin', because of both bureaucratic tradition and the Taylorist deterministic inheritance of the 'one best way'. However, in our changing society, this inheritance is outdated: as one researcher recently put it: "My own researches showed that a belief that there is 'only one best way of doing most things', is closely linked with the *inability* to maintain effective performance in changing conditions" (Pym, 1966, p. 81).

In chapter 12 we will see how the experimental data support the theory that a budget control system will have an optimal effect on motivation when there is a sufficient margin in the system within which budget fulfilment can be seen as a sport or game. This means several things: it means a motivation from within, not through pressure from outside (Bennis, 1961). Motivation through pressure from outside goes together with lower job satisfaction; motivation from within goes together with higher job satisfaction. It also means that no energy will be spilt in fighting the system: in a game people accept the basic fact that there are rules. It finally means, if the game is well played, cooperation. It is a social game, but in the sense that different departments in the organization are fellow players, not antagonists. The antagonist is the outside world: a real competitor on the market, an impending cost increase. Games are the more thrilling when played against strong odds. The only part of the game where departments are playing against each other is the game of standard-setting. Standards are often set by a game-like bargaining between line and staff. In chapter 9 it is shown that this bargaining phase can be a positive contribution to the total game, provided that certain conditions are fulfilled.

Creating the game situation demands a certain attitude of higher management and especially of the immediate superior of the budgetee. This is the really crucial factor. Technical provisions in the budget system can help to create the margin which is a condition for the game spirit. In the next chapter these will be introduced.

CHAPTER 4
BUDGETS IN SYSTEMS THEORY

Summary of this Chapter

Chapter 4 consists of five parts. In the first part, a technical control model of a budget control system is presented as 'the engineer's point of view'. In the second part, it gives a short description of General Systems Theory, and it shows how this can help us to integrate the viewpoints of various disciplines. The building of conceptual models of organizational processes is discussed in the light of General Systems Theory. These models can be descriptive or mathematical. The third part of the chapter gives five examples of mathematical models of organizations in which budgets play a role: those of Forrester and Roberts, Cyert and March, Bonini, Stedry and Charnes, and Mattessich. The fourth part shows a general descriptive model of a budget control system drawn by me, which can be seen as a map for the rest of the book. The fifth part introduces the concept of control limits, with its technical, organizational and motivational implications, and it shows how control limits are a technical tool to help creating the game situation in budget control.

The engineer's point of view

In the past two chapters, the accountant's and the psychologist's point of view about budgets were given. A third professional with a different

83

conception of our subject is the engineer. To an engineer, organizational control systems, like planning, quality control, standard cost control and budget control, all show an obvious similarity to technical controls, like the thermostat or the traditional governor of James Watt's steam engine. The block diagram of a technical control can serve as a model for these organizational controls. This model is shown in fig. 4-1. Let us take the case of a thermostat in a room heating system. Room temperature is continuously measured, and compared to a standard:

FIG. 4-1. Technical Control Model of
an Organizational Control System

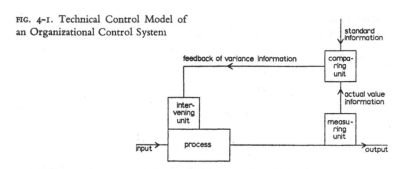

the desired temperature at which the thermostat is set, and which can be adapted between certain limits. If the room gets too cold, the comparison between measured and standard temperature shows a variance exceeding a certain limit, and a signal is sent to a device able to intervene in the heating process, for example by increasing the inflow of the water into the radiators. Now, the room temperature will increase; if it gets too high, the reverse process sets in. In this way, the room temperature will be held within narrow limits, provided that the outside temperature is not too low (in which case the capacity of the heating system is insufficient), or too high (in which case the heating system will be switched off altogether).

The essence of this control process is the negative feedback connection leading from measurement and comparison with standard to a compensating intervention. Now this is exactly what organizational control systems try to do. In our case of the budget, a standard is set; periodically, the performance of the process is measured and compared to the standard; variances are reported back to the budgetee, who is supposed to intervene to compensate for these variances, so that the next measurement of performance will meet the standard again.

The technical model of budget control is obviously a gross oversimplification. It does not show the motivational constraints of the budgetee, who is the 'intervening unit' in the system; it does not show how standards are adjusted; it does not distinguish between kinds of variances, etc.

An integration of viewpoints: the systems approach

There is a poem by Kipling about some blind men who study the elephant. The one who gets hold of a leg thinks it is a tree; the one who gets the tail thinks it is a rope; but none of them understands what the whole animal is like. Similarly limited are the viewpoints of either accountants, psychologists or engineers as I have pictured them, to understand the whole phenomenon of budget control. Somehow, we must try to integrate.

The study of organizational processes has long suffered from an atomistic approach. They have been cut into elements and these elements have been studied in the light of various specializations. Now this is necessary and right, but specialists have long been unable to get together again to reconstruct a total picture of the process studied. This again has limited the value of their specialized analysis, because elements are influenced by each other; by isolating one element, one changes it. Real progress has only been made when representatives of different scientific disciplines got together more than incidentally. This happened during World War II, and led to the new fields of Cybernetics or the science of communication and automatic control systems, and Operations Research or the application of mathematical techniques to problem-solving in organizations. Since then, several other areas have been disclosed by interdisciplinary approaches: a new Organization Theory, Information Theory, Decision Theory, a Behavioral Theory of the Firm. The most general of all these approaches is Systems Theory, a title applicable to all studies of integrated organized structures, composed of interdependent parts. Thus, it covers subjects in geography, biology, physiology, physics, engineering, economics, and social science. Its borderlines are extremely wide; it encompasses virtually everything that Systems Theorists want to include in it. More than a strict theory, it is a way of thinking: an openness to cross anv interdisciplinary borderline if necessary, and a basic appreciation of complexity.

Systems Theory is not new, nor revolutionary. It is described in the papers of Mary Parker Follett, written in 1927:

"We hear ... from both economists and psychologists of a 'want-system' by which they mean that we cannot satisfy one want or desire after another, that my different desires act on each other, and that the total want-system is different from the addition of separate wants. *Their use of the word 'system' is significant.* They are using it in the technical sense in which biologists use the word, in the sense of organized activity". (Metcalf & Urwick 1940, Dynamic Administration – The Collected Papers of Mary Parker Follett, p. 190).

In an attempt to offer a common terminology to describe general relationships for all sciences that deal with the empirical world, a General Hierarchy of Systems has been developed (based on the work of Von Bertalanffy and Boulding; my interpretation is borrowed from Johnson et al., 1963, p. 7-8 and Revans, 1964[a]).

This hierarchy has nine levels of complexity:

1. The static structure or *framework*, including not only mechanical or geometrical structures but also systems of classification like the one I am describing now.
2. The simple dynamic system with largely predetermined, necessary motions, or *clockwork*. Most of the theoretical structure of the physical sciences is at this level.
3. The closed-loop control mechanism or cybernetic system, like the *thermostat* I described. Its goals or 'standards' cannot be modified by the system itself.
4. The open or self-maintaining system, like the *cell* in biology. If external circumstances change, the system itself can adapt its goals to maintain the 'super-goal' of survival. In a very primitive sense, this is a 'learning' system.
5. The genetic level of the *plant*, consisting of a society of cells; now the system not only survives in changing circumstances but it can grow and reproduce itself.
6. The *animal* level, characterized by the brain, which creates the possibility for an 'image' or knowledge structure of the environment as a whole, to guide total system behavior.

86

7. The level of the *human individual*, who not only knows, but knows that he knows; who possesses language and symbolism.
8. The level of *social organizations*, of human communication, values and culture. Social scientists would probably prefer to split this into the level of the small face-to-face group and the level of the larger organization.
9. A level of *transcendental systems*, across the borderlines of knowledge.

Our ability to understand and predict how a system will behave decreases quickly as we go from the first level to the higher ones; while on the lower levels precisely determined mathematical formulations are possible, from about the fourth level onwards only general, statistical or vague descriptions are available. The value of the hierarchy concept is, that it shows how higher level complex systems are built from lower level, less complex subsystems. There is structure in systems; although elements are interdependent, not every element influences every other, but some elements have stronger relationships than others. Thus separate subsystems of lower levels can be identified within the larger total systems. Simon (1960) shows that the struggle for survival automatically favors the hierarchical system, composed of subsystems, above more complex ones.

The study of organizations

In studying organizations, like the present study is doing, we are operating at the eighth level of the General Hierarchy of Systems, where complexity is bewildering. Therefore, students of organizations have always tried to identify the lower-level subsystems within the total organization, which are more within our reach of understanding. The traditional organization theory of Taylor, Fayol etc. sought for second-level, clockwork type subsystems. After 1945, under the influence of the development of cybernetics, third-level, thermostat-type, subsystems within organizations were identified (not only dealing with planning and control, but also more general ones, like in Bakke's 'Bonds of Organization', 1950 and in the earlier work of Brown and Jacques at the Glacier Metal Company – see for example Oubridge, 1960). Ten years later, it became more customary to look for the fourth and fifth level, open systems[1] (Brown, 1960; Rice, 1963).

---

[1] The work of sociologists has contributed to the development of systems theories of organizations, see for example Mayntz (1964).

At whatever level one looks for subsystems, what is obtained is always a model, an abstraction of reality, not reality itself. Some models fit reality better than others, but somewhere every model has its limitations. The models that have been built for subsystems of organizations, have been used in different ways:

1. As normative models, to show what should be done. Traditional organization theory has been largely normative. In a sense, using a model in a normative way means forgetting it is a model. The applicability of normative models to organizations is to a large extent a self-fulfilling prophecy: lines of actions not corresponding to the model are never tried, and there is a tendency not to perceive results or evidence conflicting with the model.

2. As descriptive models, to understand better how a system works and to predict outcomes. The application of cybernetics to organizations has served to understand better the functioning of control and communication.[2] The engineer's technical control model for budget control is a primitive attempt in this area. 'Control' in the sense as defined in chapter 1 is always a central issue in Systems Theory. The cybernetic model works best for control inside the organization; where control involves the relationships with the outside world (Revans, 1965, p. 97 ff.) models are less easy to construct, as we are operating on the fourth or fifth level of the Hierarchy of Systems. The final purpose of improved understanding of organizational systems is, of course, to improve the decisions that must lead to desired outcomes. The levels in the System Hierarchy correspond with levels of decisions. At the second or clockwork level, we have the programmed operating decisions; at the third or thermostat level the control decisions, which can often be programmed too; at the higher levels the non-programmed decision for monitoring the lower-level processes, redesigning them, and changing parameter values (Simon, 1960, p. 49). Understanding these differences is in itself a reason for better decision-making.

---

[2] Wiener (1950) sees control as a form of communication: "When I communicate with another person, I communicate a message to him, and although this message is in the imperative mind, the technique of communication does not differ from that of a message of fact. Furthermore, if my control is to be effective I must take cognizance of my messages from him which may indicate that the order is understood and has been obeyed" (p. 16).

3. The next step is, to translate the models into mathematical language. Mathematics applied to second-level, clockwork-type systems was the area where Operations Research was very successful in the first fifteen years after World War II. The mathematical theory of simple closed-loop control mechanisms was known for a long time already. Recently, mathematics has been applied to the operation of more complex higher-level systems. Some examples of it will be described below. The use of mathematics, and Systems Theory in general, has received a tremendous stimulus from the availability of the electronic computer. Since 1955 it has become possible to actually solve problems of a complexity that made considering them only theoretical issues before. Still, the availability of the tool has a lead over its full use, and the perspective for further applications is wide. Computers can be used to actually solve mathematical equations, but an other way of using them, where analytical solving gets too complex, is for 'simulation' – a step-by-step calculation of successive rounds in time, just to see what happens. As this takes an enormous volume of calculation, it can only be done on a computer.

The use of mathematics is both a promising and a debatable issue. Lewin (1951, Chapter II) has stressed that mathematics has both a qualitative and a quantitative function: more than being a mere tool, it guides thought to a sharper analysis. This holds true very much, too, for computer use. The influence of computer logic in all kinds of scientific and practical fields has led to more accurate definitions and the resolving of ambiguities. Thus, computers have stimulated systems theory not only by being used, but by the principles upon which they are constructed and programmed. In technical jargon, the computer itself is a 'system'; and the official title of those designing computer applications is 'systems engineers'.

On the other hand, there are dangers in using mathematics. Simon (1960) has pointed to a tendency in Operations Research to simplify problems until the mathematically unmanageable elements are eliminated, and thus every similarity to reality is gone. In the same sense, McGrath (1964, p. 551-553) states that computer simulations, by entirely eliminating noise, also entirely eliminate information; that they may teach everything about nothing. In the activities of mathematical model-builders, like Stedry and Charnes (see below), I sometimes find them using variables without any reference as to how these have to be operationalized, i.e. identified in real life. Now this is quite legal in theoretical work, but if one starts to build an elaborate mathematical structure upon these 'soft' foundations, the total activity has more the flavor of play than that it has any external significance (in itself a perfect illustration of Huizinga's opinion, quoted in Chapter 3, about the play element in science).

A deeper objection against the use of mathematics is expressed by Leavitt (1964, p. 61-62), who puts Operations Research in the same category with Scientific Management: "It is the same old theme either way – the conflict between technology and humanity".

Conclusions reached with mathematical tools are often overestimated. In Holland, Monhemius (1963) has contested the belief that Operations Research is 'the science of decision-making' as it is announced to be in the Dutch language ('besliskunde'). This is exactly why people are afraid of computers. And they are right, if computers are used indiscriminately. Let us consider the following quotation:

"The cybernetical view of organization shows us the way to a more radical application of the principle of 'management by exception'. A system of reporting, based on applying this principle with an iron discipline, has become possible by the use of computers, without any reason for fear of relaxing this discipline" (Starreveld, 1965, p. 332, my translation).

In the light of the possible adverse motivational aspects of management by exception, an indiscriminate use of such a computer application could be disruptive. It is the problem of using a mathematical model without realizing its limitations.

Some examples of mathematical models of organizations, and the role of budgets in them

One rather pretentious attempt at building an extensive model of an industrial organization and using this in a computer simulation, is Forrester's Industrial Dynamics (1961). His extremely complicated models are developed to study among other things the dynamic behavior of inventories and production volumes; he calculates the flows of materials, orders, money, machine use, and men, controlled by decisions based on the flow of information. He pays special attention to the effect of time delays in the system, and of amplification (small bits of information leading to big decisions). His models and simulations are used in particular to study the effect of different *policies*, i.e. the rules governing decisions at various points. Forrester's models are predominantly rational; he bases himself on structures developed from a verbal account of the decision-making process at each critical point in the system; he takes into account non-optimal behavior because of insufficient information, but not, for instance, because of insufficient motivation.

Forrester's book does not describe any cases in which budgets are included in the model. In a paper published some years after Forrester's book, Roberts (1964) reports on the design of management control systems with the tool of Industrial Dynamics. In this case, more attention is paid to non-rational factors, like attitudes, motivations, pressure. An illustrative example is presented of the dynamic behavior of a quality control system. Although actual production quality was held constant, reject rates fluctuated considerably, due to periodic pressure on quality standards. The paper also suggests dysfunctional effects of budget practices in the case of Control of Research and Development Projects:

".... a system wich compares 'actual to budgeted expenditures' creates an incentive to increase budgets, regardless of need, and to hold down expenditures, regardless of progress; one which checks 'proportion of budget spent' creates pressures on the manager or engineer to be sure he spends the money, whether or not on something useful" (p. 115).

Two other mathematical model-building and simulation projects take still more account of non-rationality in decision-making. One is by Cyert and March, the other by Bonini. Both represent efforts to use not only technical and economic relationships, but also the relationships found in behavioral science research in the models. An inexhaustible source book for this type of model-building is March and Simon's 'Organizations' (1958), a Baedeker in organizationsland, as unreadable but as useful.

Cyert and March, in their Behavioral Theory of the Firm, have built and tested some models of industrial organizations which proved good predictors of subsequent real events; for instance, one dealing with price and output determination in a department store. Basing themselves on observation of actual decision-making, they handle decision rules that

91

are semi-rational. One of these is called '*quasi-resolution of conflict*'. Organizations have internal goals which may conflict considerably. Now the organization does *not* resolve these conflicts fundamentally, but only finds a solution in which they will no longer be so obvious. The interesting example of this is budgets themselves. Assuming an omniscient and rational organization, department budgets would be superfluous. All behavior would be directed by the one goal of profit maximization, instead of by a budget subgoal. In fact, it is quite unlikely that all budgets can be set in such a way that they together represent the case of profit maximization. Thus, by setting budgets the problem of conflicting department goals is not optimally solved, but only quasi-solved. Cyert and March call these 'aspiration-level goals' (1964). In a theoretical paper, Simon (1964), stresses that decisions are much more influenced by 'constraints' to be satisfied, than by goals to be maximized; not by lack of motivation, but just because of the cognitive inability of the decision makers to deal with the entire problem as a whole.[3]

A second semi-rational decision rule used by Cyert and March is called '*uncertainty avoidance*'. Organizations avoid uncertainty; they achieve a reasonably manageable decision situation by avoiding planning where plans depend on predictions of uncertain future events and by emphasizing planning where the plans can be made self-confirming through some control device. Here again the budget is taken as an example: it provides a negotiated internal environment. A budget is a series of contracts among the subunits of the firm; very stable during the budget period, and relatively stable from one period to another (Cyert & March, 1964). We cannot but think here of the game aspect of business as described on page 78. Here, too, it is stressed that business creates its own rules, its own rationality. I would therefore translate Cyert and March's 'uncertainty avoidance' into "creating a game environment".

Bonini (1964[a], 1964[b]) has also built a model in which he tries to use the views of various disciplines. By simulation he has studied the effect of various changes in external conditions and internal policy. An interesting variable he introduces is the 'Index of Felt Pressure' for each individual of the firm, which for example in the case of a salesman increases in-

---

[3] One could, however, also maintain that aspiration level goals which function as constraints rather than as goals, are a prerequisite for individual motivation. This is the tenor of a recent book by Hughes (1965).

versely with his sales in percent of quota. One of his experimental policy changes is particularly relevant to our subject: he tested the effect of a 'loose' vs. a 'tight' industrial engineering department in setting standard costs for manufacturing. Through the model, he checked the effect of this on sales. He found that a 'tight' industrial engineering department reduced cost in the firm. However, this led to alleviated pressure on profits and sales, and the level of total sales fell so much that the over-all effect on the firm was weak. The opposite happened in the case of 'loose' standards. This result, of course, is only obtained by working with a theoretical model of limited validity. However, it is a very interesting example of the unintended results that cost reduction campaigns, and decisions in general, might have.

In the specific area of building mathematical models for budget situations, Stedry and Charnes have done a lot of work. They have constructed three types of models:

1. A model for the one department, one goal situation.

   In dealing with levels of aspiration in chapter 3 I have pointed to the fact that the level of aspiration both depends on and, in its turn, influences performance. This is a situation which can be well expressed in a mathematical formula, which is the basis of Stedry's model. He hypothesizes various states of the budgetee: an encouraged state, three states of discouragement, and a state of failure and disappearance. He uses the model to test the effects of various rates of budget reduction. He concludes, that budgets should be reduced at a certain rate and that this should be done in such a way that an acceptable balance of positive and negative psychological reward for the individual budgetee is obtained; also, that stress upon the budgetee up to a point, is desirable, this point depending on the budgetee's individual motivation structure (Stedry, 1960, chapter 2[4]): see also my chapter 8. While this first model is deterministic, a stochastic model for the one department, one goal situation is presented in Charnes and Stedry, 1964[a].

2. A situation that Charnes and Stedry have paid much attention to is the one department, more goals case. Examples are given in Stedry & Charnes, 1962 and Charnes & Stedry, 1963, 1964[a]. Here the problem

---

[4] A review of Stedry's book by a group of accountants is given in Weinwurm (1962).

is dealt with as one of *effort allocation* depending on one of various possible reward functions. Among these is the reward function caused by 'management by exception': no reward for attainment of goals, and punishment foɪ each non-attainment (1964[a], p. 231-232). The authors remark themselves, that "some of the optimal allocation rules . . . are quite complex. It is therefore likely that although the subordinate may be seeking such an objective, he may not be capable of allocating his effort in an optimal way" (Stedry & Charnes, 1962, p. 27). So the models do not solve the problem, how to design (psychological) reward structures to obtain a desired effort allocation.

3. A third concern is about the relationship between overall company goals and department subgoals. By using a linear programming model, Stedry (1960, chapter 5) illustrates again that optimization within departments can lead to non-optimization for the total organization. One of his suggested remedies for this is "the planned use of incorrect information in setting individual standards, which would lead to an optimum in the large" (p. 143). This can hardly be taken serious, and may be is not meant to be so; one obvious comment is that in this case *somebody* should know how much and in what direction the information should be incorrect, and that therefore from a higher point of view the information could be seen as correct, or at least as correc*ted*.

Another paper by Charnes and Stedry (1964[b]) deals wholly with the issue of total company goals and department subgoals: "Perhaps an ultimate goal ɪs an organization whose control system is designed so that the attainment of goals set for employees at all levels of the organization contribute to organization goals" (p. 26).

In all the model-building of these authors, one wonders how many of the conclusions could have been reached by simple reasoning, without any mathematics at all. In the present state of practical operationalization of the variables they are dealing with, their effort allocation to mathematical model building does not look optimal.

An attempt at building 'a budget model for simulating the firm' by translating normal budget accounting practices into computer language, is made by Mattessich. His computer model "serves four main purposes:

1. To present the complete operating budget of a fictitious enterprise in form of a mathematical model together with a computer program usable for various educational purposes.
2. To provide a prototype of an operating budget that may serve in actual practice as a basis for constructing budget models and programs satisfying the individual needs of particular firms.
3. To demonstrate the connection between operations research models and traditional budgeting, and to overcome the shortcomings of the latter bij conceptual clarification.
4. To introduce accountants to the fundamental symbolism used in computer languages."
(Mattessich, 1964, p. 345, italics not used and parts between parentheses omitted).

This model may be used to test the effects of certain decisions that will be brought about by the internal consistency of the accounting system of budgeting. However, it uses only the accountant's point of view; it is traditional accounting in a computer-age wrapping.

A descriptive model of budget control for an individual budgetee

For the purpose of the present study, I will not operate at the level of mathematical model-building. The descriptive model of fig. 4-2 is not even supposed to be conclusive; it is only designed to show where various variables in the budget system fit together in a cross-disciplinary way. The technical control model of fig. 4-1 is the core of the new model; the 'comparing unit' is now the staff (controller's department); the 'intervening unit' is replaced by the budgetee with his full social network of fig. 3-3. Although the budgetee can intervene in the process himself, the main intervention path runs through his subordinates (first feedback loop). One complication in the system is that both the budgetee and his subordinates may have a role in the measuring process, and measurement can be biased. This represents a second feedback loop, which avoids intervening in the process at all. A third feedback loop consists of the influence of the budgetee (but also of the other elements in his network: staff, superior, peers and subordinates) on the standard. This feedback loop can also balance the system without intervening in the process itself; however, the influence of 'external reference points' can prevent this. The first and third feedback loop convey not only information, but also 'motivation', either positively or negatively. The feed-

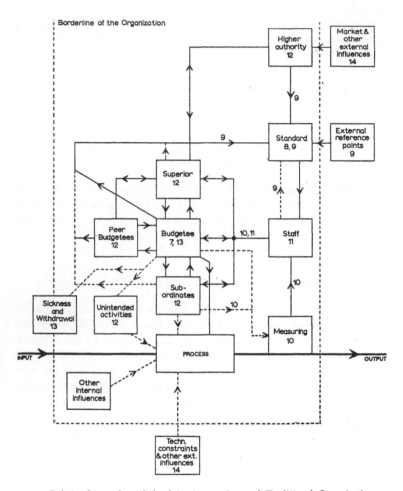

Borderline of the Organization

——— Relationships acknowledged in Accounting and Traditional Organization Theory

– – – – Other Relationships

The numbers refer to Chapters in this Book.

FIG. 4-2. Model of a budget control system for an individual budgetee.

back loops could therefore have been drawn as double loops[5], but this would have made the system still more complicated.

The model of fig. 4-2 also draws attention to the fact that although budget control in itself is a closed, third-level system, it is part of a larger, fourth or fifth level, open system. The larger environment plays a role in several places; one is, that the budgetee can 'escape' outside the system in the case of sickness (in which case he is both inside and outside the system, see Hutte, 1959-60, II, p. 285) or in the case of voluntary or involuntary separation from the organiation. Other environmental influences are technological constraints on the process; external reference points for standards, and, of course, the market situation, business cycle and all kinds of cultural influences, both on higher management and lower-level participants. The model of fig. 4-2 will serve as a guideline through the chapters in the third part of the book, whose numbers are mentioned.

Control limits in the system

A technical control system has its *control limits*. If the room thermostat at the beginning of this chapter is set at, say, 20 degrees Centigrade, its control limits may be 19 and 21 degrees. In this case there is no reason for intervention as long as the room temperature stays within these limits. Intervening with the thermostat, for example adjusting it down if the room temperature gets over 20 degrees, would quite probably only make actual temperature fluctuations worse: it would overcompensate and cause 'hunting'.

In our budget case, however, it appears that control limits are seldom set. What percentage of budget under- or overattainment is acceptable, is left to a subjective interpretation, which can vary from person to person and, moreover, from moment to moment. So it happens, that the budgetee never knows which variances he is supposed to jump upon. There is a sound statistical reason for admitting variances in actual performance around a standard. Measurements always show an amount of random fluctuation – if not, they are probably biased or faked. Some

---

[5] Stok (1959, p. 68-69) draws a double feedback cycle of this type for the case of visual presentation of quality information. Becker & Green (1962, p. 395-400) draw double cycles for both budget variance information and participation in standard-setting.

fluctuations in budget performance from period to period are to be expected for quite random reasons, without there being any indication that the process is out of control. So if we set a standard, we must be sure about what amount of fluctuation around it can be caused by chance, and set our control or tolerance limits at least as far apart. Otherwise, we might intervene while the process is still under control, and make the situation worse rather than better – like in the example of the room thermostat.

Often, the budget itself is used as a lower control limit for performance – any underattainment leads to intervention. In this case, if measurements are not faked and show normal random variances, the actual standard – in the sense of an average expected performance for a process under control – is somewhere on the better side.

The use of control limits or 'control charts' for cost and budget data has been recommended sometimes in the U.S. accounting literature: Gaynor (1944), Noble (1954), Amicucci (1965), Henderson & Copeland (1965). They all defend a statistical approach to budget variances, so that variances that could be caused by pure chance, will not lead to a (super-

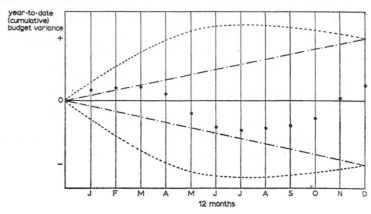

—·—·— control limit line

------- alternative control limit line

• actual variance up till the month

FIG. 4-3. Control Limits in a Diagram of Budget Variances.

fluous) intervention. Some of these papers present examples of practical use of the techniques.

In fig. 4-3 one simple example is shown of how control limits would look graphically in a diagram of cumulative budget variances (analogous to the diagram of fig. 2-2; the cumulative way of presenting budget variances from the beginning of the budget year onwards is quite customary). The thick dots represent actual year-to-date variances. The straight dash-dotted lines are control limits based on a constant percentage of tolerance. For year-to-date variances it might be more reasonable to use a percentage of tolerance which decreases over the year, which would make the control limits curved (the dashed lines in fig. 4-3). Only when the actual performance line crosses the control limits lines some kind of intervention is indicated. For economic performance measured against technical standards figures can simply be plotted on a weekly or monthly basis without cumulation over the year, and then the control limits are just horizontal lines in the diagram.

I will not try to fully describe the technical side of the use of control limits here. The literature mentioned above or rather any good book about Statistical Quality Control will help the reader who wants to experiment with these methods. Until now the use of statistical techniques and control limits for budget and cost control does not seem to be widespread.

The Sord & Welsch report of budgeting practices in the U.S.A. has collected data about intervention activities. Only one out of their 366 companies reported about explicit control limits for budgets: "Only deviations of 4 per cent over or 10 per cent under budget explained" (Sord & Welsch 1958, p. 238). In the five companies participating in the present study, I found one example of budgetary control limits. One of the plants, belonging to a larger corporation, is allowed a deviation of product cost of 2% above or below standard, before any explanation to the head office is due. Inside this plant, however, budgetary control limits are no more used than in the other companies studied. For pre-financial efficiency standards, explicit control limits were sometimes set, though also rarely. The situation is much different in the field of quality control, where almost universally control limits are used in conjunction with standards. In process quality control, even double sets of limits are frequently used: a rather tight 'warning limit', and a looser 'action limit';

these limits are based on the statistically admissible random variances in the process. The fact that control limits are used to control the quality dimensions of processes, but not the cost dimensions, can not be based on rational grounds. It is more likely that the experience of quality engineers led them to a full appreciation of measurement and statistics, and therefore to the use of control limits: while the experience of cost engineers and, especially accountants, lacks these elements; they are by tradition more concerned with 'precision' and 'exactness'. Another control area where a fruitful use can be made of control limits, much more than is usually done, is production scheduling (Schaafsma, 1963).

Higer-order-controls

Fig. 4-4 shows a model which is very much simplified in comparison with fig. 4-2, but shows more clearly the effect of hierarchical relationships in the system. A budgetee is always a member of a hierarchy. If his budget variances get out hand, most likely his superior will intervene; in other words, if he does not keep control of the situation, his superior will take over control. A technical analogy can be used here: let us represent our budgetee by a thermostat, this time in an electrical water heater. Now if the thermostat might become defective so that it no longer switches off the current at the upper temperature level, the heater would get overheated and might set the house afire. Therefore, a fuse is installed in the system, as a second order control. The theory of first- and second-order administrative control systems is well developed by Eilon (1965, 1966), from whom I have also borrowed the above-mentioned analogy.

In the model of fig. 4-4 a first-, second- and third-order control are drawn. The superior of budgetee I is himself a budgetee (II), supposed to take over control if budgetee I should fail. However, unlike budgetee I, he does not intervene directly in the process, but he intervenes with budgetee I – in the first place by asking for an explanation – in an extreme case by replacing budgetee I. Now an issue in this case is the standard II, which budgetee II uses to compare his measurements II with (here drawn as separate from measurements I, though they could be combined). In the technical analogon of the thermostat and the fuse, it will be clear that the fuse must be set at a higher temperature than the

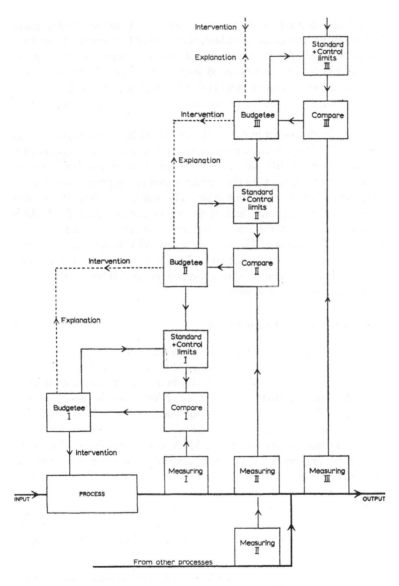

FIG. 4-4. Model of first, second and third order budget control.

thermostat – it must remain inactive as long as the thermostat functions. In the case of the second-order budget control of budgetee II, the analogy holds: his standard II must have at least the same control limits as standard I, so that he will not intervene as long as budgetee I keeps the process within the control limits of standard I; rather, standard II's control limits must be somewhat looser, to account for random measurement errors etc.

The same holds true for budgetee III, one hierarchical level higher, versus budgetee II. Only, when we go higher up the hierarchy, measurements (like measurement III) will tend to be less detailed and less frequent: higher-order-budgetees see the variances mostly integrated over various processes and over longer time spans. This integration in itself smoothes of incidental fluctuations. Still, if no explicit control limits for budgets are set, as is mostly the case, a budgetee can never be sure when his superior will intervene. He does not know what is his own free scope, and the Damocles' sword of an impredictable intervention is permanently over his head. Actually, setting explicit control limits is the logical systems implication of *delegation*.[6]

Motivational aspects of control limits

So far, the desirability of explicit control limits for budget control has only been based on a technical analogy of the control system. However, the usefulness of control limits can also be defended from a motivation point of view (Hofstede, 1964[a]). *Control limits are the formalization of the margin or 'play' within the system that is an essential condition for the game of budget control* (chapter 3, p. 75, point d).

In a recent and remarkable paper, Miles and Vergin (1966) discuss the Behavioral Properties of Variance Controls; they use this term "to include the various control charts and techniques associated with statistical quality control and covered in the accounting literature under the titles of 'Statistical Control Charts' and sampling techniques for accounting". Miles and Vergin list a number of features built into the 'variance controls' approach, which make them look promising from a behavioral point of view:

[6] Bosboom (1963, p. 13) stresses the relationship between delegation and control or tolerance limits for the subordinate.

1. They require an objective definition of performance standards, based on actual data.
2. They create a certain flexibility around standards.
3. They create control limits, within which the individual can establish his own performance targets.
4. They appear to have the potential for creating a positive atmosphere for the exercise of necessary corrective action; management's action can be viewed by both parties as problem-solving rather than punitive.
5. They are, potentially at least, both simple to apply and easy to understand.
6. Feedback can be both immediate and automatic.

The authors conclude, that "variance controls appear to offer a potentially valuable compromise between traditional control techniques and the somewhat abstract and frequently vague control suggestions made by various behavioral scientists".

Their point of view is exactly mine. It might be interesting to dwell a moment on the comparison between quality control and cost control. Unquantified experience has taught me and others, that quality control is often taken much more positively by the controlled, than is cost control. To Professor Lawrence K. Williams I owe the observation, that productivity control is generally experienced as punitive, and quality control as corrective. The more often mentioned Dutch Quality Control Study by Stok (1959) reports positive attitudes of workers confronted with visual presentation of quality feedback. Is this an intrinsic property of quality vs. cost, or is it caused by the different approach of quality control discussed before, which takes more account of what level of performance can be expected, and tolerates normal fluctuations? Can we obtain this positive effect in cost control as well? I believe we can. Defining control limits in conjunction with standards may look like an extra level of formalization in the budget procedure. In a sense, it is; but it creates room for informality. Gross (1965) introduces the 'clarity-vagueness balance': "Vagueness in goal formulation has many positive virtues. It leaves room for others to fill in the details ... Only vagueness can restore the precious element of humanity" (p. 213). Defining control limits, paradoxically, is a kind of clarity that creates vagueness.

To borrow a phrase used for the description of the ideal hospital: a budget system must have a 'calculated inefficiency' (Burkens, 1956/57).

Part II - The Research Design

CHAPTER 5
THE RESEARCH FIELD

Summary of this Chapter

This chapter analyzes how the research field was limited, starting from the aims of the study. It shows that the research was carried out in a small and non-random sample of Dutch industry. The main trades within Dutch industry were represented, but the sample was distorted towards the better-organized and larger companies, experienced in budgeting, and with a particularly open-minded top management.

The aims of the study

Just as a good entrepreneur must realize what business he is in, so a researcher must start by an examination of conscience, what the aims of his research are.

This is a study '*in width*', to use the picture of three research dimensions by the Dutch social psychologist Van Leent (1963). It starts from a part of the empirical world: budget control in Dutch business, which it tries to investigate to the fullest extent, applying relevant scientific theory of all disciplines where possible. It is not a study 'in height' (theory building) or 'in depth' (finding of philosophical bases). In another classification, it is *applied research*, starting from operating problems and working back towards theory. It is neither basic research, trying to contribute to the body of scientific theory, nor 'developmental research', a term used by Haire (1964) to describe the extension of theory into practice, starting, however, from a particular theory. Haire has introduced this concept, based on an analogy with physical science research, in an attempt to bridge the gap between the social sciences and management practices. I agree with him on the usefulness of 'developmental research' for this purpose. It tries to bridge the gap, starting from the social science side. However, I believe it is also necessary to start bridging this gap from the management practices side. This is what applied research of this kind hopes to do.

There is clearly a need for a better understanding between behavioral scientists and business managers. It is reflected in the lack of good applications of the findings of modern social science in business. It is also reflected by the hesitation of business management to cooperate in behavioral research projects. The behavioral research worker is not yet an accepted figure in business, not only in the Netherlands but also for example in Britain ('The Manager', 1964); maybe somewhat more in the U.S.A. Part of this hesitation may be due to normal defenses against any outsider (Argyris, 1952). Much of it is probably due to the failure of research workers to make themselves understood. Both industrial managers and behavioral researchers will have to go through many learning experiences in this respect (Likert & Lippitt, 1953; Argyris, 1957b; Williams, 1963; Churchman & Schainblatt, 1965; Churchman et al., 1965). I hope the present project has been a contribution to this learning process. One of the implicit aims of the study always has been interpreting behavioral science findings for managers and managerial objectives for behavioral scientists.

The first objective of my project has been *exploration*, by observing, measuring and describing the reality of the subject, looking for relationships between variables, and inducing the applicability of existing theory to the findings. Conclusions, therefore, are arrived at ex post facto – they do not have the value of scientific proof. I think that for a subject as complex as budget control, this is an unavoidable first step.

Secondly, I have tried to formulate some hypotheses, either before starting, or after the pilot phase (the analysis of the first company). These hypotheses have either been confirmed or rejected in the second part of the project; in this case, conclusions were set *ex ante*, and do have the value of scientific proof; however, only within the limited context of my five companies. Therefore, for business budget control in general, I do not pretend these ex ante conclusions to be much more significant than the other, ex post conclusions.

Limitations of the study

Chapter 1 has already mentioned the limitation of the research in 3 respects:
1. The particular kind of control: management control by operations budgets and standards.
2. The type of organizational units to be studied: 'line' departments in manufacturing organizations.
3. The hierarchical level of the people studied: first-, second-, and third-line-managers only.

Now within these limitations companies had to be found which were willing to participate in the project. From the outset, I aimed at a number of five companies. This was a compromise between two desirabilities: as much variety of research situations as possible on the one hand, and limitation of the duration of the project on the other hand. Though support and advice of several people were available, the actual research would have to be a one-man, half-time job. I decided to go for a 2-year study on this basis and I calculated that it would be feasible to study 5 companies in this period.

Selectivity in choosing companies

Selection of the companies and of departments for investigation within those companies was a crucial part of the research setup. Not only would this choice limit my analysis of the budget process to the particular methods of budget control used in these 5 companies; but also, the larger organizational context is extremely important in a research like this (Tannenbaum & Seashore, 1963) and would certainly influence the final conclusions.

The investigation units would have to be in Dutch industrial companies over a certain size, since small companies in the Netherlands were unlikely to have budget control to any extent. Let us assume that the size limit is 500 employees (this is an arbitrary choice). The total number of companies in the Netherlands over this size is about 300 (Official Statistical Data for the Netherlands, c.b.s., 1965). It will be clear that a sample of 5 out of 300 can never claim any representativity. I have, therefore, not tried to obtain a random sample.[1] The actual sample was a highly selective one in two ways:

1. The selected companies all had had a full system of operating budgets for at least five years, so their budget systems could be considered to be past infant diseases. The project therefore, did not compare situations with and without budget control. Even if such a comparison would be feasible, it would be extremely doubtful if this could prove anything. How could the effects of budgeting be separated from the general attitude of management? Therefore, I did not take up the case for or against budgeting. I think that, for the middle and large size enterprises, some method of financial management control is indispensable, and that therefore budget control is here to stay. The question is not whether or not to do it, but how to do it in the best possible way. The selection of companies with an established budget system meant in practice that only the better organized ones were chosen – each of the 5 companies had within its trade a reputation of paying much attention to its own organization.[2] My selection also meant, as I will show later, that the companies studied tended to be the bigger ones.

[1] A similar sampling problem is described in a recent study in 10 Dutch companies by Teulings and Lammers (1965).
[2] Some evidence for this is also offered by the comments the managers interviewed gave to the following written statement:

"This plant is well managed"

In a nation-wide survey in the Netherlands some years before, the same statement was used (N.I.P.G., 1958)

The comparison runs:	number of line managers	% of answers positive	neutral	negative
N.I.P.G.	388	71	20	9
our Survey	86	85	12	3

The difference, tested by chi-square, is significant at the 0,025 level. However, N.I.P.G. used a 3-point scale and I used a 3-point scale for DYNAMO 1 only and a 5-point scale afterwards; this diminishes the strength of the evidence.

2. A powerful selection criterion came about unintentionally because the companies had to be willing to share in the research. This meant showing confidential financial information to an outsider as well as allowing the interviewing of management personnel, on sometimes rather delicate subjects, and during working hours. Cooperating in such a setting demands a degree of openness and self-confidence with top management, which regrettably is not always present.

In the above-mentioned selection of better organized companies I had, to some extent, also selected the companies with the most enlightened top management. Even here, however, in two cases companies approached because they would have been valuable partners in the project, refused participation without any tangible reason.

Industrial trades represented in the sample

The 5 companies were chosen from different trades. In the Netherlands according to official statistical data (c.b.s., 1965) in 1964 1.2 million people were employed in industry; gross sales for the whole of Dutch industry were about 50 billion guilders ($ 14 billion).[3]

The main industrial trades were:

1. Metal products   290.000 people, gld. 11 billion gross sales
2. Food and tobacco 160.000   „ , „ 14 „   „   „
3. Electrical   120.000   „ , „   4 „   „   „
4. Textile   110.000   „ , „   4 „   „   „
5. Chemical   80.000   „ , „   7 „   „   „
6. All other   440.000   „ , „ 11 „   „   „

The project almost managed to involve one unit from each of the 'big five' trades. Finally, however, I was unsuccessful in finding a suitable chemical company to participate. Instead of this a company from the 'other' group was included, that is from the graphic industry. Some of the participant units belonged to corporations operating in more than one of the above-mentioned trades. I have, however, classified the 5 companies according to the trade of the units studied.

[3] In the 1964 Dutch economy, services (like commerce, insurance, banking, transport and government) accounted for about 50% of National Income, industry for about 40% and agriculture for 10%. Total population was 12,2 million people.

The five companies

The companies were:
1. A graphic company, which I shall call the *Alphabet* company. Its products are books and other printed matters.
2. A company from the metal products trade, to be called the *Buromat* company. Its products are office machines.
3. A textile company, the *Combitex* company. Its activities are twisting and weaving of yarns for industrial use.
4. An electrical company, to be called *Dynamo*. Its producing electronic components.
5. A company belonging to the food-and-tobacco industry, the *Epicure* company. It is producing high-quality branded goods.

Amongst these five, the *Dynamo* company occupies a special position within the project. It was the first to be studied and therefore served as the pilot plant. Some of the measurements and interview questions were introduced only during or after the *Dynamo* phase of the study. Therefore, comparison between *Dynamo* and the other 4 companies is not always possible. Secondly, *Dynamo* management created an opportunity for me to study two plants, located in different parts of the country, but basically similar in size, technology, and organization. This provided a unique setting for research. There appeared to be some striking differences between people's reactions on budget standards in one plant as compared to the other. As the plants were so similar, only a few causes could account for these differences. The *Dynamo* case will be described and analyzed as a case study in chapter 8.

The size of the companies and of the plants studied

Three of the companies were large corporations operating both inside and outside the Netherlands, and employing several tens of thousands of people. The two others each had a number of employees in the order of magnitude of 1000. Within the total setting of Dutch industry, the sample is clearly distorted towards the bigger companies. Including two middle-sized companies in it will hopefully prevent the conclusion that the findings only hold true for the big corporations.
The choice of the particular plants or units to be studied was generally

made by company management in the research planning stage. Within the two smaller companies, I studied the main manufacturing units; within the larger corporations, the units studied were relatively minor parts. Actual plant personnel in the six units studied (counting *Dynamo* for 2) varied from 260 to 750 with an average of 530. The six units together, therefore, only account for a minute part of total Dutch industrial employment: about 1/4 of a percent (the companies they represent, however, together account for several percent of the Dutch industrial employment: this is because of the influence of the big corporations included in our sample).

CHAPTER 6
THE RESEARCH TOOLS

Summary of this Chapter

Data were collected partly by analyzing, in the 6 plants, recorded information about budgets and standards, and the performance measured by them. Next there were extensive structured interviews of staff employees and staff and line managers. These interviews focussed where necessary on each 'measurable dimension' of the production process separately. Data processing consisted of computer calculations of product moment correlation coefficients for the total sample, plus separate factor analyses for staff and line data. Special attention had to be paid to the effect of subgroups within the total interviewee sample.

Data collecting [1]

Collecting the research data in the 6 plants of the 5 participating companies took place between March 1964 and January 1966. It was a one-man,

[1] My general guide in methodological issues has been De Groot's Methodologie (1961).
Further literature on methods I used consisted of:

Research design: Festinger & Katz, 1953
Questionnaire design: Torgerson, 1958; Blok, 1964
Study of company data: Buzzard, 1962; Acker, 1963
Interviewing: Kahn & Cannell, 1957; I.S.R., 1960; König, 1962; Trull, 1964
Coding: I.S.R., 1961
Statistical analysis: De Jonge & Wielenga, 1962; Spitz, 1965; Harman, 1960.

half-time job; only in the feedback sessions with groups of interviewees, which will be described below, was a second researcher present. The average time spent on orientation and preparation, data collection, coding, quick analysis and feedback was 6 weeks per plant, spread over a period of 3 months.

The preparatory phase

The approach for each of the 6 plants was about the same, with the exception that for the first two plants (*Dynamo* 1 and 2; the pilot phase of the study) it involved more search. In this pilot phase, a lot of information was collected which proved not very relevant afterwards, and could be omitted in the subsequent parts of the study. For instance, I scanned three years' volumes of the company newspaper to see whether 'budget' and 'standards' were referred to in them, and in what sense. It appeared that they were not referred to at all. In some cases, items were added to the questionnaires after the first or second plant; in one case even after the third plant, to replace attempts at operationalization of variables that had clearly failed.

Except for these anomalies in the first parts of the study, the approach for data collecting consisted of the following steps:

First, the c.o.p. (Dutch Productivity Committee), which sponsored the study, approached the top management of the company; a meeting of the researcher with one of the top officials of the company followed. In this contact, as well as in all subsequent contacts with the company, the researcher stressed the double confidentiality that would be maintained: company information would not go outside without management's approval, and information obtained in personal interviews would not be communicated by the researcher to anyone inside or outside the company in a way that the informant could be identified. As a result of this meeting with top management, permission was – or was not – given to conduct the study within the company; if it was, a particular one of the company's plants was chosen for this purpose.

The next contact was with the top line[2] manager of the plant to be studied.

[2] Throughout this book I am using the word 'line' to describe the departments in the plant through which production flows. 'Line Managers' are those in the hierarchy responsible for these departments. The opposite of line is 'staff', see Chapter 11.

The researcher made it clear, that as far as the project went within his company, the researcher would be reporting to this top line manager – no information would either be collected from or presented to anyone in the company without his knowledge. This was done particularly to keep the researcher from being seen as a kind of auditor or spy from some other unit within the company. It was clearly stressed that the purpose of the study was to assist Dutch industry in general to do a better job at using budgets and cost standards as a tool of management. Other topics discussed in this introductory interview with the top line manager are listed in Appendix C 1.

Subsequently, a meeting was called by the top line manager with the group of managers directly reporting to him (sometimes extended to lower levels as well), to introduce the researcher, and to allow him to give a short introductory talk (Appendix C 2). The top line manager always confirmed in this meeting that the researcher, though an outsider, was entitled to receive any confidential information in the area of standards and budgets with their performances he would ask for. The foremen and staff employees not present in this meeting were always informed by their superior, or in one case, collectively by the researcher in a foremen's meeting.

Then, further introductory interviews were held with the plant personnel manager, and with the top functional managers responsible for maintaining the budget and cost standard system, such as the plant controller, the chief industrial engineer, or the efficiency department manager. In these interviews the questionnaires reproduced in Appendix C 3 and C 4 were used loosely as general guidelines or checklists. The only 'closed' questions were those which asked the personnel manager to rate the foremen and managers in his unit on two scales, and the budget and industrial engineering staff employees on another scale. The introductory interviews with the top budget and standards staff manager(s) were also used to ask for information about budgets, standards and actual performances of the various line departments over the last one or two years.

In the same period, the researcher was enabled to see the plant and to get a broad understanding of the manufacturing process, without going into technical details.

The next step was for the researcher to study the budget and standards system, the standards and performances over the last one or two years, and the other information collected in the introductory interviews: to adapt his questionnaires for the main interviews to the specific terminology of the plant, and to decide who should be included in the main interview sample.

The main interviewing phase

The main interviews were of two types: one for staff employees and staff managers, and one for line foremen and managers. For the staff, the sample included all employees in the budget and cost standards departments having direct personal working contact with the line. Also, one or two higher-level staff employees from the quality and planning departments were included because it was expected that there would be points of contact between their work and the work of the budget and cost standards staff. For the line, the sample included all third- and second-level managers, and from the first-line or first-level managers (most often called foremen) at least one man from every department from which budget and standard information was available.[3]

The interviews were always taken in a downward hierarchical sequence, starting from the top line manager[4], so that a superior had been through it before his subordinates. The interviews were held during working hours and in a separate room on the plant premises, rarely in the interviewee's own office. Interviewees were invited to the interview through their superior. The total number of full main interviews was 140, divided as follows:

---

[3] The 'first-line-manager' is the lowest member of the hierarchy who has the responsibility for a complete part of the operation, including the appraisal of personnel and the maintenance of discipline. The second-level-manager is his hierarchical superior, and so on. We also find various 'assistants', who are specialized in one or a few aspects of the job, generally technical. These I have considered as managers of the levels $\frac{1}{2}$, $1\frac{1}{2}$ or $2\frac{1}{2}$. As titles and practices in industry vary widely, it will be clear that the management-level-classification is not always easy to make. For a more fundamental discussion of this subject see Evan, 1963b.

[4] Sometimes the top line manager was 5th or 4th level. The few 5th and 4th level interviews have been counted as 3rd level.

staff interviews: 48 – average duration 2¾ hours
line interviews – first level: 51 – average duration 2½ hours
line interviews – higher levels: 41 – average duration 3 hours.

All in all, nearly 400 hours were spent in the main interviews. All these were done by the researcher personally. The total number of interviews per plant varied from 20 to 31.

Each interview started with a standardized introduction (Appendix D 1.). The rest of the interviews were structured, but 'semi-open': some questions were 'open', so that they were just used to start the conversation on a subject; others were 'closed', in that a choice from a limited number of possible answers was asked. The main outline of the staff- and line-questionnaires is shown in Appendix D 2 and D 3.

From the point of view of method, the interviews contain 8 different types of questions or scores:

1. Fully open questions, if necessary followed up by probing questions. For example "What kind of special plans do you have for your department in the coming half year?" and the probe: "How do you mean that?" or "Could you tell me something more about that?" For these questions, answers were written down by the researcher as literally as possible.

2. Open questions for which the answers were immediately coded by the researcher. For example "How frequently do you see information about your machine efficiencies?"

   Code: (5) every day or shift
          (4) at least once a week
          (3) at least once every two weeks
          (2) at least once a month
          (1) irregularly or once a year
          (0) never, or question not applicable.

3. 'Quiz questions', or questions in which numerical information was asked from the interviewee about his budgets, standards or performances. This information was written down by the researcher as it was given, and afterwards checked with the official sources. The answer was then coded as:

          (4) in agreement with official data (within a very small tolerance depending on the question, but consistently used throughout the coding process)

(3) partly in agreement with official data (tolerance 5 times the tolerance for code 4)

(2) not in agreement with official data, or altogether unknown.

4. Scores on scales by the interviewee, such as the Control Graph scores of Appendix A.
5. Scores by the interviewee through the ranking of cards. For example, the ranking of the relative weight of various items in the appraisal by one's superior, described in chapter 12.
6. At the end of the interviews, interviewees were asked to fill out on the spot a 40-item forced-choice attitude survey questionnaire (Appendix D 4 and D 5).
7. While the interviewees filled out this questionnaire (in about 10 minutes) the researcher gave his impression about 5 dimensions of the interviews on 9-point scales:
   - openness
   - understanding
   - general cost-consciousness
   - relevance of the budget/standards
   - attitude towards the system

   For the staff interviews, the last score was for the attitude towards the line: service vs. condemnation.
8. Finally, the researcher wrote down a general impression of the interview.

The feedback sessions

Interviewees were promised feedback about the research findings in their company within a couple of months. I felt it both a moral and a psychological necessity to give this feedback to everybody participating in the project, and to do this before the final results would be available, which could be as much as $2\frac{1}{2}$ years later. Therefore, I was obliged to do a quick analysis of the findings of each plant separately, even though the full research results were not yet available. This quick analysis used very simple techniques and was primarily aimed at illustrating a general impression with some of the scoring data.

The actual feedback sessions were held between 2 and 6 months after the interviews. Per plant there were always 3 sessions: one with the higher-level (second, third and above) management group only, and two with lower-level managers and staff employees. In these last two, the second level managers were again present, so that the feedback groups were natural groups of people having a close working relationship. These sessions proved a valuable extra source of information about leadership behavior and group attitudes in relation to budgets and standards (see chapter 12). In each session, the researcher gave a presentation of the results, and tried to stimulate a discussion about them. A second researcher acted as an observer and wrote a report of the sessions, which were also tape-recorded. Both researchers afterwards recorded their impression of six dimensions of each session on 7-point scales:

team	– no team
constructive discussion	– destructive discussion
discussion well distributed	– one man or a few people dominated
lively discussion	– dull discussion
participants interested	– participants not interested
superior leads discussion	– superior does not lead discussion.

Alternative approaches

The approach of the study, as pictured, is essentially 'transversal', that is each organization was studied only at one moment in time. It would be very attractive to carry out a 'longitudinal' study of budgeting effects: to follow a particular organization through various stages of the budget cycle. However, within the available time this did not prove feasible. Another alternative would have been to have participants collect certain data themselves[5] but the subject looked too complicated to expect comparable data, if not collected by one researcher consistently.

The concept of 'measurable dimensions'

In explaining the models of the budget process in fig. 4-2 and 4-4, I have referred to only one standard for a budgetee. In fact, a budgetee has to meet several standards simultaneously; he is in the 'more goals' case

---

[5] Especially for studying aspects of managers' jobs, the self-collecting of data by participants has been tried several times: MacNaughton (1963), Cohen et al. (1965), Lupton & Horne (1965), Stewart (1965b).

described by Charnes and Stedry (see p. 93). The 'goals' in this case are the areas for which official standards are set; I will call them the 'measurable dimensions' of the production process. For the purpose of the interviews, it was necessary to discuss each measurable dimension separately with each interviewee.[6]

Although the five companies studied belonged to quite different industrial trades, there was a certain similarity in the pattern of measurable dimensions within their control systems. All their measurable cost dimensions fell into one of the following six categories:

1. Efficiency of direct labor ('direct' meaning: immediately attributable to a certain product).
2. Efficiency of indirect labor.
3. Machine hour efficiency.
4. Efficiency of direct materials use.
5. Efficiency of the use of indirect materials and tools.
6. Extra costs resulting from rejection or rework of products not meeting quality standards.

The line questionnaire was designed so as to discover which measurable dimensions were relevant to a certain interviewee, before he was asked in greater detail about them. See Appendix D3, Section C. It started with an open question (1): "What sorts of costs must be incurred to keep the department going?". The interviewer could thus check whether any costs were mentioned which were not preprinted on the cards for the next closed question (2). In this next question, the most relevant costs ("costs that can strongly be influenced in your department") were selected by picking and ranking cards. Any relevant costs not preprinted were added on blank cards on this occasion. Only after this preselecting of relevant measurable dimensions was the information for each measurable dimension (section D) collected.

It appeared that for each department within each plant, one to three of the cost dimensions mentioned above were vitally important, and two to four others of secondary interest; the remainder did not apply at

---

[6] Patchen (1963) reports on a similar research problem, in which he compared two methods of collecting data about *influence* through interviews. One was to focus questions on specific areas in the job situation, and then to reduce the answers to a general index. The other was to use a general question. He found that the specific method yielded a much better homogeneity within groups.

all. Direct labor was the only dimension which applied in all cases. In some cases, non-cost measurable dimensions could be found in meeting production schedules (time limits) and meeting quality level requirements (average quality for the products that were not rejected). The section of the line questionnaires (Appendix D 3) dealing with the specific control cycle was repeated for each measurable dimension applicable in the given situation.

Data processing

For those readers not familiar with statistical techniques the concepts of correlation and factor analysis are briefly explained in the first part of chapter 7. They are advised to jump the remainder of chapter 6.

The effect of subgroups in the total sample

The data collected consisted of descriptive information and coded information.

The coded information was collected from 140 individuals, who first of all had to be divided into 48 staff managers and employees, and 92 line managers. Within these two groups, the people from each plant formed a subgroup. Also, within the line subgroups, there were important situational differences between first-level and higher-level managers. Finally, people within a plant could sometimes be divided along departmental lines.

The correlating of scores could therefore be carried out on at least three levels:
- between individuals in the total sample
- between subgroups (taking average scores for all individuals within the subgroup)
- between individuals within each subgroup.

The effect of subgrouping on the correlation of two variables can be varied. There are three typical cases:

1. For either variable, the subgroup is a random subsample from the total sample. Therefore, correlations within each subgroup are only randomly different from the total sample correlation. Actually this is the only case in which it is admissible to add subgroups without precautions. Between-subgroup correlation is zero. The full correlation found in the total sample is due to causes working on *individuals*, within every subgroup alike.

2. With regard to both variables the split of individuals into subgroups is not random, so that there are significant differences between average scores from subgroup to subgroup, and these average scores are correlated. Within each subgroup there is no correlation between variables. The full correlation found in the total sample is due to between-subgroup differences. Causes are working on *subgroups*, not on individuals separately.

3. With regard to both variables the split into subgroups is not random. Besides, there is a correlation between scores for individuals within each subgroup. Now the total correlation found is due to the combined effect of both levels of correlation; these may reinforce or counteract each other, so that total correlation may even become zero, although within subgroups data are highly correlated[7].

For the present study, I have tried to arrive at conclusions of the highest generality by using correlation coefficients based on total sample data, but checking the effects of subgroup differences wherever these could influence the conclusions.

Calculation of correlation coefficients

Calculating product moment correlation coefficients for all relevant variables was carried out by a computer (IBM 7094/II). A program was used which accounted for missing data, and calculated correlation coefficients of any two variables using all sets of data available in the particular case. Thus, I could include the pilot plant data (from DYNAMO I and 2) in the total sample for those variables where these data were available. Methodologically, it would not be right to use the correlation coefficients thus obtained to prove any hypothesis formulated on the basis of the pilot plant data. For exploration purposes however, there is no objection to including them.

The correlations so obtained were total sample correlations. For the line interviews, I have also checked the correlations based on *within subgroup differences* only. This was done on the same computer, by first calculating product moment correlation coefficients within each of 12 subgroups (first-line and higher-level management in each of six plants); subsequently, these 12 correlation matrices were averaged using a Fisher - Z - transformation.

Finally, wherever necessary I have checked the *between-subgroup* correlation (based on average scores per subgroup) using Spearman's rank correlation test and a simple manual computation.

Factor analysis

On the basis of the total sample correlation coefficients, factor analyses were carried out on a selected number of variables; one for staff interviews (48 cases, 46 variables) and one for line interviews (90 cases usable out of 92, 60 variables). In the staff factor analysis, the six subgroups (plants) were introduced as six variables which took the value 1 if the subject belonged to the subgroup, and 0 if he did not. They were, therefore, mutually exclusive. The same was done in the line factor analysis for twelve subgroups: first-level and higher-level management in each of the 6 plants. In some cases for the pilot plants, the subgroup identification variable could not be correlated with some other variables, because for this particular subgroup all information about

---

[7] A study carried out by Indik et al. (1961) is an example how different results can be obtained when data are analyzed on a between-subgroups vs. on a between-individuals level.

the other variable was missing. Then a *zero* correlation coefficient was fed into the factor analysis.

The factor analyses themselves were carried out on the same computer as the correlation calculations. The program was based on the principal-factor-solution (Harman, 1960, p. 127 ff.) and on a subsequent orthogonal rotation according to the Varimax method (Harman, 1960, p. 301 ff.).

In an analysis like this, the number of factors to be included in the rotation can be chosen arbitrarily. On the basis of reasoning, I expected to find about six interpretable factors for the staff, and eight for the line. Both factor analyses, however, were carried out tentatively with subsequent rotations of all numbers of factors from 3 through 11. Studying a factor analysis of a set of data with a step-by-step increasing of the number of factors rotated is like focussing a microscope on an object. At first, when the number of factors is small, the picture is blurred and not understandable. Then, gradually, factors start to dissolve themselves into interpretable components. After passing the optimal number of factors, components dissolve themselves still further, but now the interpretable relationships begin to disappear and the picture disintegrates and becomes unclear again. There is an obvious subjectivity in this process, as there is in any application of factor analysis and, although it is often forgotten, in many applications of statistics. For the purposes of exploration, however, factor analysis is as useful to the student of organizations as the microscope is to the biologist. Using the subjective method pictured here, I finally chose to base my conclusions for the staff factor analysis on a rotation of 5 factors, accounting for 37% of the total variance in the data, and for the line factor analysis on a rotation of 8 factors, accounting for 45% of the total variance in the data. These percentages are relatively low, which was to be expected; because of their origin and the way they were collected, the data have been subject to many influences which have to be considered as 'noise' in the context of the analysis.

Part III - The Research Findings

HANDLING OF STATISTICAL DATA IN PART III

In the following part of the book many conclusions will be based upon a statistical analysis of data. To improve the readability of this part I have with few exceptions in each of the chapters 7 through 13 collected the details of the statistical data analysis in a separate section at the end of each chapter. Those readers who are not familiar with statistical techniques or who are happy to take my conclusions for granted can jump these statistical sections.

CHAPTER 7
INPUTS AND OUTPUTS OF A BUDGET SYSTEM

Summary of this Chapter

This chapter is the introduction to Part III, the Research Findings. It shows how the data were analyzed: some were considered as inputs to the budget system, some as outputs, while still other data helped to explain the relationship between inputs and outputs. Both inputs and outputs are classified: inputs are split into internal and external inputs, and further into the various subjects which are handled in the chapters 8 through 14. Outputs are dealing with the profitability of the enterprise and the well-being of its people; what is actually measured is the motivation to perform against the budget, split into budget relevance and budget attitude, and the job satisfaction of the budgetees. I am also testing whether performance, measured by budget variance, can serve as an output measure of the effectiveness of the system. The data show that budget variance is a poor overall yardstick; the only thing it measures in this study is whether the standards are loose or tight. The relationships between inputs and outputs are shown in a table which is based on the results of the factor analysis of line interview data. This table serves as a guide through the analysis which will be carried out in the chapters 8 through 14.

Inputs and outputs

This part of the book is devoted to the analysis of my data about budget systems, collected in actual practice. I have tried to observe the reality of budgeting in my six plants. Both in my data collection and in my data analysis I was guided by a framework of concepts which directed my efforts. It is the function of this chapter to explain this framework.

My guiding principle was the tracing of *inputs* and *outputs* to a budget system and the relationship between these. The point of departure is the model of a budget control system pictured in fig. 4-2 (p. 96). The budget control system is superimposed upon a manufacturing process; this process has its own 'input' and 'output' shown in the model. The inputs and outputs of the budget system are not the same as those of the process: they are of a different nature. They are not shown as such in the model, but they can be deduced from it. The *inputs of* the budget system are the factors which influence its functioning. They can be divided into *internal* inputs – things which can be changed by the people within the organization – and *external* inputs: the constraints imposed upon the system by the organization's environment. The existence of external inputs reminds us of the fact that the organization is an *open system*, adapting itself to the outside world, and so is the budget control system which is part of the organization. The *outputs* of the budget system are its effect upon the profitability of the enterprise and upon the well-being of the people working in it. My choice of these outputs has been explained in chapter 1.

Variables and correlation

The purpose of this study is to investigate the relationships between inputs and outputs. The data that were collected in each of the six plants through interviews, through studying company records and through merely observing what went on, are the *variables* in this investigation.

Some data could be quantified and expressed in scores for each person whom I interviewed: these are my quantitative variables. Other data were only of a qualitative and descriptive natured an the variables must be inferred from them through reasoning. The variables can be divided into measurements of inputs into the system as described above, measurements of outputs, and *intervening variables:* data which help to explain the relationship between inputs and outputs. For example, the feeling that 'trying to attain the standards is a sport' is an intervening variable which indicates why the output 'interviewee job satisfaction' is higher with the input of leadership behavior in plant X than with the input of leadership behavior in plant Y.

The relationships between quantitative variables are investigated with the tool of statistics. The essential concept is *correlation* and in order to follow the chapters in part III the reader should at least be familiar with the meaning of a (product-moment) correlation coefficient. Correlation coefficients (r) indicate the degree to which two variables vary together; they can assume values from $+ 1$ (if one variable increases, the other always increases too), through 0 (they vary independently of each other), to $- 1$ (if one variable increases, the other always decreases). When correlation coefficients differ significantly from the value 0 this means that it is very probable that there is a reason why the two variables vary together as they do; it is very *im*probable that this happens just by accident. In my case correlations between variables were computed both for exploration – finding relationships which were not predicted – and for proving some hypotheses formulated before the data were collected (the difference between exploration and proving hypotheses from a methodological point of view is described in chapter 5).

A classification of inputs

The chapters 8 through 14 in this part of the book correspond to the various *inputs* into the budget system. These inputs can be classified as follows:

A. Internal inputs.

1. Company policies: organizational rules, either expressly formulated or implicit, which guide the behavior of the people operating in the

system. Important inputs into budget systems are company policies in two fields: whether standards should be 'tight' or 'loose', and who should participate to what extent in setting standards. The effects of the 'tight or loose' policy input are investigated in chapter 8; the effects of the 'participation' policy input are investigated in chapter 9.

2. Contributions of the budgets and standards staff departments. These can again be divided into two parts: the effect of different budget accounting techniques coupled with different types of management information, and the personal impact of the behavior of budget accountants and standards engineers upon the system. The effects of the accounting techniques and management information input are investigated in chapter 10; the effects of the staff behavior input in chapter 11.

3. Different types of leadership and subordinateship behavior among line managers: frequency of communication about budget and standards results, the use of results for performance appraisal, the use of group meetings to deal with budget problems and, most important of all, the creation of a game spirit among subordinates around the attainment of budget goals, which is the main theme of this study. The effects of all of these inputs are investigated in chapter 12.

B. External inputs

1. The influence of demographic variables like the length of time in the job, the age, the education level, or the cultural background of the line managers working in the system. To some extent these inputs can be influenced within the organization, for example by 'job rotation': expressly limiting the length of time people stay in jobs; but measures like this will probably not just be taken for the purpose of improving the functioning of the budget system. From a budget system point of view, these influences are external. They are investigated in chapter 13.

2. The influence of technology, market, and economic differences between companies. The effects of these external inputs upon budget systems are investigated in chapter 14.

A classification of outputs

The outputs serve in the investigation as the yardsticks by which the effectiveness of budget systems is measured. I have already mentioned that I considered as the two fundamental outputs: the effect of the budget system on the profitability of the enterprise and its effect upon the well-being of the people in it.

1. The effect on profitability. As so many factors influence an enterprise's profitability, the chances of tracing the effect of only one factor such as budgeting on it are very slight. "To try to measure directly the effect of organization on profit would be like trying to measure the effect of a Minnesota spring shower on the flow of water over Niagara Falls" (Simon et al., 1954, p. vi). So I had to fall back on an effectiveness measure nearer at hand. Now a budget system's contribution to profitability may lie in better coordination of decisions, which will work especially at the higher levels of the hierarchy, and in improved managerial performance, which will work at all levels and maybe most at the lower levels of the hierarchy where I did my investigation. I was therefore mainly interested in the budget system's effect on the performance of budgetees (managers working in a budget system). Performance[1] against a budget can be measured by the budget variance (actual versus standard). To compare performances thus measured however, we must be sure the standards are comparable too. If not, budget variance will not be a good yardstick for performance. I could easily obtain budget variance figures from the existing records in the six plants. As the statistical section at the end of this chapter shows, the budget variance figures thus obtained show very few relationships to any other aspect of the budget systems. They appear to be mainly an indication of whether the standards are loose or tight. I had therefore to drop budget variance as a yardstick for the effectiveness of a budget system.

Higher performance by the budgetee is a consequence of higher

---

[1] Budget performance, of course, is only one aspect of total job performance. People may be poor budget performers and good performers in other respects, such as quality. Seashore et al. (1960) have tested for a large sample of non-managerial employees the hypothesis that all measures of job performance go back to the same basic factor. They had to reject it.

performance motivation. As objective measures of performance were not available, I could only trace the effect of budgeting on economic performance by measuring the motivation of the budgetees by the budget. In the information available about how budget systems function, it looked as if there were two dimensions in manager motivation through budgets (ch. 3, p. 45):

a. The *relevance* of budget standards to the manager's tasks.

b. The *attitude* of the manager towards the budget system.

Measuring relevance and attitude for each line interviewee appeared not to be easy, but usable scores were obtained. These scores serve as outputs in the investigation: as yardsticks for the effect of a budget system on the enterprise's profitability through the motivation of the budgetees.

2. The effect on the well-being of the people in the system. I measured people's general job satisfaction or morale: whether they liked their job and the department they worked in. I also measured people's feeling of being under pressure in their job and being made agitated and nervous by it. As the statistical section on p. 141 shows, there is a close relationship between high pressure and low job satisfaction. Besides being a goal in itself, high job satisfaction may also have tangible economic effects on a company, for example, lower labor turnover and a better position in the labor market. Pressure is an ambiguous item: while a certain amount of pressure may be healthy and appreciated by the individual who experiences it, too high pressure has very negative effects on the individual: anxiety, sleeplessness, an increased risk of psycho-somatic diseases like stomach ulcers and often a disruption of his family life. It has its adverse effects on the organization too: for example more absence, higher accident rates, more conflict between people and departments (see chapter 12). The measurement of job satisfaction and the reverse of the measurement of 'pressure' are the two outputs representing the budget system's effect on the personal well-being of the budgetees.

The measurement of relevance and attitude

As the concepts of 'budget relevance' and 'budget attitude' are rather basic to the analysis in the coming chapters I will illustrate them with a number of quotations from interviews.

Let us consider the following statements of line managers:
'I am referring to the standards every day. It's just indispensable. If I could start a business, I would set standards myself' (second-line-manager, plant X).
'I'd like to know the outcome, but it doesn't make any difference in the job. I don't think of standards every day. I'm just a little bit stimulated by them myself, not much. I don't believe a foreman ought to remember the standards constantly. Don't be hypnotized by the standards. Watch the job itself' (first-line-manager, plant X).
'The way the standards are used here is often quite wrong. They have a very depressing impact. If you don't make it on some job, people immediately threaten to subcontract the job. In many cases I'm just powerless against the real causes' (second-line-manager, plant Y).
'I like the standards. A man can show his results and point back to them. I am not so vain, but everybody needs an occasional pat on the back. Now with standards you know whether you did well or not, even if they forget the pat on the back. Otherwise I'd be dependent on the boss' whims' (first-line-manager, plant Y).
The second-line-manager in plant X and his subordinate disagree on the role budget standards play in the fulfilment of their tasks: they differ in budget *relevance*. The first-line-manager in plant Y and his boss disagree on whether standards are pleasant things or not; they show a difference in budget *attitude*. Other examples:
High relevance:
'I think working without standards is just impossible. You won't know a thing! Of course they influence productivity, we would not pay any attention to it without them' (first-line-manager).
'You bet they do influence productivity. They're the only decent way to jack up efficiency' (third-line-manager).
Low relevance:
'I would work as well without standards. I've always hit the standards fairly well by myself' (first-line-manager).
'I don't think I'm stimulated. It would be childish to perform less if there were no standards'. (second-line-manager).
'I don't think the standards have any influence. People just don't know enough about them' (first-line-manager).
'It's not a live system' (second-line-manager).

'It's not the standards that stimulate a man. It's inside him. Take me. I've always been fidgety. I can't sit still for a moment'. (first-line-manager).

Positive attitude:

'It's fun to try to surpass a standard, once it is set' (second-line-manager).

'I prefer standards. I have had a job as a foreman in a sheet-iron workshop before I came here. When a job was over, the manager always claimed he had lost on it. I hated that. It made me leave' (first-line-manager).

'Of course it causes a fellow problems, but I prefer budgeting. I like my job better with it' (first-line-manager).

Negative attitude:

'I would prefer to work without efficiency standards. Quality standards are indispensable' (first-line-manager).

'If you've a good reason for being substandard they can't catch you' (second-line-manager).

'Personally, I prefer a management not to set standards. A good foreman ought to take care of that himself. If I am responsible for a job, I must see to it that my people perform as efficiently as possible' (first-line-manager).

During the interviews, statements like these, which were answers to distinct questions by the interviewer, were coded and combined into scores for each interviewee: the 'questions' measure of relevance and the 'questions' measure of attitude, as described in the statistical section on page 138. Also, the interviewer scored after the interviews his impression of the interviewee's relevance and attitude: the 'impression' measures. The 'questions' and 'impression' measures were not combined, as they appeared to be not sufficiently identical for this purpose. They were used throughout the analysis as separate measures.

The hygienic nature of budget attitude

The distinction between relevance and attitude is somewhat similar to the distinction between motivators and hygienic factors made by Herzberg and described in chapter 3 (p. 53). When we consider a person's job motivation in general, the motivators or job content factors account for good feelings about the job and, most likely, for good performance (Herzberg et al. 1959, p. 114). They have only a positive potential. The hygienic or job context factors account for bad feelings about the job, can destroy the positive effect of the motivators, but have no positive potential of their own. Their best effect on motivation is zero. Positive motivation to above average performance can only be brought about by the motivators.

For motivation through budgets we can draw a parallel with the general job motivation case. Now relevance is the positive component. When the budget is not relevant, it will not do any good to performance but but it will not do any harm either. Attitude is the component with the negative potential. When a budget arouses negative attitudes, it may lead to worse performance than without any budget all. Attitude is not necessarily purely hygienic; it may have a positive potential too, but this works only when there is, first of all a certain relevance of the budget to the budgetee. Therefore we can approximately define factors in a budget system that increase relevance as motivators, and factors in a budget system that affect attitude as hygienic.

Relationships between inputs and outputs: the line factor analysis

From all the data collected from and about line budgetees (90 persons in total), I have selected the 60 most promising quantitative variables: inputs, outputs, and intervening variables. To get the fullest possible insight into their relationships I have subjected these data to a *factor analysis*.

In the method of factor analysis used, a computer processes the data to find a number of common factors which are independent of each other, and which together account for a maximum amount of the variance in the data. In our case, eight factors were found which together accounted for 45% of total data variance. Each of these factors is correlated with some of the original variables; these variables are said to 'load' on the factors. A 'loading' of 0.53 of variable no. 24 on factor no. 1 means that variable no. 24 and factor no. 1 are mutually correlated with a correlation coefficient of 0,53. Loadings can vary between − 1,00 and + 1,00; a negative loading means a negative correlation. Through the factor analysis the different variables expressing aspects of the budget system are grouped together around the different factors. Although some variables load to an important extent on more than one factor and some on no factor at all, most variables show only an important loading on one single factor. Variables loading on the same factor are those that appear to 'belong together'. They are mutually correlated, although sometimes this correlation is not evident in the original data because a third variable suppresses it there. The factor analysis technique thus finds out which aspects of the budget system 'belong together'.

In the table of fig. 7-1 the relationships between inputs and outputs are shown as they were revealed by the factor analysis of line interview data (data collected in interviews with staff people have also been factor analyzed; the results of this analysis are presented in chapter 11). The table contains with few exceptions only those variables which have loadings above 0,35 or below — 0,35 on a certain factor. This is an arbitrary limit to separate important from unimportant loadings.

The first column gives the factor number and a chosen name which best represents the combination of variables which load on these factors. Also, it contains the numbers of the chapters in this book where this factor is discussed. In the six remaining columns the variables loading on each factor are grouped into six classes. Each variable is preceded by a number corresponding to Appendix E 2 and followed by a number representing its factor loading. The six classes of variables are:

1. plant and hierarchical level, which refers to the twelve subgroups in the total sample; higher-level or first-line managers in each of the six plants.

   This is a way of tracking collectively the effects of all influences not separately measured, but which may vary from subgroup to subgroup influences that operate plant-wide, such as technology or type of market, but also influences which are overlooked by the researcher in collecting data.

2. external inputs as defined before.

3. internal inputs as defined before, measured independently from the interviewee.

4. perceptions of inputs: all inputs about which the information was collected from the interviewee themselves. It is a known fact that the same reality is sometimes perceived differently by different people, so these data do not necessarily fully represent objective reality.

5. intervening variables as defined before.

6. outputs (the only tangible output is budget variance) and perceptions

Factor no., name and chapters	Plant and hierarchical level	external input variables	internal input variables	perceptions of input	intervening variables	output and perceptions of output
Factor 1 'independence' chapters 9, 12 and 13	COMBITEX higher: 0.60 *not* EPICURE first-line: -0.36	1. higher hierarchical level: 0.43	45. frequent department meetings: 0.45	45. department meetings useful: 0.45 33. sufficient account of special problems in budget setting 0.45	60. no yes-men: -0.77 59. non-authoritarians: 0.71 58. positive attude to life: 0.64 24. cannot work without standards: 0.53 27. foreman's performance can *not* be appraised from standards -0.46 26. my department not efficient enough: 0.38	20. positive attitude (questions measure): 0.42 19. positive attitude (impression measure): 0.37
Factor 2 'budget variance' chapters 7 and 11	DYNAMO 1 higher: 0.58 DYNAMO 2 higher: 0.35 *not* COMBITEX first-line: -0.45		35. standards loose according to top line manager and staff: 0.39	51. good communication with staff: 0.37		28. budget variance: 0.78

Factor 3 'upward communication' chapters 8, 10, 11 and 12	COMBITEX first-line: 0.42 *not* BUROMAT higher: −0.48		47. boss asks his ideas: 0.61 51. good communication with staff: 0.58 43, 44. low rank order of 'department's results' and 'cost consciousness' in boss' appraisal: −0.49 and −0.36 40. high own operational control: 0.46 52. not too much paperwork: 0.44 50. information sufficiently understandable: 0.42	56. appraisal is just: 0.53	19. positive attitude (impression measure): 0.47 54. does not work under pressure: 0.44
Factor 4 'cost-conscious boss' chapters 9 and 12	BUROMAT first-line: 0.66 *not* EPICURE first-line: −0.36		46. boss discusses budget variances: 0.70 48. boss works on cost reduction: 0.65 29. high participation in budget setting: 0.37	42. does not desire more general influence: −0.48 24. can not work without standards: 0.37	18. high relevance (questions measure): 0.48 54. works under pressure −0.38 (53. low job satisfaction −0.30)

Factor no., name and chapters	Plant and hierarchical level	external input variables	internal input variables	perceptions of input	intervening variables	output and perceptions of output
Factor 5 'cost-conscious self' chapters 9, 10 and 12	ALPHABET higher: 0.59 EPICURE higher: 0.37			21. knows exactly which costs he is responsible for: 0.60 50. information sufficiently understandable: 0.42	25. thinks trying to attain the standards is a sport: 0.42 23. high score on quiz questions about general cost-consciousness: 0.37	17. high relevance (impression measure): 0.52 53. high job satisfaction: 0.40
Factor 6 'job rotation' chapters 8, 9, 10 and 13	BUROMAT higher: 0.40 DYNAMO 2 higher: 0.39 not ALPHABET first-line: −0.45	15. short period in present job −0.65 14. younger −0.59			36. expects improvement in performance: 0.51 22. high score on quiz questions about actual performance and standards 0.43 38. high correlation between own subjective evaluation of performance and budget variances: −0.35	

Factor 7 'job involvement' chapters 8, 11 and 13	DYNAMO 2 first-line: 0.52		55. plant demands the utmost of him: -0.71	57. believes that working comes natural to most people: 0.79 49. desires less general influence of staff-departments: -0.37	
Factor 8 'self-satisfaction' chapters 8, 9 and 13		39. high ability rating by boss and personnel manager: 0.37	37. high evaluation of own present performance 0.74 41. low own general influence: -0.58 31. high participation in setting technical standards 0,37 47. boss asks his ideas: 0.35	42. desires more own general influence: 0.46 32. does not desire more participation in setting technical standards: -0.40 38. low correlation between own subjective evaluation of performance and budget variances: 0.36	(53. high job satisfaction 0.34)

FIG. 7-1. Results of Factor Analysis of Line Interview Data.

of outputs: outputs about which the information was collected from the interviewee: budget relevance, budget attitude, job satisfaction and pressure.

In a wider sense all variables measured through the subjective judgment of the interviewee should be called 'intervening variables': class 4, 5 and 6 together. I am using the term 'intervening variables' in a more limited sense here, but it is true that the division of data collected from interviewees into 'perceptions of inputs', 'intervening variables' and 'perceptions of outputs' is based upon subjective reasoning and does not follow from the data themselves. In drawing conclusions on the basis of the data we should be aware of the possibility that causes and effects are not as the table shows, but that some assumed causes may be effects or the other way round. The borderline between classes 4, 5 and 6 is not absolute.

Relationships between outputs

As I mentioned already, *budget relevance* and *budget attitude* have each been measured by two measures (one based upon questions, one upon an impression of the interviewer); in both cases, the two measures are correlated with each other. The agreement between the two 'attitude' measurements is much better than between the two 'relevance' measurements. As will appear in chapter 12, the 'impression' measure of relevance is more related to motivation through forces within the budgetee, while the 'questions' measure is more related to motivation through outside pressure. This shows that I actually measured two kinds of relevance, which are only partly correlated. Budget relevance and budget attitude are independent of each other; if not a hundred per cent, then in any case to a large extent. The four correlations between the two relevance and the two attitude measures are all positive, but not very strong: they have probabilities between 5 and 14% to be caused by pure chance. In the factor analysis we find that relevance and attitude do not belong together: two of the factors are related to high relevance and two *other* factors to positive attitude.

I have also tested whether there was any relationship between relevance and attitude on the one side and *budget variance* on the other side. Theoretically higher motivation (relevance and attitude) should lead to higher performance and this should be reflected to some extent in budget variance. The data show nothing of his. In the factor analysis, budget variance belongs to factor 2 with a high loading: 0,78. I have therefore called this factor itself 'budget variance'. Very few other variables are related to the 'budget variance' factor and anyhow not relevance and attitude. We find only 'looseness of standards' as could be expected and 'good communication with staff' (see chapter 11). Besides this the budget variance factor only identifies the plants where budget variances were very favorable or very *un*favorable.

I have tried whether the relationship between budget variance, relevance and attitude would become clearer by eliminating some other influences. I have eliminated the influence of *looseness of standards* (estimated by the top line manager and the staff interviewees). I have also tested the effect of two variables which according to the theory in chapter 3 should influence the relationship between relevance, attitude and performance: *ability* of the budgetee (estimated by his boss and the personnel manager) and his *operational control*, that is the degree to which the budgetee felt he could influence the results of his department. There is some relationship between budget variance and ability ratings and also between budget variance and operational control ratings. Neither differences in looseness of standards, nor differences in ability, nor differences in operational control can explain the lack of correlation between relevance, attitude and budget variance. Only if we exclude the differences between the plants and between higher-level and first-line management (we then only look at the correlations within the subgroups), there is a positive correlation between budget attitude and budget variance. Unfortunately there is a much reason to suppose that the positive attitude is an effect as that it is a cause of favorable budget variance. Budget variances are, as stated before, poor yardsticks for our purposes. There is only one part of the investigation where they have been useful, and this is where they have been compared to people's own judgment about how well their department was running. The outcome of this comparison is presented in chapter 8.

I have already mentioned that high job satisfaction and low pressure go together. Both job satisfaction and low pressure appear to be negatively correlated with one of the measures of relevance: the questions measure; not with the other one. This relationship is caused by a number of other influences, as will be shown in chapter 12. There is no positive correlation between job satisfaction and budget attitude, contrary to what we might expect. There is even a negative correlation which has a probability of 5% to be caused by pure chance. In this case too other influences are responsible for this correlation. It is important to remember that high job satisfaction is *not* the same as positive budget attitude.

Statistical analysis of data used in Chapter 7
Measuring relevance and attitude

Operationalization of the concepts of 'relevance' and 'attitude' proved not to be easy, and even more difficult for 'relevance' than for 'attitude'. I did not want to use a direct rating by the interviewee on a 'Relevance of Budgets' scale (as I did in the case of 'Operational Control' and 'Participation in Standard-Setting', as will be shown later), because I expected that these ratings would be seriously biased by an interview situation creating a temporary 'relevance' itself. With the experience of 140 interviews, I would now be less hesitant to include a rating by the interviewee in a well-designed 'Relevance of Budgets' scale. The way I did operationalize 'relevance' and 'attitude' was:

1. By ratings by the interviewer of his impressions at the end of each interview, on 9-point scales:
   Relevance of budget/standards: low-high
   Attitude towards the system: negative-positive
   (Appendix D 3, question H 5 – H 6; Appendix E 2, variable 17-19).
2. By coding of answers on the following interview questions (Appendix D 3, section E):
   E 20: Do the standards that are set influence productivity in this plant?
   (5 = influence; 4 = some influence; 3 = no influence; 2 = perhaps negative influence; 1 = negative influence).
   E 21: Would you prefer personally to work with or without standards, or do you have no preference?
   (5 = with; 4 = perhaps with; 3 = no preference; 2 = perhaps without; 1 = without).
   E 22: Do the standards stimulate you yourself to a better performance?
   (5 = yes; 4 = perhaps; 3 = no; 2 = perhaps negatively; 1 = negatively)
   E 23: If no standards were set, but your instruction would just be to work as efficiently as possible, would this make your job heavier or lighter than it is now?
   (5 = heavier; 4 = perhaps heavier; 3 = don't know; 2 = perhaps lighter; 1 = lighter).

E 20 and E 22 were designed to represent 'relevance' and E 21 and E 23 to represent 'attitude'.

Actual scores on E 20 and E 22 appeared to be only 5, 4 and 3, i.e. positive or zero values; this agrees with my expectation (p. 50) that no negative relevance will be found in practice.

On E 21 and E 23, all values of scores from 5 to 1 were present: positive, zero and negative values: this agrees with my expectation (p. 45) that attitude can be both positive and negative.

However, all four questions were weak in obtaining a good spread in the answers: percentages positive answers (score 5) were very high: for E 20 - 81%; E 21 - 86%; E 22 - 73%; E 23 - 60%.

The intercorrelation of the answer scores (product moment correlation coefficients) are shown in fig. 7-2:

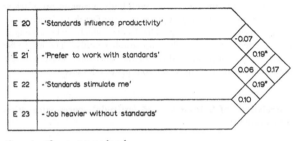

* = significant at 0,05 level

FIG. 7-2. Intercorrelations between Answer Scores on Four Open Questions

The relatively low correlations are understandable in the light of the poor spread in answer scores. Taking this into account, I felt justified to take E 20 and E 22 together, and also E 21 and E 23. I have, therefore, used the total score for E 20 and E 22 as a Relevance Index, and the total score for E 21 and E 23 as an Attitude Index (Appendix E 2, variable 18 and 20).

The intercorrelations between my four measurements of motivation are as shown in fig. 7-3:

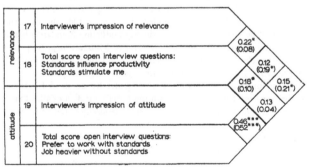

Figures between brackets are correlations within subgroups *significant at 0,05 level, ***significant at 0,0005 level

FIG. 7-3. Intercorrelations between the Two Measures of Relevance and the Two Measures of Attitude

139

Thus it appears that all measurements are slightly correlated, but that the two 'relevance' and the two 'attitude' measures are more correlated; not even for 'attitude' can the correlation be said to be very good for two measurements designed to measure the same dimension.[2] I have, therefore, not taken the 'impression' and 'questions' measurements together, but treated them separately throughout the further analysis.

The difference in the correlations with both measurements of relevance when we look at correlations within subgroups point to the fact that relevance levels are very different from subgroup to subgroup. The factors which make a budget relevant are mostly working for the whole subgroup simultaneously. The level effect works out differently for the 'impression' than for the 'questions' measure of relevance. This shows again that we are dealing with two types of relevance.

Correlations of 'relevance' and 'attitude' scores with other budget attitude measurements

In the attitude survey administered at the end of the interviews (Appendix D 5) a number of items dealt with budget attitudes. Some of these are specific, for example about the information feedback, the standard-setting process, or line-staff communication. These will be discussed in the chapters 8 through 13. Four items were of a more general nature:

2. Budgeting is first of all an accounting tool (negative).
9. I could work as well without standards (negative).
29. Taking everything into account, my department runs efficiently enough (negative).
36. Introducing budgeting (standards) has improved efficiency (positive).

The correlations of these six with the two 'relevance' and the two 'attitude' measures were as shown in fig. 7-4.

From this, it appears that generally the relevance measure through interviewer's impressions and the attitude measure through questions give the higher correlations with the scores obtained independently in the attitude survey. An exception is the correlation between item 36 ('Introducing budgeting (standards) has improved efficiency') and the 'questions' relevance measure, which is not surprising, as the questions from which the relevance measure is obtained ('standards influence productivity' – 'standards stimulate me') are rather similar to item 36.

A high 'impression' relevance score is generally obtained for those who think that budgeting is *not* first of all an accounting tool (but is, first of all, a management tool).

A high attitude score (by both measures) is generally obtained for those who think they could *not* work as well without standards.

Those who think their department does *not* run efficiently enough- and are therefore likely to search for lines of action that will make it run more efficiently – tend to have a somewhat more positive attitude ('questions' measurement) and maybe a higher relevance ('impression' measurement).

[2] It must be noted that the interviewer's impressions were rated at the end of the interview, during which he had heard also the answers on the four open 'relevance and attitude' questions.

Att. Survey item		relevance		attitude	
		17 impr.	18 quest.	19 impr.	20 quest.
2	Budgeting is *not* first of all an accounting tool	0,47***	0,12	0,14	0,26*
9	I could *not* work as well without standards	0,19	0,15	0,49***	0,50***
29	Taking everything into account, my department does *not* run efficiently enough	0,20	−0,09	0,00	0,26*
36	Introducing budgeting (standards) has improved efficiency	0,14	0,43**	−0,04	0,04

*significant at 0,05 level, **significant at 0,005 level, ***significant at 0,0005 leve‧

FIG. 7-4. Correlations of Four Attitude Survey Item Scores with 'Relevance' and 'Attitude'.

Measuring job satisfaction and pressure

Job satisfaction (variable 53) is deduced from two attitude survey items:
'I like the department I work in'.
and 'I enjoy my job'

Pressure (variable 54) is deduced from two other attitude survey items:
'My job makes me agitated and nervous' and
'I feel under pressure in my job'.
These were scored negatively, so that variable 54 actually measures the absence of pressure.

The first three of these four attitude survey items were used before in a nation-wide survey in the Netherlands (N.I.P.G. 1958). The fourth is designed especially for this study.
Job satisfaction and absence of pressure are mutually correlated with r = 0,42*** (within subgroups equally 0,42***).
The correlations between job satisfaction and pressure versus relevance and attitude are shown in fig. 7-5. The only significant correlations are negative; two of these negative correlations are caused by situations in specific plants. The third one will be investigated in chapter 12.

Variables:	correlations with:			
	17 Relevance (impress.)	18 Relevance (questions)	19 Attitude (impress.)	20 Attitude (questions)
53. High job satisfaction	−0,05(−0,03)	−0,18*(−0,18*)	−0,18*(−0,10)	−0,15(−0,06)
54. Absence of Pressure	−0,14(−0,03)	−0,22*(0,03)	0,02(0,02)	−0,09(−0,16)

Figures between brackets are correlations within subgroups.
*significant at 0,05-level

FIG. 7-5. Correlations between Job Satisfaction, Pressure and Budget Motivation

Correlations of relevance, attitude and some other variables with budget variance

For each line interviewee, I calculated his total *budget variance* over the past 3 months in percentages of his total departmental added value (total cost minus direct materials, which is a measure of total departmental activity). The period of 3 months[3] was chosen after some experimenting: it is recent enough to be currently remembered, yet it is long enough to smoothe off incidental fluctuations. For the exact coding of budget variance see Appendix E 2, var. 28.

The correlations of this budget variance with relevance and attitude are shown in fig. 7-6, which also shows the correlations of budget variance with three other variables. According to chapter 3 these might influence performance and budget variance as well. They are looseness of standards, ability and operational control.

The *looseness of standards* measurement was based on the combined judgment of the top plant line manager (50%) and all staff interviewees of the plant concerned (50%). Ratings were given on a five-point scale. See Appendix E 2, variable 35; Appendix D 2, question C 5 and Appendix D 3, question D 11. The measurement of *ability* is based on a performance rating by the boss and a promotability rating by the personnel manager. The measurement of *operational control* is described in Appendix B.

The strongest correlation appears to be between budget variance and looseness of standards, as could be expected. There is some correlation with ability ratings and with operational control. There is also some correlation with attitude, if we only look at variances within subgroups (plants and hierarchical levels). All correlations with relevance are weakly negative. I have also tried whether elimination of the influence of looseness of standards, ability or operational control made the correlation between

[3] In DYNAMO 1 and 2 a period of 2 months was used. A longer period would have included a change of standards because of the beginning of the new budget year.

budget variance, relevance and attitude stronger, but this was not the case. The conclusion is that my data do not give conclusive evidence of a relationship between motivation and performance, as measured by budget variance. There are a number of significant correlations with budget variance, but in all these cases budget variance may have been the cause rather than effect.

Variables:	correlations with 28. budget variance		
	based on total data	based on within-sub-group variance only	based on subgroup averages (rank correlation)
17. Relevance (impression)	— 0,12	— 0,06	— 0,13
18. Relevance (questions)	— 0,09	0,12	— 0,26
19. Attitude (impressions)	0,06	0,28**	— 0,36
20. Attitude (questions)	— 0,00	0,16	— 0,02
35. Looseness of standards	0,42***	— 0,01	0,70*
39. Ability	0,31**	0,11 ꞌ	0,53*
40. Operational Control	0,16	0,28**	0,17

*significant at 0,05 level, **significant at 0,005 level, ***significant at 0,0005 level

FIG. 7-6. Correlations of Basic Variables with Budget Variance

CHAPTER 8
TIGHT OR LOOSE STANDARDS?

Summary of this Chapter

In this chapter, the effect of the input: the level of the standards that are set on the output: budget motivation is investigated. First, the findings of the research projects of Stedry and Stedry & Kay on the same subject are described. Then follow my results, which largely confirm those of the other researchers. The level of standards appears to play a role in achievement motivation, apart from any other rewards or punishments connected to it.
The findings prove that:
– loose budgets are poor motivators.
– the motivating effect of budgets becomes stronger when they become tighter.
– over a certain limit of budget tightness, motivation is poor again.
– this limit, and more in general the extent to and the way in which people internalize standards, depends on factors in the situation, in management and in the personalities of the budgetees.
Interesting results have been obtained by comparing budgetees' evaluations of their departments' performance to the official performance data in the budget variance reports. In some plants the standards appear to be well 'internalized' into personal aspiration levels and to agree with people's personal evaluation standards; in others they are not at all internalized. Group management and the forces the budgetees have been exposed to collectively appear to influence

this internalizing process. This is illustrated in two case studies, the DYNAMO *and the* COMBITEX *case study.*

The role of budgets in achievement motivation: Stedry's experiment

In this chapter I will explore experimentally the implications for budgeting of the theory of achievement motivation and aspiration levels (chapter 3, p. 62 ff.). First, I will analyze the outcome of two other research projects on the same subject.

In Stedry's experiment (Stedry, 1960), 108 students as subjects had to solve six series of problems each. For each person and each series, budgets were set for the number of problems to be solved; attainment or non-attainment of the budgets was associated with small financial rewards and penalties; also, in some cases the subjects were asked 'what they hoped to perform' (their aspiration level) before the actual performing. The subjects were arranged in a 3 × 4 factorial, making all possible combinations of the following conditions:

a. No aspiration level question
b. Aspiration level question before budget statement
c. Aspiration level question after budget statement
A. Low budget (attained 69% of the time)
B. Medium budget (attained 59% of the time)
C. High budget (attained 39% of the time)
D. Implicit budget (not stated to the subject before; combined low, medium and high).

Analysis of the performance results under these various conditions showed:
- The influence of aspiration level formulation on performance was highly significant (1% level); performance was highest for those subjects formulating an aspiration level after knowing their budget, and lowest for those formulating no aspiration level at all.
- The influence of budget level *per se* on performance was not so significant (5% level); this influence appeared to be conditioned strongly by the method of aspiration level formulation, so that the interaction of aspiration level formulation × budget level was again highly significantly (1% level) correlated with performance. Performance was positively correlated with budget level for those formulating no

145

aspiration level, or formulating it after the budget statement; in these cases, only the high budget gave better performance than the implicit (unknown) budget; the low and medium budget gave a lower performance than the implicit budget, so one could conclude that stating them actually lowered performance instead of stimulating it. For those subjects formulating an aspiration level and thereafter getting their budget (condition b), performance was best with a medium budget level. High budgets in this case had an adverse effect: they led to extremely low performance, as if the subjects stopped trying.

From these results, it can be concluded that:

a. Formulating an explicit level of aspiration does influence performance. It appears that the formalization of the 'level of aspiration' procedure helps people who otherwise would not have done it for themselves to set an aspiration level and consequently perform better.
b. The influence of the formal budget level on performance is conditioned by the way in which people set their aspiration levels.
c. Only the high budgets were better than the unknown budgets.

In industry, the conventional rule is that budgets should be 'attainable but not too loose' (Stedry, 1960, p. 11); or for example:

"The standard costs and budgets are attainable but lean towards the ideal side" (Holden, Fish & Smith, 1941, p. 160).

Now it is doubtful how this must be interpreted in practice. Which of Stedry's budgets were 'attainable, but not too loose'? From the experiment we see that only budgets that had a chance less than 1 in 2 (39%) to be attained, had a positive effect on performance. Stedry therefore stresses the importance of the difference between budgets for planning (what actually will be performed) and goal-setting (optimal level from a motivational point of view).[1] In a later publication, Stedry (1962) reports that in about 60% of cases his experimental subjects who formulated an aspiration level after getting their budget, chose the budget level as their aspiration level; for the 'high' budgets, aspiration levels

---

[1] Becker and Green (1962, p. 401-402) fear that employees might dislike the idea that planning and goal-setting budgets are not the same. Personally, I cannot see why employees would not accept that an average percentage of goal-underattainment is used in the planning process.

were either on or below the budget; for the other budget levels, aspiration levels were below, on, or above the budget. Stedry apparently has not extended his budget level range far enough to discover the upper limit on the 'tight' side, above which budgets will no longer affect performance. In business practice and in some of the accounting theory of budgets, there is a clear expectation that such a limit exists:

"If people set their goals too high, they will be overstrung, disappointed and will finally acquiesce in failure" (van der Graaf, 1965, p. 9, my translation). "It will be understood that the tension in the budget loses its operational value if it leads to hypertension" (Limperg, 1965, p. 103, my translation)

Now this upper limit is most likely different for different individuals. This is shown by the results of another research study, the one by Stedry and Kay.

The field experiment of Stedry and Kay

This experiment (Stedry & Kay, 1964[a], 1964[b]) was carried out in a large US engineering plant. The experimental subjects were 17 foremen, belonging to the same subsection. They "... were divided randomly into four equal groups and assigned goals of varying difficulty by their managers in the two most important aspects of their jobs: (1) productivity and (2) quality (amount of rework required). Two levels of goal difficulty were established on the basis of past performance: (1) a 'normal' goal was set at a level which the foremen had been able to achieve 50% of the time in the previous 26 weeks; (2) a 'difficult' goal was set at a level which the foremen had been able to achieve only 25% of the time in the previous 26 weeks. Foremen in one of the four groups were assigned 'normal' goals for both productivity and quality to work on for the ensuing 13-week period. Foremen in the second group were assigned 'difficult' goals in both areas. The third and fourth groups were assigned difficult goals in one area and normal goals in the other". (Stedry & Kay, 1964[a]).

The experiment tried to prove a number of rather detailed hypotheses. In this, it was not successful. Obviously, a sample of 17 subjects split into 4 subgroups is very small to obtain statistical significance. The results, therefore, consist of statistically non-significant tendencies and ex-post hypotheses. Nevertheless they are interesting:

Difficult goals in one of the measurable areas (productivity or quality) appear to lead to either very good or very bad performance in comparison with normal goals; this is especially the case if the other area also has a difficult goal. In the case of very good results we can assume that high aspiration levels have been formed, influenced by the formal goal. In the case of very bad results, the goal has been perceived as so difficult that the foreman has withdrawn from setting an aspiration level or he has set such a level far below the formal goal. From the experiment it appeared that, where difficult goals were perceived as 'impossible' (this was assessed in interviews at the beginning of the experimental period), performance tended to be lower than when either 'normal' goals were given, or difficult goals were given that were perceived as 'challenging'. The differences between those accepting or rejecting a goal seemed to be a matter of personality differences; also, age played a part: the older men were more likely to see difficult goals as impossible (Stedry & Kay, 1964[a], also Stedry, 1964[b]).

A diagram of the effect of budget levels on performance

In line with the conclusions of the two studies mentioned above, I have tried to show the effect of budget levels on performance (all other factors, like personality effects, being equal) in the form of a diagram (fig.8-1). This is an improved version of a diagram already published before this research project in another paper (Hofstede, 1964[a]).

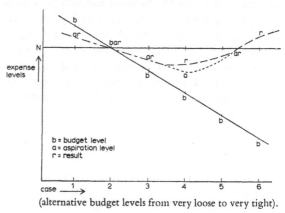

(alternative budget levels from very loose to very tight).

FIG. 8-1. Budget Level, Aspiration Level and Resulting Actual Expense Level

148

Fig. 8-1 is drawn for the case of an expense budget, so the goal is to minimize expenses. Let us assume that without a budget (Stedry's implicit budget situation) the expense level will be N. Now fig. 8-1 shows what happens if we consider various alternative budget levels from very loose (case 1) to very tight (case 6). In case 1, the budget is too loose, i.e. above level N. The budgetee will probably be aware of this and set his aspiration level a somewhat better (lower than the budget) but still above N. The result r will be equal to the aspiration level. Case 1 is the case of the 'low' and 'medium' budgets in Stedry's experiment.

In case 2, the budget just hits N. Aspiration level and result coincide with the budget. In fact, the budget does not influence performance here. In case 3, the budget is somewhat below N. The budgetee will adapt his aspiration level to the budget, but not necessarily fully; I have assumed the aspiration level on the average to be located somewhere between N and b. As the goal is not yet very tight, the result has a fair chance of coinciding with the aspiration level.

In case 4, the budget is tighter still. The aspiration level is tightened up as well, but now it has become so tight that the actual result has a strong risk of being not as good as the aspiration level. Therefore, r is shown to be above a.

In case 5, the budget is very tight; so much, that the budgetee sees it as 'almost impossible' and sets a less ambitious aspiration level than in case 4; which he may attain in the actual result.

In case 6, finally, the budget is so tight that the budgetee sees it as fully impossible, so that he stops trying; he avoids setting an aspiration level at all, and his negative attitude about the impossible budget may make his actual result worse than would have been the case without the budget. Case 6 is the case of some foremen in the Stedry & Kay experiment who got two difficult goals.

The optimal budget level from a point of view of the actual result attained is somewhere between case 3 and 4 (the minimal value of the r curve); in practice, its position will depend also on factors like the budgetee's personality, experiences in the past, and on group standards.

What the diagram of fig. 8-1 clearly illustrates is that only budget levels within a limited zone really improve performance; outside this zone (cases 1 and 6) budgets do more harm than good. Stedry & Kay (1964[b]) advocate avoiding case 1 by choosing difficult goals, and avoiding case 6 by designing a mechanism to revise the goals if the budgetee sees them as impossible. In this way, they in fact introduce some participation of the budgetee in goal-setting. A similar recommendation is given by Becker & Green (1962).

The problem is complicated when we look at successive budget cycles in time. Case 4 in fig. 8-1 may be felt as a failure to the budgetee, because his result is worse than his aspiration level; this feeling of failure may induce him to set a less ambitious aspiration level next time; case 4 may then shift to case 5. Besides, budget levels themselves will also shift in time. If not, the motivating effect of the budget will soon be gone, and special cost reduction drives will be necessary to improve cost performance (chapter 2 and 14). Stedry stresses that "*a stationary budget is not an effective control budget*. If the budget level is never attained, then some other criterion is in fact replacing it as a control element. If the level is consistently attained, the question of the possibility of consistently obtaining operation at a lower cost will never be answered, because there is no incentive to improve performance". (Stedry, 1960, p. 18; this second situation is similar to cases 1 and 2 in fig. 8-1). Stedry therefore advocates choosing budget levels so that they are attained part of the time; this percentage of the time being chosen to provide an acceptable balance of positive and negative psychological reward for the budgetee.

Achievement motivation and levels of standards in this study

Unlike both research projects described earlier in this chapter, mine is a field study. It could describe and measure aspects of the budget systems in the six plants, but it could not manipulate any variables in the systems. Let us first look at the things people say about the issue of the level of standards:

A. 'I would definitely make the standards as tight as can be attained. For example, we can plan for 20 charges a shift or for 25. If we say 20, we'll never get more. If we say 25, we'll possibly hit 24. Of course one mustn't tell the fellows' (first-line-manager).

'I prefer standards that are attainable. If not, they won't create much improvement and I wonder if they won't damage morale' (third-line-manager).

'I believe in an objective that is not attainable. The American System. That's something a fellow can pull himself up to' (subordinate of the previous interviewee).

'I think negative variances have more impact than positive ones' (third-line-manager).

'I'd be happy if the system were just a tiny bit looser' (first-line-manager).

'The large gap between the other plant's performance and ours was very depressing. Now we're closer, it's better' (first-line-manager).

B. 'If we've made it we're all happy' (second-line-manager).

'If we're not clean at the end of the day, the boys are unhappy too' (first-line-manager).

'Of course I feel swell when my department hits 135' (first-line-manager).

'At year-end we have the proud feeling we've made it' (second-line-manager).

'One feels a bit hurt in one's sence of honor if one does not attain the goal' (first-line-manager).

'We tell the fellows it's a matter of honor to attain standard time. I think this works more flexibly than piece-rates. It works better' (first-line-manager).

'I think it's easier working in a system of standards. A fellow can feel satisfied' (second-line-manager).

C. 'Standards imperceptibly penetrate into ones mind' (third-line-manager).

'A standard is something to go by' (25 managers in various keys).

'A standard is a thermometer, otherwise I would have to feel my way' (third-line-manager).

'Standards are like traffic signs, they prevent accidents' (first-line-manager).

From these quotations, it is very clear that standards can be internalized into aspiration levels; they do function as yardsticks for achievement. The level of standards is an important issue in this process of achievement motivation. In all the cases mentioned above, no direct rewards or punishments were connected to the attainment of the standards. The achievement itself was sufficient motivation.

It is interesting to compare the statements by line managers with the opinions of the budt- or standards-departments staff. One important issue in this case is whether some of the standards are used through piece-rates or other systems to directly influence workers' pay. When this happens, there is a tendency to stay on the loose side to avoid grievances and bad morale.

"I think a loose standard is better. It's my experience that with a tight standard people tend to say: 'I can't make that! It has a depressing effect. If the standard is looser, people will in fact surpass it' (work study engineer). This is the majority opinion. Yet another work study engineer says: 'I prefer a tight standard. If it's too loose, it is difficult to adjust it any more".

In the case where standards do not influence workers' pay, the general tendency is to the well-known 'tight, but attainable' standards.

'I prefer rather tight standards. Just because we don't have piece-rates here. You don't touch anybody's pay, and you give them a good goal to strive for. If we had piece-rates, there would be quite other aspects' (work study engineer).

'A very tight standard has an adverse effect, but a standard that is too loose is useless' (budget accountant).

The trouble is, that in practice 'attainable' is an ill-defined property, and ideas of attainability vary widely.

A very practical remark is:

'The most important aspect is that standards must be adjusted regularly. Every standard is only a step on the productivity ladder; there is always a danger it will stay there' (staff manager).

Finally:

'I think the essential issue is whether one has standards or not, even rough ones. I do not mind so much if they're loose or tight' (staff manager). The following pages will show, however, that this is not right.

The effect of standard levels on motivation

In all plants except DYNAMO 1 and 2, I have asked line interviewees to score whether they judged certain groups of standards to be "loose" or "tight" (Appendix D 3, question D 11).

The results are shown in fig. 8-2.

PLANT	Number of times people scored:					Average Score
	1 too tight	2 tight, but attainable	3 just right	4 fairly loose	5 too loose	
ALPHABET	3	14	12	2	1	2,5
BUROMAT	9	22	15	12	0	2,5
COMBITEX	6·	15	12	4	0	2,4
EPICURE	2	2	17	4	0	2,9

Difference between EPICURE and other plants, tested with Wilcoxon's test (one-tailed) significant at 0,01 – level.

FIG. 8-2. Interviewee's Scores for the Levels of Their Standards in Four Plants.

In three plants, the most frequent score is 'tight, but attainable'. EPICURE is the exception: here nearly all standards are considered 'just right'. The average score of a line interviewee for the 'looseness' of the different groups of standards ('measurable dimensions') important to him, is used as a variable in the statistical analysis of data (variable no. 34 in Appendix E 2). I have also asked a judgment about the looseness or tightness of the different groups of standards from the top line manager, and from the staff interviewee. Their average judgment is another variable in the statistical analysis (no. 35). I have already used this variable in chapter 7, where it appeared that there was a clear correlation between this measure of 'looseness of standards' and actual budget variance. As will be shown in the statistical analysis at the end of this chapter, variables no. 34 (looseness of standards according to the line interviewee himself) and no. 35 (looseness of standards according to top line-manager and staff employees) are significantly correlated, but the line interviewee's own judgment is only weakly correlated to the actual budget variance.

Apparently the top line manager and the staff look more at actual results to decide whether a standard is tight or loose; the line interviewees themselves describe more 'how the standards feel': their personal background and experience play a role in how they see the standards.

Another bit of information I have gathered from line interviewees expressed whether they expected improvement in performance over the next 12 months in any relevant aspect ('measurable dimension') of their department. The number of times they said to expect improvement is scored in variable 36. Expectations of deterioration are scored negatively. These scores for expectations of improvement can be considered as measures of 'goal discrepancy'. In chapter 3, p. 65, the concept of goal discrepancy has been introduced as one of the fundamentals of the Level of Aspiration Theory. It is defined as: level of aspiration minus past performance. Therefore, an expectation of improvement in performance in the coming year means a positive goal discrepancy. In the theory quoted in chapter 3 it is stated that positive goal discrepancies are generally associated with high motivation. In the statistical section of this chapter, it is shown that expected improvement in performance (goal discrepancy, variable 36) is significantly correlated with budget relevance (questions measure) and with both measures of budget attitude. As relevance and attitude together represent motivation, this confirms the expected relationship between positive goal discrepancies and motivation. *Higher motivation to fulfill standards is reflected in expectations of improvement over past performance.*

Fig. 8-1 suggests that the relationship between performance and budget level follows a curve. According to the description of fig. 8-1, motivation follows the same curve as budget levels vary. Finally, goal discrepancy follows also a curve. Goal discrepancy is represented by a (aspiration level) minus r (result). As we are dealing with expense levels, a negative a-r represents a positive goal discrepancy, that is an expectation of improvement. We see in fig. 8-1 that the expectation of improvement is greatest in a middle zone of budget tightness, between case 3 and 5. To test whether this curvilinear relationship exists in my data, I have divided the 59 line interviewees for whom I had 'looseness of standards' scores into three thirds: the top, middle and bottom third in judgment about looseness of standards. In the statistical section on page 172, the results are analyzed. It appears that all motivation measures and 'expectation of improvement' as well show the predicted curvilinear relationship with 'looseness of standards', but only a few of the differences between 'thirds' reach statistical significance. This is not surprising, as my sample was rather small. Nevertheless, the data show that *when standards are tightened up, motivation at first increases up to a certain limit of standard tightness; over this limit, motivation decreases again.* 'Standard tightness', or rather 'looseness' in this case, is measured subjectively: it is defined by the budgetee and different budgetees will differ in what they call 'tight'.

The statistical analysis shows further that *the lowest relevance is found for loose standards: the least favorable attitudes and the least expectations of improvement are found for very tight standards.*

The factor analysis (fig. 7-1) gives some additional insight into the effects of standard levels. Variable no. 34: interviewee's own judgment about looseness of standards, reaches the critical level of a 0,35 loading on none of the factors. It has nearly-critical loadings on two factors: 0,32 on factor 3 (upward communication') and − 0,31 on factor 7 ('job involvement'). 'Upward communication' is a factor which first of all represents a boss who is open to the ideas of his subordinates. It also indicates good line-staff communication and the absence of work pressure. The figures suggest that under these circumstances, standards will not easily be seen as tight. Also for this factor, budget attitudes are positive. This has practical consequences: I have stated the advice of Stedry & Kay (p. 149) to avoid loose standards by deliberately choosing difficult goals, but to avoid goals that are seen as impossible by the budgetee by designing a mechanism to revise goals if necessary. My finding that where upward communication is good, standards will not be seen as too tight, supports this advice. Only, the 'mechanism to revise goals' must function well and be perceived as functioning well by the budgetee. It is not just a simple gimmick that can be introduced; it is part of an overall attitude of management that is visible plant-wide. Chapter 12 will go deeper into this issue.

'Job involvement' is most likely a personality or cultural factor. This factor is high for those who feel that the plant demands the utmost of them: they believe that working comes natural to most people, probably also to themselves. These interviewees are mainly found among the first-line managers of DYNAMO 2, and they do feel their standards are tight, but do not show any negative attitude or de-motivation because of this. See the DYNAMO case study in this chapter, and also chapter 13.

The factor analysis also shows that variable no. 36: expected improvement in performance, has a loading of 0,51 on factor 6: 'job rotation'. This factor indicates that those who are relatively new in their jobs will expect more performance improvement. Thus, an important determinant of expectation of improvement appears to be something else than the budget level: quite simply the fact that a manager is new in his job. The interviewee's age loads also on this factor (0.59). In the experiment of Stedry & Kay, age also appeared to be a factor: it was supposed to contribute to determining the reaction of budgetees on tight standards. I have taken 'job rotation' as the key variable because it shows the highest loading (0.65), but another explanation would be that age is the key variable (see chapter 13). Of course this does not rule out the influence of the budget level which we saw before. A factor analysis just cannot show curvilinear relationships like the one between budget level and expectation of improvement.

Group differences in reacting to standard levels

The Level of Aspiration Theory in chapter 3 (p. 62) uses also the concept 'attainment discrepancy': level of actual new performance minus level of aspiration. This measure indicates the probability of feelings of success and failure. Stedry suggests, that a budget system should produce an acceptable balance of success and failure experiences for the budgetee (p. 93). In this study, I have measured feelings of relative success or failure by asking *evaluation marks*. Each line interviewee has given evaluations of the various aspects ('measurable dimensions') of his department's performance on a scale. This scale is similar to the one used for school performance in most Dutch schools: 9 = excellent, 8 = good, 7 = fairly good, 6 = satisfactory, 5 = so-so.

I assume there is a relationship between these evaluation marks and the 'attainment discrepancies' described above. People who give higher marks (7, 8 or 9) feel relatively more successful and will therefore tend to have positive attainment discrepancies; people who give lower marks (6 or 5) feel probably they performed worse than they aspired to, and will tend to have negative attainment discrepancies. Evaluation marks are averaged for each line interviewee over the various dimensions of his department's performance that are relevant, and handled as variable no. 37 in the statistical analysis.

If a budget system motivates the budgetees, there should be an agreement (correlation) between the evaluation marks and the budget variances. Where actual performance is less good than the budgetary standard (unfavorable budget variance) people should give low evaluation marks, and vice-versa. As the statistical analysis at the end of this chapter shows, budget variance (variable 28) and evaluations of own department's performance (variable 37), taken over total data, are significantly correlated (r = 0,37***). However, this correlation varies from plant to plant. It is quite interesting to compare our six plants in this respect; this is done in fig. 8-3. The data on which fig. 8-3 is based are collected in Appendix F. For every plant, Appendix F shows a number of 'cases'. Every 'case' is one evaluation mark given by one line interviewee for his department's present performance on one 'measurable dimension'. All 90 line interviewees together provided 466 cases, that is somewhat more than five measurable dimensions per interviewee. Each evaluation is compared with the official budget variance of this measurable dimension for the interviewee's department over the past three months. For each plant separately, fig. 8-3 shows the relationship between evaluation and budget variance expressed in a straight line (regression line) which is the best possible 'fit'.

The dashed lines in fig. 8-3 represent the limits between which the regression lines for each plant should fall if the differences from plant to plant were just a result of chance (0.95 confidence interval). I had predicted after the DYNAMO pilot study, that I would find significant (non-chance) differences between the other four plants. Therefore, the confidence limits are calculated on the basis of the data of these four plants only; and as COMBITEX and EPICURE fall outside the limits, my prediction is proven to be justified.

The picture of fig. 8-3 is the following: of the six plants, DYNAMO I and EPICURE show virtually no correlation between evaluation and budget variance. COMBITEX and DYNAMO 2 show a stronger than average correlation, while ALPHABET and BUROMAT take in-between positions. The difference between DYNAMO I and 2 is extremely remarkable, as both plants are so similar from a technical and organization point of view. I will explore it as a case study below. The COMBITEX case, too, will be described as a case study in this chapter.

In interpreting the regression lines of fig. 8-3, we can make two assumptions about causality: first, people tend to evaluate on the basis of the official budget variances that are communicated to them; or second, people evaluate on the basis of what they observe daily in their jobs and budget variances reflect the same thing. Most likely, both assumptions

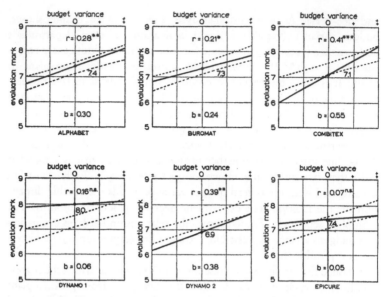

n.s. = non-significant, *significant at 0.05, **significant at 0.005, ***significant at 0.0005, b = regression coefficient.
The dashed lines are 0.95 confidence limits for subgroup regression lines based on the total sample.

FIG.8-3. Regression Lines of Subjective Evaluation of Own Department's Performance on Budget Variance.

hold true to some extent. The correlation between evaluation and budget variance points in any case to some degree of agreement between personal standards (aspiration levels) and budget standards, whichever may have been first. This means that where communications with the line on budget variance is poor, there may still be a correlation between evaluation and budget variance. If, however, the communication about standards is poor too, correlation becomes unlikely. This is the case for EPICURE (fig. 8-3). As this is mainly a staff-line problem it will be described (as a case study) in chapter 11.

The significance of the regression lines in fig. 8-3 is, that *budget or standards cannot be supposed to have any motivating effect unless they are to some extent 'internalized'*. In the case of DYNAMO I and EPICURE, as far as the motivation of my interviewees was concerned, there might as well have been no standards at all.

Fig. 8-3 also reveals that there are considerable differences as to what evaluation is given on the average to 'zero budget variance', that is a standard just made. In DYNAMO 1, this is 8,0 in ALPHABET and EPICURE, 7,4; in COMBITEX, 7,1; in DYNAMO 2 which appears to be most modest, 6,9. These figures can be considered as reflecting 'informal' budget levels for the various plants. The slope of the regression lines varies from 0,55 (COMBITEX) to 0,05 (EPICURE). This reflects the degree to which aspiration levels are set that follow the budget. ,

The evaluation variable (no. 37) shows up in the factor analysis with a loading of 0,74 on factor 8. I have called this factor 'self-satisfaction', because it shows only a low correlation (0,21) with budget variance. On the other hand, it shows a loading of 0,37 for the ability rating of the interviewee, given by his boss and the personnel manager. So it expresses a general feeling of 'being a good performer' without being actually based on the figures (see also chapter 13).

I have also introduced a variable (no. 38) to attempt to identify as individuals those who do and those who don't set their aspiration levels according to the budget (see the statistical section at the end of this chapter). This variable is scored negatively and represents therefore lack of correlation between own evaluation and budget variance. In the factor analysis, this variable loads also on factor 8: 'self-satisfaction': 0,36. This confirms that this is the factor of those who do *not* follw the budget in giving evaluation marks. Variable no. 38 has also a loading of – 0,35 on factor no. 6: job rotation. This means that the 'job rotation' people, that is those who are relatively new in their jobs, do show a better correlation between own evaluation and budget variance. We saw already earlier in this chapter, that these were also the people who expected most improvement in performance. The 'job rotation' factor explains partly fig. 8-3: why people in some plants do, and others do not follow the budget in their evaluations. Outside the factor analysis, variable no. 38 (lack of correlation between evaluation and budget variance) shows correlations with hierarchical level ($r = -0.28^\star$) and with frequency and usefulness of meetings with boss and colleagues ($r = -0,23^\star$). Correlation between evaluation and budget variance is higher for those at higher hierarchical levels, and for those having frequent and useful meetings with their boss and colleagues. This is quite understandable. The meetings issue will be further dealt with in chapter 12.

The effect of standard levels on job satisfaction

There are no indications of either a positive or a negative job satisfaction effect of any of the variables dealing with standard levels. The only exception is a $r = 0,20^*$ correlation of job satisfaction with the 'lack of correlation between evaluation and budget variance'. This is explained by factor 8 in the factor analysis: 'self-satisfaction'. It is not very important.

There are no correlations whatsoever between standard levels and a feeling of pressure. This shows that pressure is not caused by just tightening up standards. It is the personal communication which goes with it which causes the pressure – or not.

Summary of the conclusions of my study about achievement motivation and the levels of standards

1. Budgets and standards can be 'internalized' into personal aspiration levels.
2. They will have a more positive effect on motivation when they are tighter and less easily attained. This works up to a certain limit: beyond this limit, tightening of standards reduces motivation.
3. Higher motivation is reflected in expectations of improvement over past performance (goal discrepancy).
4. The relevance component in motivation is lower for budgets that are too loose than for budgets that are too tight.
5. The attitude component in motivation is more negative for budgets that are too tight than for budgets that are too loose.
6. There are important differences between plants in the way standards are internalized; plants have different 'informal budget levels' and different degrees of internalization of standards into personal aspiration levels.
7. Personality and cultural differences, like differences in job involvement, are important determinants of people's reactions to a certain level of standards.

8. Situational data like hierarchical levels, the time people have been in their jobs, and people's age, influence the way in which people react to standard levels.
9. Stimulating upward communication can help to avoid that standards will be seen as tight.
10. The use of departmental meetings facilitates the internalization of standards into personal aspiration levels.

These results confirm to a great extent the conclusions of the experiments of Stedry and Stedry & Kay. The new element in them is the role of situational data and group management in influencing budget motivation. This can be illustrated by the DYNAMO and COMBITEX case studies, which will now follow.

A case study: evaluation of own department's performance in DYNAMO 1 and 2

Both DYNAMO plants produce the same type of electronic components, with only minor constructional differences. The plants are located in different parts of the Netherlands. In the period of the interviews, both were of the same size. Technology was the same except for unimportant details. Line and budget staff organization was completely similar, so that for every manager in DYNAMO 1 a counterpart could be found with the same responsibility for DYNAMO 2. In addition, budget and standard levels were the same, except for small differences in technology and housing. It was a policy in the DYNAMO company that if the same products were made in both plant 1 and 2, there would not be any difference in cost price. In short, the plants were the most ideally matched pair of research areas any investigator could hope for. Yet, in plotting evaluation marks – given by managers to own departments' performance – against budget variance, we get totally different pictures for both plants. See fig. 8-3, regression lines for DYNAMO 1 and 2; compare also the raw data in Appendix F.[2] We read from these lines, that in DYNAMO 1 there is no correlation between subjective evaluation and budget variance whatsoever. In 87% of cases, DYNAMO 1 managers gave the marks 8 'good' or 9 'excellent'. In DYNAMO 2 there is a fairly good correlation

[2] Each of the 60 'cases' of DYNAMO 1 in Appendix F can be matched with a case in DYNAMO 2: same department, same measurable dimension.

between subjective evaluation and budget variance. 'Good' or 'excellent' marks are, moreover, given only in 45% of cases. A case with zero budget variance (standards just hit) receives on the average an 8 evaluation mark in DYNAMO 1; the same situation receives on the average less than a 7 mark (6.9) in DYNAMO 2.[8] In the periods concerned, both plants attained their overall objectives, although the positive overall budget variance was greater for DYNAMO 2 than DYNAMO 1. I have also asked for subjective evaluations from the budget staff; in this case, there was very little difference between DYNAMO 1 and 2, and the judgment was in between the DYNAMO 1 and 2 line evaluations. What could be the cause of this extreme difference in the 'internalization' of budget standards?

As both plants have so much in common, we have to look at their differences to find any clues. The main difference is one of function within the total organization. DYNAMO 1 is the parent plant. The product development department is situated there; the plant has not only to produce, but also to develop new products and to improve existing products and processes. DYNAMO 2, on the other hand, was set up four years before the interviews as a pure production plant, with as its main objective good and efficient mass production of the products developed in DYNAMO 1. This difference in function entails a different weight of budget control as a management tool in either plant. In DYNAMO 2, budget control is the major control tool; in DYNAMO 1, it is only one of several controls. In managing DYNAMO 1, stimulating creative activity is probably of more importance than budget control. The difference in function is accompanied by a difference in personalities as far as second-

[8] Once cause of possible bias cannot be overlooked. When the interviews in DYNAMO 1 were held, the new budget year had just started. As not yet everybody appeared informed of the new standards, I took the last 2 months of the previous budget year as a basis for calculating budget variances. The interviews in DYNAMO 2 were held one month later, when the new standards had had time to penetrate; here, I took the first 2 months of the new budget year as a basis for calculating budget variances. If this difference in periods has biased the comparison between DYNAMO 1 and 2, however, it can only have made the picture of fig. 8-3 less pronounced. The new standards were, if not the same, tighter than the old ones: a zero budget variance on the new standards was possibly a + variance in the old ones. Therefore, reducing DYNAMO 2 to the old standards would move the regression line to the right, and the difference with DYNAMO 1 would still be greater. On the other hand, the regression line for DYNAMO 1 on the basis of the new standards would look exactly like the one in fig. 8-3. I have tried this.

and third level managers are concerned. Although all of these managers were trained in DYNAMO 1, DYNAMO 2 managers seem to be more production-oriented and interested in organization problems. Maybe that is why they are selected for this particular job. They also stimulate each other. 'Personally, I've always been interested in budgeting, even before I came here. I am sure the interest of the department managers is influenced by mine' (third-line-manager, DYNAMO 2). In DYNAMO 1, the second-line and higher-level-managers are more of the technically creative, improvising type.

There is also a difference in personalities between first-line-managers (foremen) in both plants, but this has a different origin. In this company, second-level managers are recruited among higher-educated young outsiders, who start their career as assistants to a second-level-manager. First-line-managers mostly come through the ranks. This was at least the case in DYNAMO 1, where all first-line-managers had only primary school eduction; they had served with the company for 13-35 years and had on the average been a manager for 6 years. In DYNAMO 2, although all first-line-managers originated from the region when the plant was built, they were hired as managers when the plant was started; most of them had management experience in other industries, and most of them had some advanced education after primary school. Significantly, the first-line managers in DYNAMO 1 had lunch in the workers' cafetaria; in DYNAMO 2, they had lunch in the staff cafetaria.

'We are different from the foremen in the other plant. We had a management job before and we also have closer ties with our department managers. Their doors are open here – just give them a ring and one is welcome. It's not the same in the other plant' (foreman, DYNAMO 2).

Meetings between department manager and foremen were held more frequently in DYNAMO 2 than in DYNAMO 1; in 2, weekly; in 1, with a frequency of between 2 and 6 weeks. We will meet the DYNAMO 2 foremen again in chapter 13.

In the past four years, DYNAMO 2 had had a tough time to meet the standards. In accordance with company policy, standard levels for both plants, after a starting-up period of about one year, had to be the same; this meant in practice that standards were set according to the situation in the leading parent plant, DYNAMO 1. 'We're tied to the best result they can find' (second-line manager, DYNAMO 2).

The management of all levels in DYNAMO 2 felt it as a challenge to beat the parent plant.

'This is a new plant. We are growing with it, we're building up something. It gets close to one's heart' (foreman, DYNAMO 2).

After four years of hard work, just about the time of the interviews, they had made it. As a matter of fact, shortly afterwards they became more efficient than the parent plant.

'We had excessive rejects for years. Now they're on standard. I'm very proud. I do like standards' (second-line manager, DYNAMO 2).

'Some of the foremen in the department meeting were not convinced the standards helped to increase productivity, but I've convinced them. Of course one has to use them. It is my custom to write standards and variances on the blackboard in the meetings' (second-line manager, DYNAMO 2).

On the other hand, DYNAMO 1 management had had little trouble in meeting the standards. Their variances were nearly always favorable.

'Our standards do not influence productivity. If there are any significant variances, there is always something wrong in the calculation' (second-line manager, DYNAMO 1).

'My task is made easier by the standards. Maybe it would be different if they were very tight' (foreman, DYNAMO 1).

The feedback sessions (see Chapter 6) in DYNAMO 1 and 2 were also rather different. In DYNAMO 2, the discussions were generally more lively, although there were differences between groups. The critical factor seemed to be the way in which the group leaders dealt with standard matters. Standards had to be relevant to them personally, but also they had to have the social skills to involve the group of their subordinates in these issues. Both conditions were fulfilled to a larger extent in DYNAMO 2 than in DYNAMO 1.

In summary, to explain the difference of internalization of standards in DYNAMO 1 and DYNAMO 2, we can find the following clues: Firstly, DYNAMO 1 was a development plant where creativity was probably more important than budget control, while 2 was a mass production plant where budget control was the main control tool. Secondly, this difference in 'function' led to a number of differences in 'functioning'; also, there were differences in personalities reinforcing this effect. Finally, DYNAMO 1 had been in a position where it was the leading plant. Standards were mostly set after its performance so that overall variances were always positive and hardly any effort was needed to meet overall cost objectives. This led DYNAMO 1 management to give high evaluation marks to their departments' performance throughout even though actual budget variances showed losses in various cases. DYNAMO 2 had been in the challenging situation of building up a new plant with a wholly new team. The pioneering situation (in a small country town) perhaps helped to forge team unity. DYNAMO 2 managers were probably selected because they had the organizational and leadership skills necessary for such a situation, which meant they had more of an innate interest in budgets; also, they reinforced each other's interest. The standards they were up against were very real to them: they knew they had been achieved in the parent plant. They knew they had a lot to learn, which made them humble; they were eager to improve, which made them study and discuss standards and variances frequently and furthered the standards internalization process.

The evaluation differences shown in fig. 8-3 lead to the question whether DYNAMO 1 judgments would have followed the standards more if these had been tighter. This might have meant using a different set of standards for either plant. There are methods in budget accounting to apply different standards for different plants and balance out differences through an equalization account[4] to get equal cost prices. If this would have been done, goals might have been set that meant a challenge to DYNAMO 1 too, without making them impossibly high for DYNAMO 2.

One other feature of the DYNAMO case must be mentioned. In this company, there was a clear conflict between the measuring and the planning function of a budget, as described in chapter 2 (fig. 2-1). It was in the company's interest that parts of the company, like plants, met their budgets as precisely as possible ('uncertainty avoidance' – see chapter 4). Neither positive, nor negative budget variances of any size were desirable. But of course top plant management felt measured by the standards too, and as one staff interviewee lucidly remarked 'People prefer to be scolded at year end for a budget gain over being scolded for a budget loss'. Many standards are of such a nature that possibilities for a favorable

---

[4] In fact there existed such an equalization account in the DYNAMO accounting system. It was only used for balancing out small differences in equipment, housing and other technical matters, however, not for balancing out psychological differences.

variance are limited, while possibilities for an unfavorable variance are much larger. We can think here for instance of the production volume in an automated process, which cannot exceed the limit it is set at, but which can drop to zero if the equipment breaks down. It is known that every now and then such explosive unfavorable variances will occur. In order to avoid unfavorable overall plant results, top plant management will be tempted to set standard levels below the maximum attainable. In this way, nine out of ten variances will be somewhat on the favorable side, and this will balance the unpredictable catastrophe on the tenth variance. This was the case in the DYNAMO plants. In DYNAMO 1, there were several complaints about the looseness of standards, and even in DYNAMO 2, where they had been behind for a long time, people begain to note it after the introduction of the latest budget:

'For me they could have tightened up the reject standard for this year by $\frac{1}{2}$ percent still' (first-line-manager, DYNAMO 2).

'Sometimes reality is lost in the standards, they're just too loose. Top plant management wants it that way: I can only guess what their reasons are. They ought to set two standards, one for financial purposes and one as an objective. Now, sometimes, there is no challenge whatsoever' (second-line-manager, DYNAMO 1).

This last manager suggests what is the only good solution to a problem like this: using different standards for measuring and planning purposes (fig. 2-1). In general in industry, there seems to be a resistance on the part of both accountants and managers to do this. Greater awareness of the motivational issues in standard-setting may help to overcome this resistance.

A case of extremely unfavorable budget variances: the COMBITEX situation

COMBITEX is the plant with the most unfavorable budget variances in my sample. In the year before the interviews, total unfavorable budget variance was 16% of total added value (all costs minus materials). 12% was due to volume variances (chapter 2) and 4% to the combined effect of efficiency variances and expense variances. Standards were felt to be tight at COMBITEX, but more so by the top management and the staff than by line interviewees themselves. The relevance of the standards was fairly low.

'Too tight standards can have a negative effect. That is exactly the situation we're in at this moment' (staff interviewee, COMBITEX).

The unfavorable COMBITEX budget variance was the unplanned result of change in two respects. One was technical change. The plant had been extended considerably shortly before the interviews, and the extension had only recently been consolidated. The increase in production volume because of the expansion had been planned but not fully realized, and this is how the unfavorable volume variance had been created. Interestingly, there did not seem to be much pressure on COMBITEX management to change this situation. If relevance were higher, there would probably have been more pressure on the standards and a greater chance of getting them adjusted to a more realistic level.

The other type of change COMBITEX management had to face was social change. The plant is located in a small province town with an agriculturally oriented population. During the first fifteen years of the plant's existence, COMBITEX people were a rather closed group. People were eager to work for COMBITEX and to earn a good piece-rate in it. A management style adapted to the agricultural tradition developed, based on benevolent authority and the acceptance of it. With the extension which almost doubled the plant, COMBITEX had to attract new people. The new generation was less easy to manage and less willing to accept dependence. COMBITEX corporation management was aware of this and, both through its well-managed personnel department and through the management hierarchy, set the stage for democratization. Piece-rates were abandoned and this was done so thoroughly that even individual production data were no longer registered. 'Job enlargement' was the watchword.

COMBITEX' foremen, however, were ill prepared for these changes. They were all old-timers who started as operators when the plant was founded sixteen years ago, and who acquired their industrial experience in the old-style COMBITEX plant over fifteen years. Although they had been sent to management development courses and, in general, intellectually accepted the new approach, they just lacked the skills and the tools to manage their people the new way. The organization had been based on maintaining productivity by piece rates. Piece-rates were gone, but nothing was there to replace them. Thus, productivity started to drop. Standards that had been attained before were no longer attained. Foremen had a feeling of failure; in 47% of cases evaluation marks 5 or 6 were given, more than in any other of the six plants. Ability ratings (variable 39) were low.

'Things don't look rosy just now. The causes are varied. We've been a closed group, the plant was the mother to people. Now that we're overgrown, we have attracted other people of a different mentality. It used to be less complicated, now it's larger, less clear. We've got job enlargement and less supervision. Then there's the labor market. People get independent, they do not want to work at machines that are not attractive. Productivity is dropping, our standard used to be 75 units, but we 'll have to lower it' (staff interviewee, COMBITEX).

Looking at the regression lines of evaluation on budget variance in fig. 8-3, we see the COMBITEX line is the steepest of all. This is because of the very low evaluations given to the negative variance cases. Yet relevance is low, because the low raters have a feeling of failure – and failure has a demotivating effect (chapter 3). The cause of the failure is *not* in the standards themselves, but the standards serve to make it evident. 'The standards are fairly loose. That is, in theory they're loose, not in practice. That we don't attain them is not the standards' fault' (foreman, COMBITEX).

In spite of the failure feelings, the attitudes of interviewees towards the budget and standards system are rather positive at COMBITEX. Personal relationships are good; there is an excellent man to-man communication, and people do not feel anything like injustice in the way are treated. COMBITEX is an example of budget motivation that is exactly opposite to that described in Argyris' 'Impact of Budgets on People'.

Statistical analysis of data used in Chapter 8
The variables to be considered

The new variables in this chapter are (see Appendix E 2):

34. Interviewee's own judgment about the looseness of his standards, scaled by him on a five-point scale: 1 – too tight; 2 – tight, but attainable; 3 – just right; 4 – fairly loose; 5 – too loose. Each relevant measurable dimension is rated separately and an average is taken over all relevant measurable dimensions.

36. Expected improvement in performance in the coming year (scored by interviewer: 2 – deterioration expected; 3 – about stable; 4 – improvement expected); scored for each measurable dimension separately and totalled for the three most relevant measurable dimensions.

37. Average evaluation of present performance of own department, scored by interviewee on 5-point scales for each measurable dimension and averaged over measurable dimensions: (5 – so-so; 6 – satisfactory; 7 – fairly good; 8 – good; 9 – excellent). Interviewees were asked to rate 'present' performance. If they asked over what period, the answer was: the past month.

38. Lack of correlation between the evaluation of no. 37 and official budget variance of no. 28 calculated for each interviewee separately and averaged over all his relevant measurable dimensions.

The coding was as follows:

Ideal correlation was considered to be:

     Budget variance code 1 (>5% loss) – evaluation code 5 (so-so)
     Budget variance code 2 (1-5% loss) – evaluation code 6 (satisfactory)
     Budget variance code 3 (even ± 1%) – evaluation code 7 (fairly good)
     Budget variance code 4 (1-5% gain) – evaluation code 8 (good)
     Budget variance code 5 (>5% gain) – evaluation code 9 (excellent)

For every evaluation by every interviewee for each measurable dimension, points were given for deviations from the ideal correlation. For instance, if a situation with budget variance code 1 was evaluated 7, (7-5) = 2 points were given. If a situation with budget variance code 4 was evaluated 5, (8-5) = 3 points were given. Thus, zero points represents ideal correlation; four points is the maximum lack of correlation possible.

Relationships between variables

In fig. 8-4 the intercorrelations between budget variance and the other variables dealing with the level of standards issue are shown.

In fig. 8-4 we can consider budget variance and looseness of standards as inputs, expectation of improvement as an output and evaluation as an intervening variable. Two of the three intercorrelations between input variables are significant. The top line judgment about looseness of standards follows actual variances closer than the budgetee's own judgment.

Variable no. 37 (evaluation) shows a correlation of $r = 0.37^{***}$ with budget variance (no. 28). The within-subgroup-correlation is $r = 0,28^{**}$ and the rank correlation for 28 and 37 based on subgroup averages (plant + hierarchical level), is $r_R = 0,65^*$. This could be expected because of differences in budget variance level from subgroup to subgroup.

Variable no. 37 (evaluation) is also significantly correlated with looseness of standards (no. 35). People will apparently give higher marks in plants where the standards are looser.

Variable no. 38, lack of correlation between own evaluation and budget variance, is significantly correlated with no. 37, evaluation. This means that those who give their department high marks on present performance tend to neglect the budget variance figures. Conversely, it means that *if unfavorable evaluations of own department's performance are given, they tend to be based on budget variance.* Variable no. 38 is significantly negatively correlated with budget variance, no. 28. This does not mean, however, that

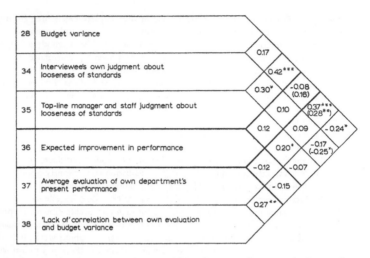

28	Budget variance				
34	Interviewee's own judgment about looseness of standards	0.17			
35	Top-line manager and staff judgment about looseness of standards	0.42*** 0.30*	-0.08 (0.16)		
36	Expected improvement in performance	0.10 0.12	0.37*** (0.28**) 0.09	-0.24*	
37	Average evaluation of own department's present performance	0.20* -0.12	-0.17 (-0.25*) -0.07	-0.15	
38	'Lack of' correlation between own evaluation and budget variance	0.27**			

Figures between brackets are correlations within subgroups; they are only shown where they differ to any important extent from overall correlations.

*significant at 0.05 level, **significant at 0.005 level, ***significant at 0.0005 level

FIG. 8-4. Intercorrelations of Variables Dealing with the Level of Standards Issue.

those who evaluate according to the budget figures have more favorable variances: it is a fictive correlation, caused by the way variable 38 is scored. The explanation of this is as follows: Points are scored representing deviances from the ideal evaluation for a given level of budget variance. Now we have noted the tendency of those who neglect the budget variance figures, to give high marks. In the case of positive budget variances, they will then hit the ideal evaluation just by accident; in the case of negative budget variances, they will be far off. Thus there is a greater chance of high 'lack of correlation' scores for the negative budget variances; this explains the negative correlation. It has no real meaning.

The correlations with motivation and job satisfaction are shown in fig. 8-5.

Looseness of standards is not significantly correlated with the motivation variables: we will see that the relationship is curvilinear. If the top line sees standards as loose, there tends to be less pressure.

Expected improvement in performance is significantly correlated with three of the four motivation measures. It looks therefore a fairly good measure of overall motivation. Evaluation is negatively correlated with attitude. In plants where a positive attitude towards the system prevails people appear to be more often willing to give a critical evaluation of their department's performance. Finally we find a positive correlation of variable no. 38 'lack of correlation evaluation-budget variance' with job satisfaction. This can be explained through the factor analysis. In the factor analysis the factor which

170

Correlations with:

Variables		34 interviewer's own judgment about looseness of standards	35 top line mgr. and staff judgment about looseness of standards	36 expected improvement in performance	37 average evaluation of own dept.'s performance	38 lack of correlation evaluation-budget variance
17	Relevance (impression)	−0.05(−0.04)	−0.08(−0.05)	0.09(0.03)	−0.12(−0.06)	−0.09(0.03)
18	Relevance (questions)	−0.15(−0.14)	−0.06(0.09)	0.19*(0.25*)	−0.01(0.09)	0.06(0.00)
19	Attitude (impression)	0.10(0.10)	−0.07(0.07)	0.33**(0.16)	−0.15(0.02)	−0.14(−0.07)
20	Attitude (questions)	−0.06(0.07)	0.04(0.13)	0.19*(0.23*)	−0.24*(−0.07)	−0.08(−0.05)
53	Job satisfaction	0.06(−0.14)	−0.06(0.11)	0.04(0.13)	0.10(0.11)	0.20*(0.36***)
54	Absence of pressure	−0.01(−0.15)	0.17(0.18*)	0.06(0.09)	0.08(0.06)	0.03(−0.10)

Figures between brackets are correlations within subgroups.

* significant at 0.05, level, ** significant at 0.005 level, *** significant at 0.0005 level

FIG. 8-5. Correlations of Level-of-Standards Variables with Motivation and Job Satisfaction.

shows highest loadings for both variable no. 38 and job satisfaction is 'self-satisfaction'. This represents an attitude in people which makes hem feel they like their job but which also does not encourage them to evaluate their performance in terms of the figures.

Fig. 8-6 represents the check on the predicted curvilinear relationship between variable 34: 'interviewee's own judgment about looseness of standards' and motivation plus expectations of improvement. Interviewees in the ALPHABET, BUROMAT, COMBITEX and EPICURE plans were divided into three groups: the top, middle and bottom third in judgment about 'looseness of standards'.

Division of line interviewees into:	17 relevance (impression)	18 relevance (questions)	19 attitude (impression)	20 attitude (questions)	36 expected improvement in performance
1/3 who judged their standards 'tightest'	6.1	9.4	6.8	7.7	0,9 ×
significance of difference	n.s	n.s	0,05	0,01	n.s
1/3 who took a middle position as to tightness or looseness of standards	6.8	9.5	7.6	9.4	1.5 ×
significance of difference	0.02	n.s	n.s	0,05	n.s
1/3 who judged their standards 'loosest'	5.9	9.2	7.3	8,0	1.2 ×

Scale for 'impression' scores: 1 to 9
Scale for 'questions' scores: relevance 6 to 10
                                              attitude   2 to 10
Scale for 'expected improvement in performance': 0 to 3 ×
Significances of differences between cells are tested with Wilcoxon's test for comparing samples, one - tail. n.s = not significant.

FIG. 8-6. Check on Curvilinearity in the Relationship between Looseness of Standards and Output Variables.

CHAPTER 9
PARTICIPATION IN STANDARD-SETTING

Summary of this Chapter

This chapter offers evidence of a positive effect of participation in standard-setting on motivation. It begins with an application of the theories about "participation in decision-making" on the budget case. It shows how participation was measured. For studying participation, it is necessary to distinguish between budget or financial standard-setting and technical or non-financial standard-setting Only participation in financial standard-setting has a direct effect on the motivation to fulfill the budget: of all quantified aspects of a budget system studied, this is the one with the strongest effect on motivation.

External reference points for standards are important for motivation: this is shown through a number of quotations from interviews. Authority of persons higher in the hierarchy also obviously plays a role in standard-setting. Attitudes towards authority were measured for the line interviewees, and these appear to influence the effect of participation on motivation. The data also show that low participation in budget setting does not automatically lead to a desire for more. Participation must be experienced before it becomes attractive. In the plants studied, with one exception, first-line management did not participate in budget setting. The issue is raised which level of management should participate in the setting of a budget.

Participation in the setting of technical standards has no apparent overall effect

173

on motivation, but it is considered a prerogative of any manager. Managers' job satisfaction is affected if they do not participate enough in the setting of their technical standards.

Standard setting too has a clear game aspect; this is demonstrated through quotations.

Finally, the BUROMAT *situation is presented as a case study of high budget participation and low participation in the setting of technical standards.*

Participation in perspective [1]

'I like working with standards, but with standards I've got a say in myself' (second-line-manager).

'Standards are something to go by. But having a standard that is set by consultation and then trying to surpass it; that is the greatest fun' (second-line-manager).

'My budget makes my task easier. It would be different if it were imposed without consultation. In that case the job would be very tough' (second-line-manager).

'I like standards if both parties agree about them. That is not always the case' (second-line-manager).

'I see no use in us gabbling in the choir when they are setting the standards. It is difficult enough without us' (first-line-manager).

'If they had to consult with all of us, where would they be? I've got no idea how the standard is set. I don't care so much' (first-line-manager).

'It is a healthy situation that the objectives are set from above. Maybe if we would do it ourselves we would take it too easy' (second-line-manager).

To several writers on the subject, the human side of budgeting *is* participation in standard-setting. In this book I hope to have shown that this sole concern is not justified and that budgeting has many other human aspects. Yet the participation issue is important. We have met 'participation in standard-setting' in chapter 1 as the spot where the control vs. autonomy conflict in budgeting was expected to be best visible. We have met it in chapter 2 through the assumption in at least part of the accounting theory of budgeting, that goal-setting by the organization

---

[1] This heading is borrowed from McGregor (1960, chapter 9).

improves people's performance, but having people participate in this goal-setting improves their performance still more. In chapter 3, participation in decision-making has been related to autonomy need satisfaction and also to other motivational processes in the budgetee. Finally, in chapter 4 we have seen the influence of the budgetee on the standards as a feedback loop in the control system (fig. 4-2). This feedback loop can balance the system without intervening in the actual process to be controlled, but the influence of 'external reference points' can prevent this.

Applying to the budget case what has been stated in chapter 3 about the positive effects of participation in general, we can predict the following:

a. Participation in standard-setting leads to improved communication, to better standards; it makes the standard-setting system a learning system (see also chapter 4).

b. Participation in standard-setting up to a certain limit increases higher management control: it decreases the probability of distorted information and other undesirable 'alternative actions' subordinates sometimes resort to in the face of non-participatively set standards.

c. Participation in standard-setting increases motivation to fulfill the standards. This is because participation satisfies autonomy needs, affiliation needs in the case of group participation, and achievement needs. The latter, because it may stimulate the 'internalization' of the standards for self-appraisal purposes, as a level of aspiration. Participation may offer the formalization of the level of aspiration procedure which appeared so important in the Stedry experiment (p. 146). Participation will tend to make the standards more relevant to the participant's task and therefore increase the relevance component of motivation; it may also lead to other desired outcomes, like a feeling of belonging, and thus influence the attitude component of motivation. Finally, participation in standard-setting serves as a safety device against goals that would be felt as impossibly difficult – it is a mechanism for guaranteeing a certain amount of balance and fairness in the system (compare p. 150).

Several limitations to the positive effects of participation in standard-setting can also be predicted:

a. A specific limitation to the positive effects of participation in standard-setting, not applicable to participation in decision-making in general, is that performance is measured by precisely the same standards that are set. Therefore, an apparent positive effect on performance may be just fictitious, and based on a lowering of the standard instead of on a real performance increase (Stedry & Charnes, 1962, p. 3, footnote). 'Any fool can learn to stay within his budget. But I have seen only a handful of managers in my life who can draw up a budget that is worth staying within' (N. Dreystadt to P. F. Drucker, quoted in Drucker, 1954, p. 74).

b. Personality traits of the participants may limit the benefits of participation: authoritarians and persons with weak independence needs will maybe perform better on standards set by higher authority.

c. National culture and business subculture may be counteracting forces to successful participation in standard-setting (e.g. foremen in a plant may not think it their legitimate role to have a say in budget standards).

d. Participation can not be incidental; it will work only when an experience of successful participation throughout is built up in the subordinate.

e. Several situational constraints limit participation in standard-setting. One of these is operational control as defined on page 10; the budgetee must perceive to have influence on the results the standards are about. There is no use for a manufacturing foreman to participate in the budget for his share of personal department costs, for example. Another situational constraint is the availability of external reference points for the standard to be set, like:

    – technological data: machine speeds, etc.
    – studies by acknowledged specialists, like quality engineers and work study engineers.
    – comparison with the performance of other, similar units within or outside the organization.

Such external reference points limit the amount of free scope left for participative standard-setting.[2]

f. A final limitation is based on the function of a standard as a checkpoint for achievement. A standard that is self-generated may have *less*

[2] In a study by Philipsen and Cassee (1965) the availability of external reference points for productivity standards is related to the type of leadership that will be found in an organization.

authority and challenge, and reaching it may give less success feelings than a standard based on unshakable external evidence (see chapter 3, page 63). In the process of setting and performing to standards, satisfying autonomy needs through participation may conflict with the satisfaction of achievement needs later on.

Limitation a is quite serious. It points to the vital importance of external reference points, like those mentioned under d, in the process of standard-setting. In the usual stress on participation in standard-setting they are often overlooked.

The way the effect of participation in standard-setting is usually described is about like model A in fig. 9-1. Basing myself on the theoretical analysis in these pages and on the findings which will be presented, I think model B in fig. 9-1 is a better, although less simple picture of the effects of participation in standard-setting. I have split motivation into its components "relevance" and "attitude", and introduced two other sources of data for standards which are quite realistic: external reference points, and authority of persons higher in the hierarchy. All three can serve to make a standard relevant to the budgetee: 'It is not clear from recent evidence . . . that participation in goal-setting is so advantageous as to preclude the inclusion of non-participatively set goals in behavioral models' (Charnes & Stedry, 1963, p. 6).

The mere presence of external reference points is not sufficient to make a standard relevant to a budgetee. He must perceive these reference points as applying to his situation.[3] A participation process may help to find external reference points that the budgetee perceives as valid. We can call this 'participation in standard finding', following van Doorn (1964). The effect of higher authority on motivation, or rather the effect of the mix of participation and higher authority that is used to set standards, will depend on personality and cultural elements in the budgetee. For example, the budgetee's being more or less authoritarian may have an influence: authoritarians may more readily accept non-participatively set standards. Positive effects of a mix of higher authority and participation in setting goals for Research and Development Scientists have

[3] In Festinger's more-mentioned Theory of Social Comparison Processes (1954), he analyzes under which circumstances people consider external reference points for comparing opinions and abilities as valid; for example, the difference with their situation must not be too great.

A. The Traditional View of the Effect of Participation in Standard-Setting

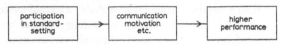

B. Improved Model of the Effect of Participation in Standard-Setting

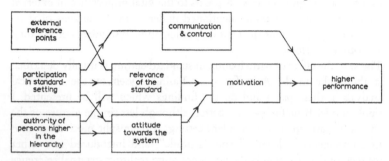

FIG. 9-1. Two Models for the Relationship between Participation in Standard-Setting and Performance.

been published by Pelz (1964). He proved that those setting their own goals autonomously were not the best performers, nor were those whose goals were set by higher authority alone. The best performers were the engineers and scientists for whom three or four 'echelons' contributed in the goal-setting process: themselves, their colleagues, their immediate boss, and either higher executive levels or some outside client or other body.

When the right mix of external reference points, participation and higher authority has not been found, standards will be felt by the budgetee as not legitimate, and this will impair his motivation to perform, at least the attitude component of it (Miles and Vergin, 1966).

The participation scale

To test the effects of participation in standard-setting in the present study, I had to measure participation. After pre-testing, I arrived at the following participation scale: (fig. 9-2).[4]

---

[4] A general participation scale is described in Likert (1961), p. 243.

	a myself	b staff	c myself	d staff
Decision taken by me/them without consultation	8	8	8	8
Proposal by me/them, followed by consultation; my/their opinion generally prevails	7	7	7	7
Proposal by me/them, decision made jointly	6	6	6	6
Proposal sometimes by others, sometimes by me/them; decision made jointly	5	5	5	5
Proposal by others, my/their opinion asked, and has a lot of weight	4	4	4	4
Proposal by others, my/their opinion asked but does not have much weight	3	3	3	3
My/their opinion not asked, but decision explained to me/them	2	2	2	2
My/their opinion not asked; decision not explained to me/them	1	1	1	1

line a + b: as it is
line c + d: as desirable

FIG. 9-2. Participation Scale

This scale places a stress on who makes the proposal, rather than who takes the final decision. It does not, for example, have a scoring possibility for 'proposal made by me, decision made by higher management'. Although this is often the formal procedure, the practical impact of this situation depends fully on whether higher management usually accepts proposals without change or not. Even if proposals are changed, the proposer has a lead. Interviewees were invited to score on the scales *as the process really functioned*, not as it was designed formally.[5]

On scales a and b the actual roles of interviewee and budgets or standards department staff were scored, and on scales c and d the roles the inter-

[5] Although the scale was designed to be scored by the interviewees rather than by the interviewer, especially in cases where the interviewees' role in the standard-setting process was slight, it proved a difficult and time-consuming task for them to understand the scale and score. Therefore, if such a situation could be expected, the interviewee was only asked to describe his role in the standard-setting process verbally, and the scoring was done by the interviewer.

viewee considered desirable. The scores for the staff role were only used to check whether the scale was well understood; there obviously must exist a balance between the roles of the interviewee, his superiors (not rated) and the staff.

The following quotations can illustrate the various line roles on the participation scale:

8. 'For supplies they just take the figures we quote'.
7. 'I do the budgeting myself. Wages, tools, everything. I'm doing it for the fifth time now. Up till now I've always got approval'.
6. 'I don't have much trouble with the budget. I make it myself, but the controller exerts a lot of pressure in the subsequent discussions'.
5. 'The budgets are made most often in a joint effort by my colleagues and me. We get some instruction how to calculate for example labor cost increases. Also, which items we have to budget ourselves and which not. Then we hand them in, and get them back three or four times. Most often they've made streaks in them, indications where we have got to economize. Sometimes they're just cut and imposed, we've got to accept that'.
4. 'We are consulted throughout'. 'We can change the standards if we don't agree with them'.
3. 'If I do not agree with the standards they are applied all the same'.
2. 'The figures are explained to us. Personally, I do not desire another role'.
1. 'I couldn't tell you exactly who sets the objectives, somebody in the plant or somebody in the head office'.

Comparison between scales c and a in fig. 9-2 showed whether more participation was desired. Some quotations from interviews with line managers where this was the case:

'The objectives are set from past years' data; the budget people make a proposal. What I don't like about it is that they have a couple of months to prepare their proposals, and they want us to decide in one day'.

'Reject percentages are taken from the other plant. Our opinion is not asked. I don't agree with that. If the materials are bad, how can we avoid rejects?'

'I definitely think I ought to be consulted when materials standards are set. It's quite possible there are changes in production methods which they do not take account of now'.

'I would like to join the standard-setting team. We foremen usually know more details than our boss.'
Some quotations from interviews with line managers of cases where more participation was considered unnecessary:
'I think they ought to play a tight game. Somebody must coordinate: the boss and the specialist. Just those two, no need to consult with the foremen'.
'I wouldn't like another role myself. I don't know if the roles are well divided at the higher levels, but basically I think it is OK that objectives are set from above'.
'Personally, I don't claim a role in setting the budget. Maybe I'm wrong, but I've got a job to do which keeps me busy enough not to bother about other things'.
'I do not think it should be different. As a foreman I don't need to do the work study engineer's job'.

The effect of participation on motivation

When I collected the scores of my line interviewees on the participation scales, it became evident that participation in the setting of financial standards (budgets) was much less general for first-line managers than for second and higher-level managers. On the other hand, participation in the setting of technical (non-financial) standards was fairly evenly distributed over all levels of management. This is illustrated by fig. 9-3.[6]
I therefore decided to analyze the effects on motivation of 'budget participation' and 'technical standard participation' separately.
My hypothesis when I set up the research project was *that higher participation leads to higher motivation to fulfill the standards*. As is shown in the statistical section at the end of this chapter, I found significant correlations of budget participation (the scores of the interviewees on the participation scale) and all four measures of budget motivation: two measures of 'relevance' and two measures of attitude. For the case of participation in the setting of financial standards my hypothesis 'higher participation leads to higher motivation' is thus confirmed. Of all variables studied, budget participation is the one with the strongest effect on all measures

[6] In fig. 9-3 for every subgroup the score is shown that represents the 'typical' case, not an average as this would be meaningless on an ordinal scale like the participation scale.

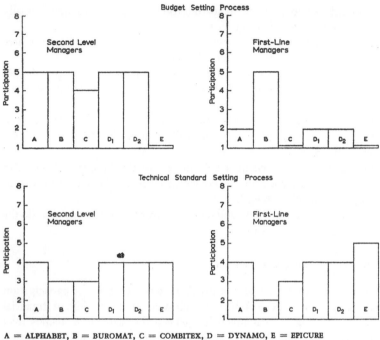

A = ALPHABET, B = BUROMAT, C = COMBITEX, D = DYNAMO, E = EPICURE

For the meaning of the participation scores see fig. 9-2.

FIG. 9-3. Typical Scores on Participation Scales for the Six Plants

of motivation. For participation in the setting of technical, non-financial
standards the picture is different. No correlations with budget motivation
were found. Although technical standards are essential components for
a budget system, those who participated in their setting will not automatically be motivated to try to fulfill the budget.

To get an overall picture of the effects of participation we have to go to
the factor analysis results (fig. 7-1). It appears that budget participation
(variable 29) has a loading of 0, 37 on factor 4 'cost-conscious boss'. This
factor is strongly influenced by the BUROMAT data, which are collected
in a case study on page 192. In short, factor 4 shows us a situation where
there is high budget participation and high budget relevance, but also

high pressure from above for results. The next highest loadings for 'budget participation' are below the 0,35 limit; they are on factor 5 'cost-conscious self' (0,31) and on factor 1 'independence' (0,28). The 'cost-conscious self' factor accounts for high budget relevance without pressure; it is the 'game' factor, which will be analyzed in more detail in chapter 12. The 'independence' factor accounts for favorable attitudes towards the system; I will devote a special section of this chapter to it below.

We can conclude from the above that budget participation leads to higher motivation, but that in this process many other aspects are also important, and will determine what kind of motivation people will feel. Technical standard participation (variable 31) does not show any loadings on the same factors as budget participation. It has a loading of 0,37 on factor 8: 'self-satisfaction'. This is the factor of those who rate their own performance high, and are considered by their boss as more able. It appears that these people feel they are consulted more than others in the setting of technical standards. There are no motivational variables related to factor 8.

The influence of external reference points for standards

We have now tested the main relationship shown in fig. 9-1 (model B): the influence of participation on relevance and attitude. The model also shows 'external reference points' as influencing the relevance of standards. External reference points guarantee that the participation process does not lead to low performance because of loose standards. From a point of view of motivation, they may have the positive effect of making standards more valid checkpoints for achievement (point f, p. 176). However, external reference points must be seen by the budgetee as valid for his situation. An example of valid external reference points can be found in the DYNAMO case study in chapter 8. To DYNAMO 2 budgetees, the fact that they knew that standards were based on DYNAMO 1 achievements made these standards valid and relevant, even though they had participated little in setting hem. I have not been able to quantify the impact of external reference points on standards in the six plants. Only rarely is the source of standards so clear as in the DYNAMO case. Most often external and internal sources are mixed inextricably.

183

The meaning of external reference points to interviewees can best be illustrated by quotations:

'The positive effect of standard-setting depends on the number of measurable versus non-measurable factors in the line department' (staff interviewee).

'The impact is strongest for machine-tied standards, when people know exactly what is expected from them. Where standards are well known, not only by one man but by everybody. Standards that are best measurable and visible are the best incentives' (staff interviewee).

The role of the specialist in standard-setting:

'I cannot but be happy with my role in standard setting. Otherwise, I'll have to do time- and motion studies myself. I'm just dependent on the specialists' (second-line-manager).

'The standards are quite fair. Two weeks ago the work study man explained them to us, they've taken account of everything. Some time ago we had a dispute with the work study department. Then we timed the job ourselves. Our times were tighter than theirs' (first-line-manager).

'The standards are most often too tight. Those fellows are too theoretical. I've asked the engineer to check them. One has to be a Fred Kaps[7] to do those calculations' (first-line-manager).

Sources of standards outside the plant:

'Those standards are data from a similar plant. What another plant can do, we can do too. That's how I see it' (first-line-manager).

'The standards are set after the situation in another plant with larger lot sizes and other tooling. I've been busy showing them that those standards don't apply for us. I'm working with the work study engineer to make better ones. Kind of a hobby of mine' (first-line-manager).

'For product B the standards are just pressed upon us because of competition's selling price' (first-line-manager).

'Quality standards are based on customer demands. They're quite tight. If we could set them somewhat looser we would work easier. But that is just our point of view, of course the customer is right' (second-line-manager).

From these quotations, it is clear that external reference points can have a very real meaning to budgetees, but they can also be rejected.

[7] A well-known Dutch illusionist.

In the statistical analysis I have used as variable 33 the scores on the attitude survey item 'Budgets are set here without taking sufficient account of my department's special problems'. This tells whether a budget is seen as 'legitimate'. Answer scores on this item (scored positively) show a significant correlation with both measures of budget attitude, variables 19 and 20 (0,24* in both cases); not with budget relevance. So if external reference points are rejected, the attitude component of motivation will suffer. Legitimacy of the budget is a 'hygienic' factor in motivation.

The participation-authority mix

Model B in fig. 9-1 shows 'authority of persons higher in the hierarchy' as another input which will influence the relevance and attitude. If there is less participation, the role of authority in standard-setting will generally be heavier. Now it may depend on the people involved which situation they prefer. After the pilot study in the DYNAMO plants, I was struck by the difference in desire for participation between the DYNAMO I foremen and the DYNAMO 2 foremen (compare the case study in chapter 8). I realized, that there would probably be a difference in authoritarianism between those two groups, and, following Vroom (1959, p. 327), I hypothesized that this would be a conditioning factor in the relationship between participation and motivation. For the other four plants, non-authoritarianism was then measured through attitude survey items in the small attitude survey administered at the end of the interviews. The method of measuring it is explained in the statistical section on p. 196. Scores of interviewees on 'non-authoritarianism' are used as variable no. 59 in the correlation and factor analysis.

An alternative hypothesis is that *hierarchical level* (variable no. 1) is a conditioning factor in the relationship between participation and motivation; for instance because first-line managers do not think it their legitimate role to have a say in standards. This hypothesis is difficult to separate from the previous one, as *hierarchical level and non-authoritarianism appear to be significantly intercorrelated* ($r = 0,42$***). This can also be seen in fig. 9-4, where average scores for 'non-authoritarianism' are shown per subgroup, including staff subgroups. The higher-level managers and the staff score higher throughout than the first-line managers. Besides, staff scores vary less from plant to plant than line management

PLANT	Average 'non-authoritarianism' score (59) for:		
	higher-level managers	first-line managers	staff interviewees
ALPHABET	11.2	8.6	12.2
BUROMAT	13.0	11.6	12.6
COMBITEX	15.3	10.8	12.3
EPICURE	10.5	9.0	11.4
TOTAL 4 PLANTS	12.7	10.1	12.2

Differences between higher-level and first-line managers and between staff and first-line managers, tested sith Wilcoxon's test, one-tailed, are both significant at 0.0005-level.

20 = maximal non-authoritarianism 4 = minimal non-authoritarianism

FIG. 9-4. Average 'Non-Authoritatianism' Scores for Subgroups

scores: there seems to be more of a 'standard staff attitude' than a 'standard line attitude' in this respect. See chapter 11. It is tempting to speculate about causality in the case of the correlation between hierarchical level and non-authoritarianism. Do people get less authoritarian and more independence-oriented when they are in a higher-level job, or are the selection criteria for higher level jobs such that less authoritarian people are preferred? An interesting case are the BUROMAT foremen, who are the least authoritarian (although the difference between them and the other foremen in non-authoritarianism is not significant), and are also the only foremen who participate actively in setting their budgets (fig. 9-3).

The most plausible assumption is that there is something in the psychological climate or subculture of a company which leads to both attracting people with certain characteristics for certain jobs, and moulds them to adopt these characteristics still more once they are in their jobs.[8]

'Non-authoritarianism' appears in the factor analysis of line data (fig. 7-1)

[8]. Cassee (1965) has published data about hospitals showing that here first-line management shows stronger task-oriented leadership while higher-level management leadership is more employee-centered, emotionally balanced and open to change. Crozier (1965) has shown that in a bank organization the preference for authoritarian superiors increased down the hierarchy.

with a high loading (0,71) on factor no. 1, which is called 'independence'. Not surprisingly, also 'hierarchical level' loads on this factor. Furthermore it is the factor of those who dare to give disagreeing answers in the attitude survey (variable 60, 'no-yes-men', see p. 196). They have a positive attitude to life in general (var. 58) and to the budget system in particular (var. 19 and 20). They have more frequent department meetings and think these are more useful (var. 45). They feel their budget is legitimate ('sufficient account of my department's special problems', var. 33). Finally, as we have seen already, there is some indication that they participate more in the setting of their budget (a loading of 0,28 of var. 29). To interpret this factor I assume higher hierarchical level to be an important cause, which brings along more 'non-authoritarianism'. However, department meetings (meetings of the boss with his subordinates as a group) help to mould people in this direction, and this works also for lower-level management. It looks like these people have learned to use standards and therefore have begun to like them. It is rather significant that they are at the same time those who are less impressed by authority. Standards as objective yardsticks replace to some extent subjective and arbitrary authority in managing the job.

As the statistical analysis on page 197 shows, the influence of 'non-authoritarianism' on the relationship between participation in budget-setting and motivation, as it appears from my data, offers some surprises. My expectation was that for non-authoritarians the positive correlation between participation and motivation would be stronger than for authoritarians. The data show that this tends to be true for budget relevance, but that exactly the opposite is true for budget attitude: here, the correlation between participation and positive attitudes exists only for the authoritarians, not for the non-authoritarians.

The explanation of this unexpected result can be found by analyzing individual cases. It then appears that in plants where there are more non-authoritarians, people have positive attitudes throughout, whether they participate in their budget or not. They are basically positive to the idea of using standards, instead of more arbitrary ways of managing. They see standards as tools which make their managerial task lighter: 'I can use them so well downward in the organization' (second-line manager). 'Standards can be passed on. Together with our subordinates we can say: this is our task' (first-line manager). The only effect of participation to these people is that it makes the standards much more relevant to them. On the other hand, in plants where are more authoritarians, people are often initially somewhat hostile to the idea of using standards as managing tools; they undergo them passively instead of actively.

'If the standards are rather tight they make my job heavier' (second-line manager).

Their use of standards downward is also different:

'My task is heavier through the standards. I have to supervise more closely, to use the whip more' (first-line manager).

When these people participate in setting their budget, they learn to work with standards in a different way and their hostility disappears. The standards also become more relevant to them, but to a lesser extent than is the case for the non-authoritarians.

The desire for more participation in standard-setting

The desire for more participation can be read from people's scores on the participation scale (fig. 9-2, by comparing the scores on line c and line a). We must again distinguish between budget participation and technical standard participation. One would suppose that those who do not participate much in budget-setting desire to participate more, but this is not the case. To be more precise, it is not the case in general, when we look at all six plants simultaneously. Within the subgroup of each hierarchical level in each plant, we do find this supposed relationship: low participation in budget-setting leads to a desire for more, but the level of participation that is desirable varies strongly from subgroup to subgroup. First-line managers for example, who are in most cases not accustomed to participate in budget-setting, seldom desire it.

This lack of desire for more participation in budget-setting does not mean that, once people do participate, this does not motivate them. We have already seen that it does. Only, as proposed on page 176 point d, participation cannot be incidental: an experience of successful participation has to be built up. It is not surprising, therefore, that for participation in *technical standard-setting* there does exist a strong tendency for those who do not participate to desire participation. In this case, there is a commonly accepted norm that a manager, also a first-line manager,

188

should have a say in his standards. Compare also the BUROMAT case study later on in this chapter.

The factor analysis shows that a desire for more budget participation (var. 30) is found to some extent (loading 0,28) in the job 'rotation' situation (factor 6). The younger people who are newer in their jobs tend to desire more budget participation: the norm of what amount of participation is desirable may shift for the next generation.

This brings us to the question:

Who should participate in budget setting?

Fig. 9-3 has illustrated the common practice not to give first-line managers a role in budget setting, to which only BUROMAT does not adhere. Who *should* participate in setting a budget? In chapter 2, dealing with management information systems, I have stated the logical proposition that decisions have to be taken at the level where the outcome can best be influenced. In this study I have tried to measure the degree to which the outcome can be influenced by 'operational control'. Now operational control tends to be higher at the lower management levels. In my data, this can be demonstrated by the fact that variables 1: hierarchical level, and 40: perceived operational control are significantly negatively correlated: $r = -0.28**$) *This means that probably in many cases the main participation in budget setting could fruitfully be lowered to the first line of management.*

To get full participation (for example score 5 on the participation scale) for first-line managers, the accounting system must be designed such that each department run by a first-line manager becomes an expense center, if not a profit center (p. 30). This is not always possible, for example when first-line managers work in shifts and shift results are not separately measurable. Then the lowest superior multiple shift supervisor is the natural budget participant, but *he must pay a lot of attention to communicating with his shift foremen;* the crucial parts of the budget probably have to be set in a joint meeting with the shift foremen.

In some cases the decisions that affect outcomes are made at higher management levels. For example, I have seen a case were several departments were linked by the same conveyer belt which dictated production speed. Here only the superior supervising the total unit could be the chief participant in production volume budgeting, but in this case, too, he should consult with his subordinates.

The game of standard setting

All of the foregoing analyses miss the flavor of the standard-setting process in one important area: the game aspect. If budgeting is a game, it is a game in two phases, not unlike bridge. First comes the bidding: the standard-setting process. Then comes the actual playing: trying to accomplish the bid. The game aspect of standard setting can be illustrated with many quotations:

'It is a game. We tighten up the proposed standards beforehand and then we drop some of it and so does the line manager. It's quite passionate bargaining, but in a friendly way. It's the greatest fun of my job' (staff interviewee).

'It's a kind of a bargain. The budget man is in it and sometimes my boss too. It's quite a sport that way' (second-line manager).

'To set the standard for the number of workers we have quite a discussion with the line. It's a game, defense and attack, to find the right standard level' (staff interviewee).

'I'm planning to save one man each shift. You won't show this to the controller's department, will you? We had quite a fight about the standard last year, but I've still been able to win. If I give in myself I'm done for' (second-line manager).

'We romp around with several people about materials and number of people and reject percentages before. Then we propose a standard and the line manager checks it. We usually have a fight about the waste percentage' (staff interviewee).

'They proposed 81 people. Pending the meeting I've brought it to 86. The way it works is not quite all right, it's not my ideal. I'm the real producer, am I not? They always come with a fully documented proposal and with united efforts. It's a strong front against me; I'm always a minority. I want a role in the proposing phase' (second-line manager).

'The extremely favorable variances show us where we've been deceived' (staff interviewee).

'When we have developed a more efficient way of packaging we only introduce it after the new budget has been set' (second-line manager).

It appears that the game-aspect of standard-setting is experienced as a positive feature as long as players are about on equal footing. If one party is more powerful than the other, negative attitudes and evasive practices arise.

The effect of participation in standard-setting on job satisfaction

In the 'cost-conscious boss' factor of the factor analysis we find a combination of high participation in budget-setting with an indication of low job satisfaction. This is not a causal relationship; other influences are responsible for it, as chapter 12 will show. There is no direct correlation between budget participation and either job satisfaction or pressure. This indicates again what we saw already: participation in budget setting is not desired by most people until it has really been experienced. Those who do not have it don't feel dissatisfied with their jobs for that reason. The situation is different for technical standard-setting; there is a significant ($r = 0,30^*$) correlation between participation in technical standard-setting and job satisfaction. This means that *not* participating in the setting of his technical standards diminishes a manager's job satisfaction. Pressure is not correlated with any of the variables dealing with participation.

Summary of conclusions about the effects of participation in standard-setting

From the previous pages, it appears that:
1. People's reactions to participation in budget setting are different from their reactions to participation in technical standard-setting.
2. Participation in budget setting is most often found at the higher management levels. Participation in technical standard-setting is equally found at all management levels.
3. Participation in budget-setting leads to higher motivation to attain the budgets. Participation in budget-setting affects both the relevance and attitude component of motivation positively, but it will depend on other factors which one will be affected most.
4. External reference points for standards play a vital role in budget motivation to the extent that they are perceived by the budgetees as valid and legitimate.

5. A feeling of illegitimacy of the budget does not affect its relevance, but it does affect the attitude component of motivation.
6. Standards as objective yardsticks replace to some extent subjective and arbitrary authority.
7. The effect of participation in budget setting on the relevance of the budget is stronger for non-authoritarians than for authoritarians.
8. Those who do not usually participate in budget setting mostly don't desire it. Participation becomes attractive only after it has been experienced.
9. People who are relatively new in their jobs, and younger, tend to desire more participation in budget-setting.
10. Low participation in technical standard-setting tends to lead to a desire for more participation.
11. In many cases the main participation in budget setting could fruitfully be lowered to the first line of management.
12. Standard setting is a game; this is experienced as a positive feature as long as the players are about equally powerful.

Extremes in participation: the BUROMAT case

The BUROMAT plant is a fairly new plant in one of the bigger cities of the country. BUROMAT employees are city dwellers, and maybe this fact alone already makes them less traditional and more open to change than the employees in most of the other studied plants. This is definitely reflected in the mentality of BUROMAT foreman, who came through the ranks but are of a more independent nature than the foremen in the other plants with the possible exception of DYNAMO 2. Higher level management in BUROMAT has not come through the ranks; as in the DYNAMO plants, it consists of higher-educated people attracted from outside. As the plant is fairly young and has been growing steadily, managers are relatively young too.

The BUROMAT plant is a production unit of a larger organization. There is a much bigger parent plant where products are made production ripe before being transferred to our plant. The situation is again somewhat ' like DYNAMO, in that the parent plant has a lead in efficiency over the subsidiary and there is a tendency to measure the subsidiary by the standards of the parent plant.

BUROMAT plant management is cost conscious and so is the head office management to which the plant manager reports. BUROMAT management believes in the responsibility of the line manager and this induces them to consider the foremen as members of the management team to a greater extent than is generally the case in the Netherlands. The foremen also consider themselves as members of the management team. This is shown by their scores on the Control Graph (Appendix A, fig. A-2B). While in other plants first-line managers produce rather flat Control Graphs which indicate a 'worker's attitude', the Graphs for BUROMAT foremen are much steeper and very similar to those of higher-level management in the other plants. A consequence of their belonging to the management team is that BUROMAT foremen each have their own expense budget: the accounting system is designed to accomplish this. The budget setting game is played consistently with the foremen; their bosses have a coordinating and supporting role.

'We must make a budget each year. Some data are given: what is the cost of a kilowatt? What is the new man hour rate? What percent increase in social security? When we've made it we take it to the department manager'.

'The department manager discusses my proposal with me, where it's too high, where too low. He then takes it to the plant controller' (foreman).

The budget is taken very serious at BUROMAT. Among other things, people believe budget performance has a considerable influence on total job appraisal. Budget discussions are held in an atmosphere of grim earnestness and pressure: there is no play element. This pressure is considerably reinforced by the attitude of the budget staff. The BUROMAT budget staff has a big finger in the pie and although it formally does not propose budgets, it uses its power in a way that is not accepted by everybody and considered rather arbitrary:

'I prefer a tight standard. There's more push in it'.

'Of course standards must be tight. They must have an element of coercion' (BUROMAT budget staff interviewees).

'We put the various items in the budget. Then we discuss it. You probably can imagine how such meetings with budget people go. Then they cut the budgets without consultation' (second-line manager).

'Some items are cut drastically, others they just leave untouched. Sometimes I've been told: 'please make a new budget, you're too high'. If it is very clear it is impossible to do with less, they accept. It is somewhat puzzling what criteria they use'.

'I have the experience that my budget is usually cut by 10 percent. Therefore, if I've made a realistic budget, I increase it by 10 percent. The system is OK except for those 10 percent cut'.

'If you can't make it, the best thing is to surpass the budget drastically; that will show those guys that they won't get the economies they want anyhow'.

'I think the system is OK. That's the way it's done everywhere. It's obvious they have to set a standard, and for budgetary reasons it is better they make it fairly tight'.

'We make the budget ourselves, but sometimes we're given an instruction that we have to stay 10 percent lower than last year. When the budget people get it they start discussing it with us but sometimes then they just cut it without consulting us. Yet I think the budgets are set in a realistic way: Everybody can voice his opinion. It's quite instructive'.

'Consultation is OK, but I object against the way they do it. If we insist a lower budget is not justified, they must accept it'.

'I will never accept that they sometimes strike out parts of the budget without discussion. I think that's wrong' (line interviewees).

BUROMAT managers ask for a different staff role: they want more support in setting the budget:

'Wanted: More contact with the budget staff when we make the proposal; more two-way communication of exact data'.

'Making this budget gets on your nerves; the time is always too short'.

'The way we support each other as colleagues is OK. But I would like more contact with the accounting department in making the budget, because we're technicians' (line interviewees).

From these quotations it will be clear that the budgets thus set are not always met, but as the staff in this case does use different standards for measuring and planning, the overall planning budget is usually realized. A special case are the technical standards of BUROMAT. A few years ago, production has switched to new products for which standards like direct labor hours and rework percentages were set in the parent plant. However, as conditions in the satellite plant – like lot sizes and tooling – are different, these standards were not immediately valid; they were not accepted by line management either. For lack of time, estimated objectives have been set by higher authority, without consulting the lower levels of management.

'They just set the objective we have to comply with. There is hardly any possibility to change them. Up till now this system was OK, because the objectives set could be met. For next year we're in trouble'.

'They won't change the standards once they are set. But if they wanted to do it another way, they would need quite a crew of work study engineers' (line interviewees).

Technical standard setting in BUROMAT, therefore, has been using only the 'external reference points' and 'authority of persons higher in the hierarchy' sources drawn in fig. 9-1. It has used hardly any participation. This contrasts strongly with the situation for the expense budgets, where participation is used throughout. BUROMAT management has realized the undesirability of this situation, and a strong effort was made to overcome the shortage of good standards. When the interviews were held, several departments had already been reached:

'The engineers supply the times and I supply the practical data. It's a matter of cooperation. It is OK now. It used to be different'.

'Consultation with the work study engineer is OK now. Formerly we didn't have that' (line interviewees).

The basic weaknesses of the total standard setting process at BUROMAT as pictured here are its lack of accepted external reference points for standards, its lack of play, and its ill-understood staff role. BUROMAT is the plant where the feeling of pressure is highest. The basic strengths of the BUROMAT system are the cost-consciousness of its management and the active role of the foremen in budgeting. The BUROMAT case can also serve as an illustration of the effects of the staff attitude and the boss' attitude which will be described in the chapters 11 and 12.

Statistical analysis of data used in Chapter 9

The variables to be considered

The main variables in this chapter are (see Appendix E 2):

29. Budget participation, that is own estimate of maximum role in budget setting process ('maximum' referring to the measurable dimension for which participation was highest).

30. Discrepancy between desired and actual role in budget setting process.

31. Technical standard participation, that is own estimate of maximum role in non-financial (technical) standard setting process.
32. Discrepancy between desired and actual role in technical standard setting process.
The participation scores (29 and 31) are derived from line 'a' in the participation scale (fig. 9-2).
The scores for 'discrepancy between desired and actual role' (30 and 32) are derived from the positive differences between the score on line 'c' and the score on line 'a'.
Other variables to be considered:
33. Perception of legitimacy of the budget, measured by attitude survey item: 'Budgets are set here without taking sufficient account of my department's special problems'.
59. Interviewee's non-authoritarianism index, as an average score on four attitude survey items:
'A clear order is better than consultation' (Appendix D 5 no. 21).
'Young people sometimes get rebellious ideas, but as they grow older they ought to get over them and settle down' (24).
'Subordinates ought to accept their boss' decisions without reserve' (31).
'People can be divided into two distinct classes, the weak and the strong' (34).
The 'non-authoritarianism index' needs some more explanation. Attitude survey items 24 and 34 are borrowed from the third F-scale by Adorno (1950, p. 252 ff.). No. 21 and 31 were designed by me. The attitude surveys I used included two other F-scale items:
'Obedience and respect for authority are the most important virtues children should learn'. (Appendix D 5, no. 14).
'If people would talk less and work more, everybody would be better off' (39).
On the basis of the first statistical exploration using subgroup average scores the numbers 21, 24, 31 and 34 were selected to compose the index as having the highest intercorrelations. The correlation calculation on the full data showed afterwards that excluding no. 21 and including no. 14 would have been slightly better. The 6 intercorrelations would have been between $r = 0.19^*$ and 0.37^{***}. In the four items actually selected, they are between $r = 0.16$ – nearly significant – and $r = 0.36^{***}$). No. 39 shows low correlations throughout.

A drawback of the F-scale, and of my additions as well, is that all items are stated negatively. As a check, I have scored:
60. 'Yes-men-index', that is simply the total number of 'always' or 'mostly' answers in the attitude survey out of a total of 40 items (Appendix D 3). Indeed, the 'yes-men-index' and the 'non-authoritarianism index' are highly correlated: $r_{59/60}: - 0.59^{***}$. So when rephrasing the F-scale items in the positive sense one will get quite different results. With the existing negative statements, the yes-men-effect reinforces the differences in F-scale scores.

Relationships between variables

Fig. 9-5 shows correlations of budget motivation and job satisfaction with participation.

		correlations with	
Variables:		29 budget participation	31 technical standards participation
17	Relevance (impression)	0,56***(0.30*)	0.13(0.08)
18	Relevance (questions)	0.34** (0.22*)	−0.05(−0.33*)
19	Attitude (impression)	0.28** (0.22*)	−0.07(−0.01)
20	Attitude (questions)	0.29** (0.12)	−0.18(−0.06)
53	Job Satisfaction	−0.13(0.09)	0.30*(0.13)
54	Absence of pressure	−0.17(0.15)	0.06(0,00)

Figures between brackets are correlations within subgroups.
* significant at 0.05 level, ** significant at 0.005 level, *** significant at 0.0005 level

FIG. 9-5. Correlations of Participation with Budget Motivation and Job Satisfaction

The conclusion is a positive effect of budget participation throughout and no effect of technical standards participation.

Variable no. 33 (legitimacy) shows the following correlations with budget motivation:

17 relevance (impression) $r_{30,17} = 0.11$ 19 attitude (impression) $r_{33,19} = 0.24*$
18 relevance (questions) $r_{33,18} = -0.11$ 20 attitude (question) $r_{33,20} = 0.24*$

Only attitudes are affected by the degree of legitimacy of the budget, not relevance.

Fig. 9-6 tests the influence of non-authoritarianism (variable 59) as a conditioning factor on the correlations between budget participation and motivation.

		correlations with variable 29: budget participation, for		
Variables:		18 interviewees with lowest non- authoritarianism	21 interviewees with average non- authoritarianism	23 interviewees with highest non- authoritarianism
17	Relevance (impr.)	0.47*	0.64**	0.76***
18	Relevance (quests.)	0.33	0.47*	0.33
19	Attitude (impress.)	0.40	0.36*	0.15
20	Attitude (quests.)	0.58*	0.20	−0.03

* significant at 0.05 level, ** significant at 0.005 level, *** significant at 0.0005 level

FIG. 9-6. The Influence of Non-Authoritarianism on Correlations between Budget Participation and Budget Motivation.

The expectation is that the correlations will be stronger for those with the highest non-authoritarianism scores. Fig. 9-6 shows that this expectation is confirmed for the impression measure of relevance. The difference between the first and third correlation is significant at the 0.07 confidence level. The effect on the questions measure of relevance is ambiguous; but both attitude measures show clearly the opposite tendency: the correlation between participation and attitude is strongest for the more authoritarian interviewees. The difference between the first and third correlation for the question measure of attitude is significant at the 0.02 confidence level.

Finally, we have to test whether low participation leads to a desire for more. That is, whether 29 (budget participation) is negatively correlated with 30 (role discrepancy), and the same for 31 and 32 (technical standard participation).
We find:

budget participation: $\quad r_{29,30} = -0.05(-0.25*)$
technical standard participation: $r_{31,32} = -0.63***(-0.38**)$

Figures between brackets are again within-subgroup correlations.

For budget participation, the relationship between low participation and a desire for more exists only within subgroups. For technical standard participation it exists throughout total data.

CHAPTER 10
MANAGEMENT INFORMATION AND ACCOUNTING TECHNIQUES

Summary of this Chapter

There is a regular flow of written information within every budget system. This has been one of the objects of an earlier study by Simon et al. The conclusions of this earlier study deal with the use of figures by line management. They also deal with decentralization of account structures. My results confirm Simon's results about the importance of person-to-person relationships for the use of figures, but more of the relationships within the line than of those between staff and line. My study also confirms the importance of decentralization of account structures. It investigates the practical advantages and disadvantages of 'full profit centers' vs. 'expense centers', and the importance of the choice of the types of budget and cost variances that are reported.

Feedback information can be classified along different lines; two such classifications are given. Actual knowledge of figures by line interviewees was measured and their scores can be shown to be correlated with other aspects of the budget system. The people who are more recent in their job and younger have the best ready knowledge of performance and standards data. There appears to be much over-information in actual practice, which diminishes the impact of more important data. The question of whether foremen should receive financial information is considered. Finally, this chapter shows what was found with

199

regard to the accuracy, understandability and timeliness of feedback information. All these factors can, if missing, spoil an information system, but only the person-to-person communication that goes with it can make it succeed.

The Simon study of controller's departments

A budget system causes a flow of written information: measurement data from line departments to staff departments, and variance reports from staff departments to line departments. We have met this information flow in chapter 2 among the key issues in the Accounting Theory of Budgets. The part of chapter 3 mostly concerned with it is the section about 'knowledge of results' (p. 63), where it is shown how receiving information about one's results can be an important instrument for motivation. Finally in chapter 4 the written information flow is shown in the models as an essential part of the system.

From an accounting point of view there are many ways to design a budget system and to deal with the written information in it. Part of this is of no interest to the non-accountant, but part of it will directly influence the effectiveness of the total budget system. Which aspects of the written information flow within a budget system influence its effectiveness?

In the past to my knowledge one serious attempt has been made to evaluate budget systems systematically in this light. It is the U.S. Controllership Foundation Study 'Centralization vs. Decentralization in Organizing the Controller's Department' (1954), which was already mentioned in chapter 3. Researchers were Simon, Guetzkow, Kozmetsky and Tyndall, from the Graduate School of Industrial Administration, Carnegie Institute of Technology, Pittsburgh. I will shorten the references to this study to 'the Simon study'.

The Simon study used open-ended interviews with over 400 line and staff managers in manufacturing, sales and staff departments in 7 different companies. It wanted to evaluate the issue of the organization of the Controller's Department against its impact on the enterprise's profitability; and this final yardstick being too far away, it used as direct criteria to evaluate the effectiveness of controller's departments:

1. The extent to which the controller's department provides informational services of high quality;
2. The extent to which it performs these services at a minimum cost;

3. The extent to which it facilitates the long-range development of competent accounting and operating executives.

Measuring against these criteria the researchers came with a number of conclusions and recommendations. Those which refer to written information systems are interpreted freely below; other conclusions from the Simon study will be quoted in chapter 11 (staff-line-communication).

The conclusions of the Simon study relevant to this chapter were:

1. Direct and active channels of person-to-person communication between staff and line are more important for management's use of figures than the way the figures themselves are presented.
2. It is highly desirable that account structures are decentralized to individual manufacturing and sales units.
3. This decentralization need not go so far, however, as to make separate profit-and-loss statements for each of these units.
4. Accessibility and reliability of source records are the decisive factors in deciding upon the geographic decentralization of the controller's department.

The importance of interpersonal communication for the use of periodic accounting reports

Most people are poor readers. Written communication is therefore not a very effective way of transferring a message, if we leave the legal aspect out of consideration. In a small experiment in a Dutch company, Naus (1963) showed how poorly for example bulletin board messages came through to the people at whom they were directed. The effectiveness of written communication depends strongly upon the additional oral communication which goes with it.

In the factor analysis (fig. 7-1) it appeared that 'information (reports) sufficiently understandable' (var. 40) had a loading of 0,42 on factor 3: 'Upward communication'. This same factor represents a favorable opinion of staff behavior. All this suggests that it is the possibility of a free person-to-person communication with the boss and with the staff which makes the written information understandable. For example, the subordinate must be able to ask questions. The staff must receive 'feedback' on its reports. 'When I receive the budget variance report I take it immediately to the controller. He must explain to me why for example my maintenance expenses are so high and my supplies expenses so low' (third-line-manager).

'The reports are OK; if not, we ask questions' (first-line-manager).

The objective of the periodic reports is not only that they are understood, but also that they are used. As the correlation analysis on page 217 shows, there is very little correlation between 'reports understandable' (var. 50) and budget relevance (var. 17-18) as part of motivation. Relevance, by its definition on page 45, should indicate to what extent the figures are used. It is not just understanding the figures which makes for an effective use of them. There is some correlation between understandability and attitude, indicating that *understandability of reports is a hygienic factor in a budget system.*

In the six plants there were tremendous differences in the way people used (or did not use) periodic reports:

'Yes, I got that report; I put it in my drawer' (second-line-manager).

'I've seen it but not yet studied it' (second-line-manager).

'I don't know what the plant manager does with these figures; I never hear anything about it' (staff interviewee).

'When the budget variance report arrives I mark the interesting data with a red pencil; then I send them to the foremen, who must give an explanation within a week' (second-line-manager).

'I pass the report on to the foremen with a number of questions on a slip of paper. They take it to the budget accountant to find out where the figures come from' (second-line-manager).

'We mostly know the results a few days before they are published. Around the 4th to 7th of the new month I walk into the accounting department. I can then make some occasional remarks to the plant manager about our budget gains and losses before he sees them on paper' (second-line-manager).

'I get the information myself in the controller's department. I mostly know it earlier than my boss' (first-line-manager).

Although none of these remarks identifies any precise action taken, the latter ones at least indicate interest in and discussion of the figures, which is about the maximum one can expect. I have no examples of actions that are directly triggered by figures in periodic reports. The reality in a plant is mostly too complicated for that: there are always a number of reasons leading to a particular action.

All in all, there is agreement between this study and the Simon study as to the decisive role of person-to-person communication in the process of using reported figures. Except that where the Simon study mentions just staff-line communication, my data indicate that communication between superior and subordinate within the line organization is probably even more important to the use that is made of the figures.

The influence of accounting techniques on the impact of the system; decentralization of account structures

In the six plants I found three issues in the accounting techniques used which had an impact upon the effectiveness of the whole budget system. The first two of these were also stressed in the Simon study. The issues were:

1. Decentralization of account structures according to the responsibility areas of individual managers.
2. The choice between full profit centers and expense centers.
3. The choice of the types of budget and cost variances that are reported.

It appears in the statistical analysis of data that the scores of interviewees on the attitude survey item "I know exactly which costs I am responsible for' are significantly correlated with budget relevance as well as budget attitude (p. 217). The fact that people see their cost responsibility clearly defined is an important input into a budget system which affects budget motivation. It is even correlated with people's job satisfaction. In the factor analysis (fig. 7-1) 'knows exactly which costs he is responsible for' is the highest loading variable on factor no. 5 'cost-conscious self'. This factor represents high budget relevance and high job satisfaction, and in this case the information reports are also seen as sufficiently understandable. There is more in the 'cost-conscious self' factor, which has to do with the leadership style; it is not only the clear cost responsibility which explains the high job satisfaction. We will meet factor no. 5 again in chapter 12.

'Knowing exactly which costs one is responsible for' is also correlated with actual knowledge of performance figures and general cost information (these variables are explained in the statistical section on page 215).

It is interesting that understandability of reports in itself is *not* correlated with knowledge of figures. This suggests that only the man who not just understands the figures, but also sees his responsibility for them will pay enough attention to them to know them by heart.

Few accountants will deny the importance of following lines of managerial responsibility in their account structure. Yet in my six plants I found several cases where responsibilities were not covered fully by accounting reports. The reason was either the dynamics of the management structure which kept changing until the accountant gave up trying to follow it; or the more fundamental cause, that in modern business separating responsibilities is becoming a more and more difficult task. The increasing dependence of the effectiveness of 'line' operations on 'staff' support leads to a situation where it is very difficult indeed to identify what is 'line' and what is 'staff', and where responsibilities are just joint responsibilities. See also chapter 11. To some extent, the ideal of 'responsibility accounting' becomes more and more difficult to realize.

Full profit centers versus expense centers

The second point where accounting techniques have an impact on the effectiveness of the budget system is in the choice between full profit centers and expense centers for line departments. The Simon study has concluded that either system works, and that there is definitely no reason to go over to the often more complicated 'full profit center' system. The definitions of these systems are given in chapter 2. Of my five companies, three used full profit centers and only two used expense centers for their manufacturing departments. In the case of full profit centers, transfer prices between one department and the next obtain a tremendous significance. These prices are often felt by line managers as not quite real; the U.S. term for it is 'wooden money', and in the DYNAMO-plant I heard several times: 'We have to distinguish between real guilders and DYNAMO-guilders".

Transfer prices are only one of the reasons why systems of full profit centers are difficult to understand for line managers. I heard many complaints from staff interviewees that the line did not really understand as much about the system as they should:

'Line management accept whatever we do'.

'I really doubt whether the department managers have a sufficient understanding of budgeting and calculating'.

One of the plants used full profit centers and reported regularly the budget variances, split into volume variances and efficiency + expense variances (see p. 31). None of the first and second-line-managers whom I interviewed, however, was able to explain the difference between these two types of variances to me. This means that where full profit centers are used, considerable efforts must be spent to educate the line management in understanding the system and using the possibilities it offers for improved decision-making.

In the case of expense centers there are other pitfalls. In this case only expenses are budgeted per department, and direct production costs are controlled by standard cost control. The tendency here is to 'responsibility accounting' (see p. 30), whereby the elements of direct costs which can be attributed to a given department, are shown to the manager of that department, but more often in technical units than in money. The drawback of the 'expense center' approach is that the department manager has no longer one economic objective: maximizing his total departmental profit, but a number of separate targets, at least two: minimizing direct production cost and staying within his expense budget. This may lead to conflict situations for the manager and to decisions which are non-optimal from the point of view of the total economic result; for instance, in the case where direct production costs could be lowered by purchasing better tools, but the cost of these tools would set the expense budget off balance. From a motivational point of view, a total departmental profit expressed in one money value or percentage offers more challenge than a series of sub-targets whose interrelationship is unclear.

The conclusion is, that if expense centers are used, the system must be made sufficiently flexible so that, for example, expense budgets can be adjusted or surpassed when this cuts direct costs with a larger amount. Competent staff assistance should be available to solve micro-economic problems like these in cooperation with line managers. In this case, too, an effort at line education is indicated, though of a somewhat different nature. Most of all, this system demands an open two-way staff-line communication.

The third issue where accounting techniques have an impact on the effectiveness of the system deals with the choice of the types of budget and cost variances that are reported. In chapter 2 the differences between volume variances, efficiency variances, expense variances and accounting system variances have been described. Above we met the first- and second-line-managers who were not able to explain the difference between volume variances and efficiency + expense variances. Yet, from a practical point of view this difference is essential. Taking all six plants together, what a line manager could do most about in general were his *efficiency variances;* next came his expense variances. Volume variances are often quite uninteresting to the line manager, as he cannot do anything about them: it is for example the sales department which determines his volume of production. Where we have no full profit centers for departments, volume variances cannot even be computed for departments without special effort. Yet, as soon as a certain department becomes a bottleneck in the manufacturing + sales system, it suddenly acquires a tremendous influence on the volume variances of the plant as a whole. This is a tricky issue in feedback reporting. Accounting system variances, finally, are of no interest to the line manager at all.

With few exceptions, therefore, *efficiency variances should be the core of the feedback reporting system.* In most plants they were. The system must of course be built to compute these variances; what difficulties may be encountered in doing this, was shown by the ALPHABET case. ALPHABET, like most graphic companies in the Netherlands, is a typical job shop: it has many small short-run orders which need many different operations each. For this reason most jobs are not costed beforehand, as the clerical effort of doing this would be almost more expensive than the job itself. The only preparation given to such jobs is determining their routing through operations. The operators register both the type of operation done (by a code number) and the time and materials consumed on some job document. After completion of the job the standard cost elements for the coded operations are compared to the cost actually incurred, and thus an efficiency percentage is found. The drawback of this system is obvious. Efficiency thus defined will seldom improve: the figure can improve only by people working harder or cheating more in filling out their job cards. Real efficiency improvements are seldom due to working harder: they depend on methods improvements. In the ALPHABET system unfortunately the effect of methods improvements remained invisible, as both the standard and the actually incurred cost were adapted. ALPHABET management saw this as a serious shortcoming in their cost control system and were looking for a better solution: when efficiency improvement is not measurable, there is no 'knowledge of results' and less motivation to improve.

Classes of feedback information

The Simon study concludes that from a management point of view, accounting information is used to answer three different kinds of questions (Simon et al. 1954, p. 2, 3):
1. Score-card questions: 'Am I doing well or badly?'
2. Attention directing questions: 'What problems should I look into?'
3. Problem-solving questions: 'Of the several ways of doing the job, which is the best?'

The score-card function of accounting information is important from a motivational point of view. In chapter 7 I quoted one line interviewee: '...everybody needs an occasional pat on the back. Now with standards you know whether you did well or not, even if they forget the pat on the back.'

This means that accounting information need not bring any sensational new insight. It seldom does; often it only confirms what people expected already:

'The most important thing to me is whether my overall result is positive or negative. I have certain expectations, because I make notes of all jobs we have completed ourselves. In the beginning of the new week I phone the accounting department: I am curious and when we are positive, I am happy' (first-line-manager).

'I want to see the outcome. I know myself beforehand whether I am working at a loss or not' (first-line-manager).

'The only surprises in the figures are when there is some mistake in them' (second-line-manager).

When accounting information has only a score-card function, receivers need not be helped by explanations (see chapter 2, p. 34, point 2). When it is used for attention-directing purposes on the other hand, explanatory notes with the information may be imperative. For score-card use it is quite right to have line-managers update their own graphs, they will probably like it.

In chapter 2, I gave another classification of feedback information, into:

1. Information required for making decisions (all three of Simon's classes belong to this group).
2. Information which does not lead to immediate decisions, but which gives useful background data and influences the general attitude and esprit de corps of the reader.
3. All other information, which is superfluous and acts as 'noise', diminishing the impact of 1 and 2 type messages.

During the line interviews I have measured actual knowledge of information of type 1 in this classification – performance and standards figures[1] – and type 2 information – general cost information. These measurements are represented by the variables 22 and 23 (see the statistical section, p. 215). In the factor analysis (fig. 7-1), variable 22 – knowledge of performance and standards figures – has its highest loading on factor 6: job rotation. The people who are more recent in their jobs and younger, know more figures. This may represent a development in management style from the older to the younger generation: modern management becomes much more information-dependent and learns to use information. In the correlation analysis (p. 217) we find, not surprisingly, a positive correlation between knowledge of performance and standards figures and budget relevance. The relationship with budget attitude is more complex.

Type 2 information – not required for making decisions, but giving background data – appears to be important too. Having a good knowledge of these figures, for example, about the cost of production machines, of raw materials, etc. (variable 23) appears in the factor analysis with a loading on factor 5: 'cost-conscious self'. This factor, as we have seen, represents a favorable situation from a point of view of budget motivation. In the correlation analysis (p. 217), actual knowledge of

[1] There is a tendency for people to have more ready knowledge about actual performances or variances than about the standards. Once they know there is a standard, they often do not bother so much about it.

general cost information is positively correlated with both relevance and attitude, though not always significantly.

Type 3 information – noise – is, unfortunately, rather widespread. In one of the plants, for example, there existed 74 different types of periodic management information reports, partly internal, partly on behalf of the head office; some of these could definitely be considered as just 'noise'. Fig. 10-1 shows which percentages of interviewees in the five companies agreed with the statement 'there is too much paperwork in this company' (Appendix D 5, no. 35). Obviously, 'paperwork' means not only periodic accounting reports, but when the paper workload is high in general this will be reflected on the periodic accounting reports too.

Company	'There is too much paperwork' according to:	
	% of line managers	% of staff interviewees
ALPHABET	43	13
BUROMAT	47	67
COMBITEX	14	0
DYNAMO	64	33
EPICURE	20	13

FIG. 10-1. % of Interviewees who think there is too much paperwork in their company ('always' or 'mostly' scores).

Most complaints about 'too much paperwork' are voiced by line managers:

'The greater part of the figures are of no use to me' (third-line-manager).

'These reports are terrible. They were explained to us four years ago, but now there's only one line in them of interest to me' (second-line-manager).

'Those graphs contain so much information that a lot of it I just let go by. What I check is whether I can meet the performance and quality requirements' (first-line-managers).

In one company, the monthly budget variance report contained 19 different tables and graphs. I asked line interviewees expressly which of these they usually read. Only 3 out of the 19 were read by more than 25% of the interviewees. In this case, the optimum amount of information has clearly been surpassed.

'People do not see the wood for the trees, they don't use the information sufficiently' (staff interviewee).

When the staff complains about ' too much paperwork', this is often because in the larger companies they must supply the head office with information. Sometimes the system of management information is largely prescribed from the head office:

'I spit at those head office instructions. They are extended to the impossible, to the preposterous' (staff interviewee).

'Our reports contain several items which are requested by the head office instructions, but which are useless' (staff interviewee).

The basic problem is mostly an insufficient split between information required for the accounting consolidations and management information:

'This report is designed to inform line management as well as the Headquarters accounting department. It is a Janus face' (staff interviewee).

The same type of conflict as we have seen for a budget between its measuring and its planning function (chapter 2), exists for accounting reports, between their management information and their accounting information functions. The only good solution is to make a radical split between these two. Besides preventing overinformation, this also makes it possible to select the best personnel for each job; those best at supplying accounting information may not be the best management informers (Bos, 1955; Hall, 1964; see also chapter 11).

Variable no. 52, expressing 'not too much paperwork', has a loading on factor 3 in the factor analysis: 'upward communication'. Where written information is part of a smooth person-to-person two-way communication system, there is less danger of a feeling of over-information. In the correlation analysis we find a significant correlation (0,33**, within subgroups 0,38***) between 'not too much paperwork' and 'information reports sufficiently understandable'. This confirms what I have suggested already, that over-information reduces the effectiveness of a report: conversely, low understandability may lead to a feeling of over-information.

Who should receive periodic feedback reports?

As in the case of participation in budget-setting described in chapter 9, financial feedback-information is largely confined to second-level and higher management. In the six plants studied the distribution of financial feedback followed about the pattern of the upper half of fig. 9-3, though in DYNAMO 2 a conscious effort was made to have the first-line managers involved as well. There is some rationale in giving first-line-managers only technical performance data feedback. After all, this is closer to what they are dealing with in practice: '. . . the action which first-line supervisors take to control costs is not in dollar amounts at all. They think in numbers of people and in quantities of material and yields in processing' (N.A.A. 1963, p. 9). Money is a common denominator to balance different factors in economic decision-making. If there is only one main economic factor like keeping the production going, money information may not be necessary at all.

We must keep in mind, however, the difference between type 1 (decision-making) and type 2 (background data and attitude influencing) information. While financial information may not have much decision-making value to the first-line-manager, a good dose of it will influence his attitude to economic problems and his general cost-consciousness. 'I would definitely like to know more about costs, whether I am working too expensively or up to cost standards. If I knew, I could think of improvements. As long as one is ignorant one can do nothing but go on in the same way' (first-line-manager).

My conclusion is that in many cases a well-selected amount of financial information could have positive effects on the motivation of first-line-managers who beforehand did not receive any. Obviously this information should be preceded by adequate instructions. Also, it is only valuable if there is a climate in which first-line-managers will feel free to ask questions to the staff and to their boss to help their understanding of the figures.

What holds true for first-line-managers holds true also, but to a lesser extent, for workers. In some of the six plants some technical results of departments were made visible to workers through graphs in the department; only in one case financial results.

'I think I would be interested in knowing our results in guilders, so I could tell my people. Just now I know the labor efficiency, but not whether we made money or not' (first-line-manager).

Here we meet other factors, however: joint consultation, management-union relationships, productivity sharing plans and the like, which I will not go into. This is definitely a vast field for further study.

Accuracy of feedback information - the measuring problem

In the model of fig. 4-2, representing a budget control system, I have drawn dotted lines from the budgetee and his subordinates to the 'measuring' block. This means that in many cases the budgetee and his people are themselves the source of much of the information used in the feedback process.[2] As they are interested in the outcome as well, this may have a rather strong impact on the accuracy of measurements.

'... in business enterprise, the act of measurement is ... neither objective nor neutral. It is subjective and of necessity biased ... For a long time, in many companies forever, realizing the budget figures becomes more important than what the budget is supposed to measure, namely economic performance' (Drucker, 1964, p. 288-289).

Jasinsky (1956) gives an extensive selection of examples of distortion and manipulation of measurements used in management control systems. This is one of the main reasons why an excess of pressure in a budget system has an adverse effect. *People are always smarter than systems* and if the system is functioning in such a way that it pays to make figures 'look right' instead of doing something about the underlying causes, this is what will happen.

'Our system is based on trust. If it were not, data would not be reliable' (first-line-manager).

A few extreme examples of distortion of information were found in this study: In one of the plants the production of one department when moving to the next department was counted mechanically. Suddenly there appeared differences between what was supposed to be delivered by the first and received by the second department. After considerable detective work it was discovered that the foreman of the first department

---

[2] I heard several complaints from line managers about the amount of work involved in supplying this information 'The foreman used to be more of a clerk here than somebody who looked after his people' (second-line-manager).

secretly manipulated the mechanical counters so as to make his department's production look higher. One would expect these things to happen where, for instance, somebody's salary depended on the figures, but this was not the case here. This foreman just wanted to look better than his colleagues. Not surprisingly he was fired as a result of his excessive motivation.

In another plant I met a machine operator, who remarked: 'The foreman is very keen on us not stopping our machines. But if a machine is broken, he tells us not to hurry'. After investigation I found out that the key variable in the production reports in this plant was machine efficiency, but that machine repair time was excluded in computing it. So the foreman used machine repair time to give his men a rest.

The least accurate information is found where measurements are the basis for somebody's pay, as in the case of piece rates. Any measurement which would make a rate too high or too low is corrected or faked. *Data used for determining pay are basically unfit for efficiency measurement.*

'With a little bit of skill one can make his performance units look just as he wants' (first-line-manager).

Similar manipulations of information can be found when a subsidiary reports to the head office. 'Our weekly information system is not quite realistic because the head office is copied on it. We do not hang our soiled linen in the street' (staff interviewee).

The most reliable measurements are those which deal with actual flows of cash. All efficiency measuring systems should finally be anchored to such cash flow measurements. One should beware of "management by ratios". Altogether, obtaining reliable information remains an art. It is not surprising that the Simon study considered accessability and reliability of source documents to be the decisive factors in deciding upon the geographic decentralization of the controller's department (p. 201).

Another source of unreliability of feedback data is plain errors. When the system becomes too complicated, errors become difficult to discover and still more difficult to correct, and consequently the confidence of line management in feedback information is lowered:

'We have quite some doubts about this information. It is almost impossible to check anything. My boss recently wanted to investigate some figures; it took him a full day' (first-line-manager).

With increased automation of data processing the procedure for tracking errors may become more complicated. From a motivational point of view it is important that the system should remain as clear as possible.

Understandability and timeliness of feedback information

We met the factor of 'understandability of reports' as a hygienic factor in the budget system earlier in this chapter. Why are reports not understood? The accountant's language is different from the manager's language and this impairs the understandability of feedback information by the manager:

'Wanted: a complete revision of the budget variance reports. It is absolutely not understandable. Our controller does the utmost to explain it to us, but the whole way of presenting data is so specialized that many people just can't follow it' (third-line-manager).

'The budget variance report is unreadable. If I had time I would follow a course in accounting to understand it' (third-line-manager).

'The only way to improve the understandability of these reports is to make us all accountants. Just forget about it' (second-line-manager).

'The reports are rather unclear. Maybe they are crystal-clear to an accountant, but not to a metalworker like me' (first-line-manager).

'They do not understand it fully, because the results are published in accounting jargon. We have made it too difficult' (staff interviewee).

'They do not really try to understand it' (superior of the former interviewee).

There is room for creative solutions to expressing accounting information in the language of the manager (N.A.A. 1963; Eshbach & Shene 1964; Ydo, 1965). One of the recurring issues is whether reports should show only variances which can be influenced by the receiver, or overall variances, inclusive attributed costs. I have not been able to discover a clear operational advantage of either of these two approaches, provided that it is made clear in the reports which costs are attributed. A difficulty about showing only variances that can be influenced is that is it not easy to decide who can influence what. In economy, as in physics, solids become liquids if pressure is increased.

Timeliness of reports is a problem about which I found the controller's department more concerned than the line. Line managers mostly see to it that they get their really crucial decision-making information in time.

For score-card use (p. 207), information needs not to be immediate. Like understandability, timeliness belongs to the 'hygienic' side of feedback communications. One can spoil communication by producing reports that are absolutely unclear or far too late. One cannot, however, guarantee good communication by clear and timely reports. It is the person-to-person communication which goes with it which determines the use and meaning of periodic accounting reports.

Statistical analysis of data used in Chapter 10

The variables to be considered

Two variables deal with how the line managers perceived the written management information:

50. Attitude Survey Item: 'The management information reports I get are sufficiently understandable'.
52. Attitude Survey Item: 'There is too much paperwork in this company' (scored negatively).

A third variable deals with knowledge of figures:

21. Attitude Survey Item: 'I know exactly which costs I am responsible for'.

I have not only asked for line *opinions*, but also checked personally the *ready knowledge of figures* which were communicated through the management information reports. This was done through 'quiz questions' (marked with* in Appendix D 3). I have used two sorts of 'quiz questions', the results of which are summarized in the variables 22 and 23 in the Correlations Computation and Factor Analysis:

22. This variable summarizes how well the line interviewees knew figures about actual performance and about the standards. These figures were asked for during the interviews and afterwards checked with the official records. Answers were scored as 'right', 'partly right' or 'wrong or unknown', according to whether they fell within preset tolerance limits. Variable 22 represents for each line interviewee the average answer score for both knowledge of actual performance and of standards over the three best known measurable dimensions. A high score on variable 22 means that the interviewee knows the figures by heart, a low score means that he does not know the figures.

23. This variable summarizes similar scores for the answers on five quiz questions dealing with 'general cost-consciousness', like: 'How many guilders' worth of products passes through your department in a year?' and 'What is the total investment in machinery within your department?' These data are not periodically reported, but a knowledge of such figures proves a general interest in cost information.

Testing the correlations between the variables

The correlations between the variables 50, 52, 21, 22 and 23 are shown in fig. 10-2. The interpretation of fig. 10-2 runs as follows: Those who think they get more understandable reports also think that there is not too much paperwork, and that they know better for which costs they are responsible. However, there is no relationship between understandability of reports and actual knowledge of figures.

There does exist a relationship between 'knowing exactly for which costs one is responsible' and actual knowledge of figures, but this is apparently not caused by clearer written information.

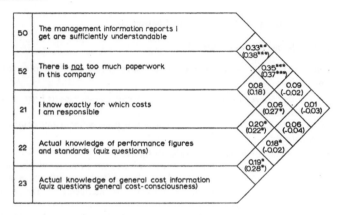

Figures between brackets are correlations within subgroups.

* significant at 0.05 level
** significant at 0.005 level
*** significant at 0.0005 level

FIG. 10-2. Intercorrelations between Variables Dealing with Written Information and Knowledge of Figures.

To what extent now is written information important for budget motivation and job satisfaction? To check this, the above-mentioned variables should be considered as input variables and correlated with the 'output variables': relevance and attitude, job satisfaction and pressure.

If we do this, we get the data of fig. 10-3.

It appears that 'information reports understandable' correlates most with attitude; 'knows exactly for which costs responsible' correlates with both relevance and attitude, 'actual knowledge of performance + standards' correlates with relevance while the correlation with attitude is ambiguous, and 'actual knowledge of general cost information' tends to correlate with both relevance and attitude, though not always significantly.

216

'Information reports understandable' and 'knows exactly for which costs responsible' are also correlated with job satisfaction. This can be explained through factor 5 in the factor analysis: 'cost-conscious self', on which these variables all have high loadings. The interpretation of it will be postponed till chapter 12.

	Variables:	correlations with:			
		50 information reports understandable	21 know exactly for which costs responsible	22 actual knowledge of performance + standards	23 actual knowledge of general cost information
17	Relevance (impress.)	0.03(0.03)	0.31**(0.11)	0.26*(0.17)	0.23*(0.35***)
18	Relevance (quests.)	0.15(0.07)	0.28**(0.23*)	0.17(0.33**)	0.11(0.02)
19	Attitude (impress.)	0.07(0.20*)	0.22*(0.25*)	0.21*(0.14)	0.24*(0.09)
20	Attitude (quests.)	0.21*(0.33**)	0.28**(0.13)	−0.03(−0.25*)	0.17(−0.06)
53	Job Satisfaction	0.29**(0.27**)	0.22*(0.25*)	0.06(0.12)	0.16(0.17)
54	Absence of pressure	0.20*(0.17)	0.10(0.14)	0.08(0.18*)	0.06(0.11)

Figures between brackets are correlations within subgroups

* significant at 0.05 level, ** significant at 0.005 level, *** significant at 0.0005 level

FIG. 10-3. Correlations between Budget Motivation and Job Satisfaction and Variables Dealing with Written Information and Knowledge of Figures.

CHAPTER 11
STAFF - LINE - COMMUNICATION

Summary of this Chapter

This chapter first discusses the validity of the concepts of 'staff' and 'line'. Maintaining them for lack of something better, it then tests the impact of staff – line communication on the effectiveness of a budget system as measured through budget motivation. Feelings of undue domination by the staff exist among some line interviewees, but they do not seriously affect their budget motivation. The general evaluation of the communication between line and staff by the line is correlated with the attitude component in budget motivation, showing that staff – line communication is a 'hygienic factor'. A factor analysis of staff attitudes is used to investigate what the staff can do about stimulating good communication. It appears that the competent specialist is best received, and that a stress on tactfulness by the staff man's boss also helps; this can be stimulated by giving the line counterparts a voice in the appraisal of the staff man's performance. The different staff attitudes are illustrated with case material.

The attitude survey and interview data show some significant differences between staff and line people. Staff people show more of a 'spectator' role in the business. They also find different rewards and frustrations in their job than the line does. The latter part of the chapter is devoted to internal organization problems of the staff. It is important that enough time is allowed for communicating with the line. A sound cooperation between financial and technical standards people is essential. Staff people appear generally less well managed from a personnel point of view; they feel a need for a career path. The data do not indicate that one particular type of basic training for budget and standards staff people is superior to another. The chapter ends by showing how a staff man can overcome the frustrating situation that his role in the budget system is just 'hygienic': by being an educator.

Do 'line' and 'staff' exist?

There is considerable doubt in present day literature about the validity of the staff-line concept. The traditional picture of the line which controls and the staff which advises does not correspond to reality in modern business, and it is doubtful if it has ever been true. 'Staff' departments wield considerable control (Irle, 1963[b]), sometimes more than 'line' departments, so that there are cases where the traditional picture would be almost restored by calling the staff 'line', and the line 'staff'. Or the influence and responsibilities of staff and line are so interwoven that the best fitting definition is one of equivalent partners in a project team. In chapter 10 I have indicated the difficulties this may give for 'responsibility accounting'. It adds to the confusion that the word 'staff' is used for different types of non-direct jobs, for example those with an advisory ('pure staff'), auditing or auxiliary function (Van der Schroeff, 1958). Although the line-staff distinction is therefore clearly obsolete (Logan, 1966), there is nothing to replace it yet. We are all caught in the first-level systems model (chapter 4), of organization offered by the organization chart, which is invalid not only by its being static but also by its trying to picture multiple relationships in a two-dimensional framework.

Recognizing many reasons to be careful with using the words 'line' and 'staff', in my case I felt justified in doing it. In the budget systems which I investigated there were clearly two types of roles: manufacturing management and the people in the budgets and cost standards departments. I am designating them by 'line' and 'staff' as collective nouns for lack of better terms (Luyk, 1963). Within each group people may differ widely in their actual role conception.

Staff - line communication in the Simon study of controller's departments

The study of Controller's Departments by Simon and his co-workers

(Simon et al. 1954) quoted in chapter 3 and 10 gave a thorough analysis of staff-line communication problems. Its conclusions on this subject can be summarized as follows:

1. It is essential for the controller's department to develop direct and active channels of communication with line management.
2. Development of staff and facilities for special studies is more important than elaboration of periodic accounting reports.
3. Within the controller's department it is advisable to separate personnel into (a) bookkeeping and reports publishing, (b) assistance to the line in current analyses of accounting information and (c) special studies in project teams together with line- and other staff-people.[1]
4. It is relatively unimportant whether the plant controller reports to the plant manager or to the company controller, as long as he has the authority to provide reports to the plant management as requested.
5. There should be a plan for the development of accounting personnel.

Simon's main concerns were therefore the channels of communication between staff and line management (point 1, 2) and the internal organization of the controller's department (point 3, 4, 5). My concern in this chapter covers about the same area. I want to test the impact of staff – line communication on the effectiveness of a budget system as it is measured through the motivation of the budgetee (relevance and attitude). Then I want to check what the staff can do to improve staff – line communication. Finally I want to see what this means for the internal organization of the staff department, taking into account what kind of people staff employees are and how they differ from line managers.

Line - staff conflict: the dominating staff

There is a lot of folklore in business about the informal conflicts which the formal line-staff organization appears to create. A good example is given in McGregor (1960, ch. 11). The conflict seems to be fostered by the stereotypes line and staff have about each other. The line sees the staff as impractical, trying to dominate and empire-building; the staff sees the line as unimaginative and unwilling to follow good advice. The line is irritated by the staff and the staff is frustrated by the line.

[1] Recommendations of a similar nature are already given in Holden, Fish & Smith, 1941, p. 158 ff.

I have used the Control Graph Technique to find out to what extent the line felt dominated by the staff. See Appendix A, fig. A-3[2]. My reasoning was that if a line manager felt staff influence as illegitimate he would indicate this by scoring 'ideal' staff influence lower than 'actual' staff influence. The figures show that among higher-level line managers the number of those who score ideal staff influence below actual approximately balances out the number of those who think the staff should have more influence. Higher-level managers in ALPHABET on the average think the staff should have less influence than it has. I will come back to the ALPHABET case later. First-line managers in majority think the staff should have more influence than it actually has. The interviews reveal that this is sometimes meant to express a desire of more support from the staff: 'We seldom see them. They don't come as often as they should' (first-line-manager).

The staff itself also thinks it should have more influence, with the exception of the COMBITEX staff, which will be dealt with as a special case later in this chapter. Also, the staff tends to estimate both actual and ideal staff influence higher than the line does. This is most likely the normal human characteristic of seeing your own task as more important than somebody else sees it. There is a fair agreement among staff interviewees of all four plants in fig. A-3 as to what influence the staff should have.

Individual feelings of being unduly dominated by the staff (or the reverse) were treated as a variable in the statistical analysis of line interview data (var. 49 in App. E 2). In the factor analysis, this variable is only related to factor 7 (job involvement), which has little to do with the motivation through the budget system. The statistical section at the end of this chapter shows that feelings of *not* being dominated by the staff are significantly correlated with budget attitude, but only within plants and hierarchical levels; between plants it is the other way round. It is not true in the plants where the line sees the staff as the most dominating that they have the worst attitude towards the budgets and standards system. The conclusion from my data is that undue domination by the staff is sometimes felt by higher-level line management and by the staff itself,

---

[2] In the Control Graph, 'staff' included all indirect departments the line managers were dealing with. I wanted to include the possibility of domination by non-line departments other than the budget or standards department.

but that it does not seem to be a major problem in budget motivation.

Line - staff communication

The interview questions to the staff 'How wholesome is the relationship between your department and line management?' (App. D 2, question E 13) and to the line 'How wholesome is your relationship with these (staff) people'? (App. D 3, question E 11) led to many comments.
Positive comments dealt with line and staff involving each other mutually in joint problems:
'We have good contacts with the industrial engineers. They always consult us when setting standards' (first-line-manager).
'We used to disagree, but now things go smooth. They have listened to the advice of the foremen' (first-line-manager).
'When something is changed in the process we warn the cost engineers' (first-line-manager).
'The relationship is good, they take us serious, they respect us and ask our advice' (staff interviewee).
Many comments described resolution of conflict in a friendly way:
'We do not always agree, but things go fine. We know each other' (first-line-manager).
'The contact is smooth. There may be some friction but it is always resolved. We have our practical problems, they have their figures. We have to bridge that' (first-line-manager).
'We crack some hard nuts, but in a friendly way' (second-line-manager).
'We bicker sometimes, but that's part of the game' (staff interviewee).
'The atmosphere is good, they are always ready to listen to you. They do not always follow up your advice. They're not very efficiency-minded' (staff interviewee).
Several comments dealt with the antithesis between practice and theory:
'We have a good-natured contact. We realize they are not practical people' (first-line-manager).
'I think they appreciate our work, although they think we are bureaucrats and theoreticians' (staff interviewee).
'I sometimes wonder if the efficiency department is not one big madhouse. Do they really know the practical side of our job'? (first-line-manager).
'People with 20 or 30 years of practical experience must often go for

information to staff fellows who have just been hired' (first-line-manager)
'The relationship is poor. The deeper reason may be this: our people
can look into the staff office through the glass walls. They say: Those
fellows just do nothing all day long while we work ourselves to death'
(first-line-manager).
Sometimes the staff feels it is used as a bugbear by the line:
'The department managers sometimes use the controller as a bugaboo.
If one of their subordinates is over his budget they tell him to go and
bring the message himself. Then the poor fellow is over his nerves for a
day' (staff interviewee).
'Some managers blame the controller's department for matters they
should blame on their bosses. For example if they are insufficiently
involved in the setting of the budget. That is simply the problem of
their higher line boss being autocratic' (staff interviewee).
Finally, there are the outright conflict cases:
'We try to consult with the efficiency department, but it generally ends
in a row' (first-line-manager).
'Yesterday still we had strong words about a change in a standard' (first-
line-manager).
'My experiences with the cost standards departments are not so pleasant'
(first-line-manager).
'On our level we have quite some differences of opinion. Not on the
human plane, although this may also be part of it' (second-line-manager).
'The relationship is tense, we disagree about certain calculations. I think
I don't have pleasant contacts with any of them. When the foremen get
me involved there is always something rotten' (second-line-manager).

The measurement of line attitudes towards the staff was done through
three attitude survey items, which together supplied one 'communication
with staff' score (see the statistical section on p. 245). In the line factor
analysis (fig. 7-1) 'communication with staff' had a loading of 0.58 on
factor 3: 'upward communication' and a loading of 0.37 on factor 2
'budget variance'. The latter is rather unimportant. It only shows that
where standards are loose there is less risk of a clash with the staff. The
relationship of 'communication with staff' with the 'upward communication' factor is of crucial importance, however. It shows that good
staff-line communication does not arise out of a vacuum. It is found

where there exists also a good upward communication within the line. When people are subject to the influence of the staff without being able to resolve possible grievances arising from this with their boss, attitudes towards the staff will become negative. A similar case on workers' level is described in Dunnington, Sirota and Klein, 1963.

The 'upward communication' factor shows that good communication with staff is also related to 'not too much paperwork' and to 'information sufficiently understandable'. This confirms Simon's conclusion that direct and active channels of person-to-person communication between staff and line are important for management's use of figures (chapter 10). In the statistical section of this chapter it is shown that 'communication with staff' is not or is negatively correlated with budget relevance and positively related with budget attitude. Good communication with the staff is therefore a 'hygienic' factor in a budget system. It is indispensable to avoid negative motivation, but it does not guarantee that the system works. It may even be more difficult to realize when the system does work.

The specialist and staff-line communication

What can the staff do about it? My guess was that there would be elements in the staff people's attitudes towards the system and in their role conception which would help to create wholesome relationships with the line, and therefore avoid negative budget motivation.

The relationships between staff and line as seen by the line ('communication with staff') are better in three plants (DYNAMO 1, DYNAMO 2 and COMBITEX) than in the three others.[3] What differences in staff attitudes could account for this? My expectation was that three staff characteristics might be important for the line's perception of line-staff communication:
1. Whether the staff tried to dominate the line
2. Whether the staff saw its role as one of giving service or rather as one of measuring and evaluating
3. Whether the staff behaved tactfully.

However, there might exist other staff attitudes which explained better

---

[3] The difference in 'communication with staff' scores from the one group of plants to the other is highly significant. Testing with Wilcoxon's test we find $T = 3.5$, meaning significance below 0.0005-level.

the difference in line reaction. To take the fullest possible inventory of staff attitudes, I used the Staff Factor Analysis (fig. 11-1). The explanation of fig. 11-1 is given in the statistical section at the end of this chapter. I found five factors representing basic attitudes of my staff interviewees:

1. The specialist attitude
2. The piece-rate-setter attitude
3. An attitude of not condemning the line
4. An attitude of high job satisfaction and giving service
5. An attitude of not dominating

Of these five, the only one showing a clear split between the three plants with better and the three plants with less good line-staff communication, was factor 1, *the specialist attitude*. Fig. 11-2 B shows that the three plants high on the 'specialist' factor are COMBITEX, DYNAMO 2 and DYNAMO 1[4]); the same are also high on line-staff communication (fig. 11-2A).

I chose the description 'specialists' because factor 1 in fig. 11-1 pictures them as those who:

– have no line experience (11)
– have a sense of independence (46)
– think their department is well organized (30)
– are considered high performers by their boss (37)
– do not see budgeting as an accounting tool (16)
– do not desire more influence of the staff (14),
   which means that they do not want to dominate more, but they think the staff has high influence already (13)
– do not desire more influence of the line (15) and do not think the staff should leave more to the line (17)
– finally, are convinced that line management follows their advice (28).

Thus the data suggest that *line-staff communication is better and conflict is less where the staff people are competent in their specialization*. Line people seem to accept staff influence if they can see the staff as experts.[5]

There is no sign that the specialists try to be 'nice' to the line. There is one aspect about them which has not yet been mentioned: they think that working does *not* come naturally to most people (43). They look rather pessimisticly at this aspect of human nature. Nevertheless, the line

---

[4] The difference in factor loadings between the first three plants taken together and the latter three plants taken together is significant at the 0.05 level.

[5] An analysis of the role of the expert in the staff is given in Blau & Scott, 1963, p. 172 ff.

Factor no., and name	plant	external input variables	internal input variables	perceptions of input	intervening variables	perceptions of output
Factor I 'the specialist'	COMBITEX 0.61	37. high total job performance rating by boss: 0.36	11. no line experience: −0.45		46. no yes-men: 0.67 30. in my department efficiency can not be improved: 0.62 16. budgeting is not first of all an accounting tool: 0.60 13-14 does not desire more general influence of staff −0.55 (thinks staff has high influence already: 0.34)	28. line management follows our advice 0.44 (25 cooperation between my department and the line good: 0.28)

Factor 2 'the piece rate setter'	ALPHABET 0.59 *not* BUROMAT −0.45	9. long period in present job: 0.43	10. lower educational level: −0.53	34. low role of my department in standard-setting: −0.45 32. not too much paperwork: 0.43 31. my department not undermanned: 0.42	44. less positive attitude to life: −0.51 30. in my department efficiency can not be improved: 0.45 24. line management not quality-conscious: 0.37	43. does not believe that working comes natural to most people: −0.51 15. does not desire more general influence of line: −0.49 17. staff departments should not leave more to the line: −0.45	38. would prefer another job: 0.48

Factor no., and name	plant	external input variables	internal input variables	perceptions of input	intervening variables	perceptions of output
Factor 3 'no condemnation'	not EPICURE −0.60	9. short period in present job: −0.60		33. sees standards as tight: −0.46	22. line managers sufficiently cost-conscious: 0.68 19. reports not for showing subordinate failure: 0.62 24. line management quality conscious: 0.60 21. line managers aware of the job of my dept: 0.57 14. desires more general influence of staff: 0.45	
Factor 4 'high job satisfaction and service'	EPICURE: 0.41 not DYNAMO I −0.36	8. older: 0.41		31. my department undermanned: −0.42	23. line-managem. sufficiently conscious of the need for reliable clerical data: 0.58	39. high job satisfaction: 0.65 (25 cooperation between my departm. and the

Factor 5 'no domination'	1. does not belong to budget accounting department −0.56	10. lower educational level: −0.36	41. plant does not demand my utmost: 0.70 20. much time spent communicating with the line: 0.55 34. high role of my dep. in standardsetting: 0.50 35–36 high rank order of 'understanding production problems' 0.43 (and 'tactfulness' in boss' appraisal: 0.30)	17. staff departm. should leave more to the line: 0.55 21. line managers aware of the job of my departm. 0.46	42. appraisal is just: 0.51 12. service attitude: 0.49	40. do not work under pressure: 0.49 (25 cooperation between my departm. and the line good: 0.30)	line good:' 0.32)

FIG. 11-1. Results of Factor Analysis of Staff Interview Data

229

230

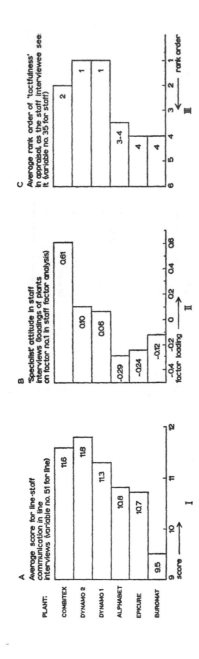

Rank correlation between plants in I and III, tested with Spearman's Rank Correlation Test, two-tailed, significant at 0.05 – level

FIG. 11-2. Comparison between Line Attitude Towards Staff and Staff Attitudes Towards Line

managers have a good communication with these specialists probably because they have something real to offer.

'I am happy with my role. I rely on the specialist. Otherwise I would have to do their work myself' (third-line-manager).

This effect of 'specialization' was not predicted and the data are just an indication that it may exist – no statistical proof. It seems an important proposition and a fruitful area for further investigation. For staff management its message is clear. There is no substitute for staff competence.

Tactfulness for the staff

The three staff characteristics which I expected to be important for line-staff communication were staff domination, the service versus evaluation dimension, and tactfulness. Of these, staff domination was negatively included in the 'specialist' factor. The specialists are those who do not want more influence; they tend to think they have a lot of influence already. To be quite clear, this is the *staff* attitude about staff influence; we have already seen that the *line* attitude about staff influence was not a major issue in budget motivation at all. Line feelings of being not unduly dominated by the staff are not correlated with line opinions about staff-line communication.

The second assumed staff characteristic was: seeing its role as service to or as evaluation of the line. The importance of this factor is suggested by Argyris' study about budgets (1952[a]). Staff attitudes towards service and evaluation did not come out as one single dimension in the staff factor analysis. Parts of it can be found in the factors 3, 4 and 5, but none of these seems to be correlated with the line attitude towards the staff. Maybe this has been a matter of not finding the right measurements. Individual statements by staff interviewees suggested that there are differences in staff role conceptions between service and evaluation, but the figures do not show an overall impact on staff-line-communication.

The third staff characteristic we should investigate is tactfulness. It is not related strongly to any of the five factors in the staff factor analysis – it has a loading of 0.30 on factor 5: 'no domination'. What I measured was not tactfulness itself, but the order of importance of 'tactfulness' for performance appraisal, as seen by the staff interviewee. I asked him to rank 10 cards with appraisal criteria (Appendix D 2, question F 2). One of these cards was 'tactfulness towards line people and colleagues'. Interviewees were asked to rank these cards as they thought their boss would do when actually appraising their performance. 'Tactfulness' came out fairly high. In DYNAMO 1 and 2, it averaged first. Its lowest average position was in EPICURE and BUROMAT: fourth.

Its important position is confirmed when we look at which characteristics of staff interviewees correlate best with their boss' appraisal of their overall performance (Appendix E 1, variable 37). We find:

45. Non-authoritarianness ($r = 0.44^*$)
25. Good cooperation with line ($r = 0.41^*$)
35. Rank order of 'tactfulness' in boss' appraisal ($r = 0.34^*$)

So the staffman's boss gives highest overall ratings to non-authoritarians who are tactful and cooperate well with the line.

The distribution of the rank order of 'tactfulness' in the boss' appraisal between plants is shown in fig. 11-2 C. The rank correlation between line-staff communication and rank order of 'tactfulness' is significant. Thus differences in the importance attached to 'tactfulness' in the staff offer an explanation for the difference in line attitudes towards the staff.

We have found two alternative explanations of the differences in line attitude now: 'Specialization' of the staff and importance attached to 'tactfulness'. They are independent of each other ($r = -0.02$). The influence of tactfulness was predicted, the influence of specialism was not. The two explanations do not exclude each other, however. It is even quite likely that both factors cooperate in improving staff – line communication: specialization and tactfulness. As to the characteristic 'service versus evaluation', the data suggest that the line can accept the staff in either role, provided that it is competent, it does not try to dominate and it behaves tactfully.

The way the 'tactfulness' scores were obtained suggest that staff management can improve staff-line relationships by paying more attention to tactfulness in their subordinate's appraisal. It is not by accident that the DYNAMO company offers the highest rank-order for tactfulness (and about the best overall staff-line communication). In this company, appraisals of the staff for salary increase purposes are based on the joint judgment of the staff manager and the line managers with whom the staff man is supposed to communicate. All staff interviewees were conscious of this fact. This system which I met in none of the other plants, seems to have a strong impact on improving staff-line communication.

Case material about staff roles and attitudes

When comparing the interviews with staff people in DYNAMO I and 2 and COMBITEX with those in the other three plants, we find a difference in atmosphere. In both DYNAMO plants and COMBITEX, staff people are concerned about their role and the role of the line. In the interviews they stress the formal aspect that they are staff without formal decision-making power, and they express their concern about the power they have informally. This illustrates their 'not wanting to dominate'.

'I don't make the budget. I only assemble it. Of course an accountant can't make a budget; this would upset the whole purpose of budgeting. The budget is made jointly by budget department and line management. The official procedure here is that all standards are set by line management, the accountant only does the registering. In practice, however, things are often different'.

'I think the department managers, who are the real producers, don't participate enough. The plant manager takes too much of a share himself'. 'The purpose of the budget variance reports is feedback, not audit. We do not want to be criticizing them, it is our job to help them. That is my private opinion' (DYNAMO staff interviewees).

'The foremen see our people not only as a help but also as reporting underattainments of standards; this may lead to a rebuke by their boss' (COMBITEX staff interviewee).

Unfortunately there are no Control Graph data for DYNAMO. In COMBITEX, where they are available, we find that staff interviewees on the average see their influence as higher than it ideally should be (fig. A-3). 'We have exerted too much pressure on the line. We should give all levels of line management a greater share in decision-making, it is them who must do the real job'.

'Every now and then we from the staff are dominating too much which gives one a pleasant feeling of personal satisfaction, but also of being a kind of dictator'.

'Officially we have an advisory role, but our finger in the pie is nearly a hand' (COMBITEX staff interviewees).

233

It is interesting to see in fig. A-3 that COMBITEX line management on the average does not share this concern for undue staff domination. Maybe just because the staff feels this way, at least the higher-level line managers are less concerned about staff influence than their counterparts in ALPHABET, BUROMAT and EPICURE. The COMBITEX first-line managers agree with those in the other plants about the ideal staff influence, but see the actual staff role nearly on the ideal level.

'If the standards are too tight, it is my own fault. Then I should protest. We are lucky this is a small plant. We can walk into the staff office if we want to. These things can be settled quickly. We definitely have sufficient influence. If our reasons are good, we always win' (COMBITEX first-line manager).

In ALPHABET, BUROMAT and EPICURE the staff is les concerned about its impact on the line.

'We often see that the staff function is not clearly advisory, it is not well defined' (*line*-manager).

'Of course the standards have an impact. We sometimes compel the line people. They'll have to accept them'.

'When the standards are not met we show the reason in the report. But we don't always see a result. My colleague has once put the same final remark on the report during a full year' (staff interviewees).

One of the questions in the staff interviews dealt with: 'When you get the figures and you see a serious underattainment of a standard, what do you do'? (Appendix D 2, question E 4). The most frequent reaction in all plants is to warn the lower-level line manager, or just to check for possible mistakes. However, in the latter three plants some staff interviewees show low sensitivity about line reactions by answering for example: 'We analyze the figures further and put it in the report with comments'.

'We go to the plant manager. If it's very important, we write it down. If you signal it to the department manager he will not take it serious and will not take action. As a staff man I cannot give hell to a department manager. This can much better be done by his boss'.

ALPHABET is a special case altogether, because it was the only plant where part of the workers were paid on individual piece-rates. This thoroughly influenced the staff role and attitudes as well as part of the line attitudes. We find the attitude of ALPHABET staff people as a special factor (no. 2) in the staff factor analysis (fig. 11-1). ALPHABET has gone through a lot of conflict about piece-rates in the past:

'The present relationships are fairly good. They have been very poor. It has never come so far that an industrial engineer was knocked off the department, but I am sure people have planned to do it' (staff interviewee).
'Standards used to be imposed, we just had to accept them. There have been made mistakes, it has created a big antagonism in people' (line interviewee).

Many of these conflicts are as much as ten years old, but people find it hard to forget. ALPHABET top management is very conscious of this problem, however, and big advances had been made to a better staff-line communication. One of these is budgeting: not being burdened by the piece-rate past, this was very positively received by the line. Another was a new, creative solution to workers' compensation through a kind of collective productivity sharing, which was in its pilot phase.

'The relationships with the budget department are excellent' (line interviewee).
'The relationships between workers and industrial engineers have improved since we have productivity sharing. Of course there are some people with private resentments' (line interviewee).
'Generally the industrial engineer is well received now, maybe not with enthusiasm but good, if he realizes which things he can say and which things he can't say' (staff interviewee).

Thus the roots of the problem in ALPHABET were in the past, and there was a clear development towards better staff-line relationships. The BUROMAT situation has been analyzed already in chapter 9; the EPICURE situation will be described in more detail later in this chapter.

Differences between staff and line people

Are staff people different from line people? It is often said they are. I have checked the evidence in my data for significant differences between staff and line, in cases where the same questions were asked both to staff and to line interviewees. My data suggest that staff and line people tend to be quite similar in most respects. Yet there are some differences: In the first place staff people tend to put themselves at a certain distance from what actually goes on in the business. This conclusion is based on

235

a number of indications. One of them is that although most of my staff interviewees were closer to first-line management by status, they tended to identify with higher-level line management. Their views on the distribution of control in the hierarchy (Appendix A and B) are more similar to those of higher-level line managers than to those of first-line managers. Their scores on 'non-authoritarianism' in fig. 9-4 are about the same as those by higher-level line management as opposed to first-line managers (and there seems to be more similarity from plant to plant between staff people than between line people in this respect).

Staff people differ significantly from line people in their attitude whether 'working comes naturally to most people' (attitude survey question 3 in Appendix D 5; correlation with line-staff difference $r = -0.19^*$). We have already seen that the more competent specialist within the staff (without line experience) is even more convinced that working does *not* come naturally to most people. One staff interviewee expressed it: 'We sometimes base ourselves on the assumption that the worker is lazy by nature. Maybe that's not right.' In spite of this man's insight, most staff people, at least those from the budget and standards staff, have more of what McGregor calls a 'Theory X' attitude (see chapter 13). This often goes together with a 'they' attitude': 'they' are lazy by nature – we, of course, are excluded. We will see in chapter 13 that it also goes together with less involvement in the job. Budget and standards staff people have a tendency to play the spectator role, to look at the plant turmoil from aside (and also somewhat from above). I have asked for the evaluation marks of line department performance, which where used to correlate with budget variance (fig. 8-3) also from staff people. Although the staff is used to working with figures, their evaluations correlated nearly always less well with official data than those from the line. Staff people seemed to be more concerned with the method of measuring than with the content of what was measured (compare Blau & Scott, 1963, p. 174). In the second place, the intrinsic rewards and frustrations in a staff job differ from those in a line job. I have asked all interviewees at the end of the interviews two questions:

– Which part of your job do you enjoy most?
– And which part of your job do you dislike most?

(Appendix D 2-3, questions G 6-7). I have divided the answers to both questions into four classes (this analysis can be considered as a very much

simplified replication of Herzberg's experiment quoted in chapter 3).
The four classes are:
1. Elements in the job itself:
   – the technical side of the job
   – working on new developments
   – organizing, planning
   – specific parts of the job, for instance bookkeeping in the case of
     an accountant, time and motion study in the case of a work study
     engineer
   – variety and routine.
2. Job results:
   – getting production out on time
   – having everything running smoothly
   – achieving improvements
     (as well as their opposites)
3. Social contacts in the job:
   – leadership, getting things done through other people
   – resolving conflict
   – education of others
   – appraisal
   – stimulating teamwork
   – giving support to others
     (as well as their opposites)
4. Paperwork, meetings and working conditions:
   – clerical work for line managers
   – meetings between line and staff
   – too much or too little work
   – fatigue and stress

The distribution of both the 'enjoy' and the 'dislike' questions over the
four classes is shown graphically in fig. 11-3, separately for 92 line
managers and 48 staff interviewees. There are various significant differences between 'line' and 'staff' as to what they enjoy or dislike about
their jobs.

On the 'enjoy' side, the main difference is that line people more frequently
mention job results as a source of satisfaction. The staff seldom sees results
– they miss this fundamental reward (Morris, 1963, chapter 17).

On the 'dislike' side, the line has more trouble in social contacts – it has

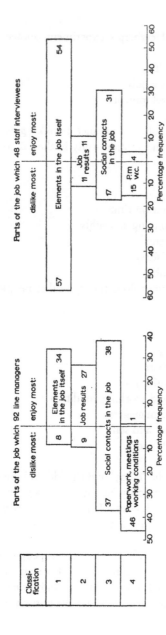

Figures in the blocks are % of total "dislike" statements or "enjoy" statements for line respectively staff

FIG. II-3A. Comparison between line and staff as to which parts of the job they dislike most and enjoy most

238

CLASSIFICATION	CLASS TITLE	"DISLIKE"	'ENJOY'
1	Elements in the job itself	0.0005	0.025
2	Job results	n.s.	0.025
3	Social contacts in the job	0.025	n.s.
4	Paperwork, meetings, working conditions	0.0005	n.s.

FIG. 11-3B. Statistical significance of differences between line and staff, tested with chi-square.

to manage people which may be rewarding, but also may give conflicts and frustrations. The biggest thorn in the flesh of the line is class 4: paperwork, meetings and sometimes working conditions (there are only a few cases where working conditions are involved). The typical line manager hates clerical work. He often hates meetings with the staff too. 'It is a pity that a standards system brings along so many meetings with the efficiency, quality and budget people' (second-line-manager). 'People talk too much. I always try to avoid meetings. I prefer working' (first-line-manager).
Staff people do not hate meetings: these are seldom mentioned as a source of negative feelings by them. They do dislike clerical work sometimes, but for them this is classified as class 1: elements in the job itself. Most budget accountants dislike bookkeeping; most efficiency engineers dislike time and motion studies. Staff people find more frustrations in the job itself. What they like is organizing, planning ahead, new developments.
So we have seen that, after all, staff and line people are different. The background of these differences is in their different organizational roles. Certain roles attract certain people; but people also develop the attitudes which their roles demand.[6] When we put a line man in a staff role he changes, as one foreman complained:
'I have lost several good assistants to the efficiency department. They used

The classical example of attitude changes under the influence of role changes is the study of Lieberman (1956).

to be practical people but as soon as they are there they suddenly veer round. It is a great pity'.

Organization of staff departments: time for interaction with the line

A hypothesis when starting the project was that staff-line communication would be better where the staff had more time for it. I have asked staff interviewees to estimate the percentage of their working time spent in person-to-person contact with line people (Appendix E 1, var. 20). Estimates varied from 0 to 50% with an average around 25%. In the staff factor analysis (fig. 11-1) we find 'time spent communicating with the line' belonging to factor 5: 'no domination'. It does not seem to influence line attitudes, but it should be stressed that with a few exceptions I only interviewed staff people who do spend a fair amount of their time communicating with the line.

For staff employees in departments dealing with technical standards, line contacts are self-evident. When these departments produced their own feedback reports or graphs it was always done by the engineers themselves. In budget departments the basic data were always supplied by the accounting departments, but the periodic reports were mostly made by the budget specialists who also had the line contacts. Where reports were produced by the accounting department directly for management use there were complaints about mistakes and low understandability. Also it was important for the budget specialist to be thoroughly familiar with the figures in order to be able to assist the line managers in their interpretation. The separation between reports publishing and line assistance advocated by Simon (p. 220) was thus not carried out fully in any of the plants.

The actual amount of assistance given to the line in interpreting feedback data varied largely.[7]

'People come daily for explanations or clarifications, from the foreman to the plant manager'.

'Four out of ten department managers come once every month to discuss the budget variance report. Also frequently during the month. If I see some outcome which looks abnormal I immediately go and see *them*'.

[7] See also Hall, 1963.

'Line managers come to see me when they have budget losses, not when they are better than the budget'.

'Every month a few customers'.

'Probably it is more me who sees them than the other way round. The initiative is mostly mine'.

'People do not come and see me. I go and see them, or I send them the data and have a chat with them afterwards'.

'We seldom have contact about the reports. It used to be more'.

I have not been able to quantify these contacts in a meaningful way per line manager, but if they are frequent, they indicate that the budget or standards are relevant to the line manager. The reasons for the line managers coming or not coming for assistance are outside the reach of the staff; the staff people cannot make the line managers come, but they can prevent them from coming back when the desired assistance is not given. Thus again the staff role is 'hygienic'.

In the staff interview data a high estimated percentage of time spent communicating with the line (var. 20) is significantly correlated with (the numbers refer to Appendix E 1):

21. Line managers are aware of the job of my department ($r = 0.34^*$)

40. I do not feel under pressure ($r = 0.33^*$)

41. This plant does not demand my utmost ($r = 0.31^*$)

31. My department is not undermanned ($r = 0.29^*$)

17. Staff departments should leave more to the line ($r = 0.26^*$)

35. Rank order of 'tactfulness' in boss' appraisal ($r = 0.26^*$)

These correlations suggest that (to the extent that people's estimates of time spent were unbiased) allowing much time for staff-line interaction breeds favorable attitudes towards the line and a stress on tactfulness; they also suggest that undermanning and pressure in staff departments threaten the time available for communication with the line; this is apparently what is sacrificed first. The practical implications of this for staff management are that sufficient staff people should be available who have the time (about 25% of total time), the status and the skills to interact with line management and to assist it in interpreting data.

For a complete budget system there should be cooperation between technical standard setting engineers and budget accountants. Now historical reasons, status differences and differences in attitude tend to bar communication between these two groups (compare chapter 2, p. 27). The differences in attitude are reflected in the differences in answers on the question 'Which part of your job do you consider the most important?' (Appendix D 2, question B 6). Budget accountants most frequently answer 'setting budgets' or 'setting standards' or the like; standards engineers more frequently answer 'improving efficiency'. In five of the six plants these barriers were well overcome and inter-staff-cooperation was good. In two of these plants both groups reported to the same controller, though through different group managers. In three other plants they reported to different managers, but this was no problem for cooperation.

The exception was EPICURE. This plant had started budgeting before it had technical standards. For the manufacturing departments only expenses were budgeted (they were 'expense centers'). The only person involved from the line was the manufacturing manager. Department managers and foremen were only dimly aware of the existence of the budget. They had no contacts whatsoever with the budget department (see fig. 9-3). Technical standard-setting was started in the EPICURE plant five years ago in an efficiency department which was a staff function to the manufacturing manager. The prime objective of its creation had been an incentive scheme for production workers using group bonuses. Later on it had extended its operations to the measurement and improvement of other aspects of productivity. It produced various productivity reports and maintained close contacts with manufacturing management of various levels.

In EPICURE the integration between technical standards and budgets had not yet taken place. Budgets were based on historical data, and only for new products a hesitating contact was beginning. People from the two departments seldom met; they did not receive each other's reports. 'The supply of information we get is limited. I can only see what's going on in my own area. I wonder where the efficiency department stands in the organization' (efficiency department interviewee).

This situation explains why EPICURE line managers show no correlation between subjective evaluation marks and budget variance (fig. 8-3). It also offers an explanation of the low scores of EPICURE higher-level line managers for their own and other's control (Appendix A, fig. A-2 A): they are not involved in the financial side of it. Finally we have seen that there is little challenge in the technical standards as seen by EPICURE managers (fig. 8-2). This is probably the consequence of standards not being tied to cost control, but mainly used for workers' incentives. The EPICURE case gives evidence that the necessity of integration of financial and technical standards is not just a theoretical issue. It really matters.

The management and training of staff people

The attitude survey data suggest that the staff is generally less well managed than the line. Staff interviewees scored significantly less favorable than line interviewees on three attitude survey items (see p. 246):
- This plant is well managed
- In this plant my private interests are taken account of as much as possible
- My career opportunities here depend first of all on myself

In interpreting these differences we should realize that all line interviewees were managers and most staff interviewees were not. Still the data suggest that from a point of view of personnel management the staff is less well off than the line. The career path especially seems less clear to the staff. Simon's call for a development plan for accounting personnel (p. 220) applies well to this situation.

Why is the staff less well managed? One explanation is that staff managers are ex-staff employees and their staff attitude of spectatorship makes them less successful in managing subordinates. Also the role of a staff manager will often be less clear than the role of a line manager. The staff manager is often half specialist, half manager.

The career path for staff seems to be a critical issue. Where should budget and standards department people come from and where should they go? The staff factor analysis shows that line experience of staff people is not an asset. The best line-staff contacts are found for specialists without line experience (factor 1). Accounting training, however, does not seem to be a very good background either (Barr, 1964). Formal educational level in general does not seem a crucial condition (it was treated as a variable in the staff factor analysis and showed up negatively only on factors 2 and 5). What really counts is competence in the specific job and a basic ability of communicating with other people, even of educating them. Where can this be learned? I think that a sound on-the-job training with a staff boss who sets the good example is still the best school.

As to future possibilities for staff people, I have asked the staff interviewees 'If you could choose another job within this company, what type of job would it be?' (Appendix D 2, question G 2). 31% said they would choose a manufacturing management job; 49% would stay in a staff function of the same type, and 20% would choose something else (personnel, sales, design). We see that we not only have to consider career paths withing the staff function itself. About one half of the interviewees were attracted to other functions, and mainly to the line. In some cases staff experience may be a good training for a line job. Some of the most able line managers I interviewed had it.

The staff man as an educator

The message of this chapter may sound somewhat disappointing to the staff man. I have tried to show that the staff role in the functioning of a budget or standards system is basically 'hygienic': he can spoil the system in several ways, but the main succes of the system depends on factors outside his reach; mainly the relationships within the line organization which will be discussed in chapter 12. This looks like a rather frustrating situation for the staff and it justifies the picture of staff frustration shown earlier in this chapter.

There is however a way out of this frustration. A role the staff man can play which is truly creative is the one of systems architect and educator. He is in the best position to have a view of the total system and to identify its weak points, both technical and human. The technical side is his specialization anyway, but he could become a specialist in the human side too, which means he should educate people. The most successful staff people I found in this study were those who conceived of their role as one of eduction and who used their contacts with their colleagues and with the line for this purpose.

Statistical analysis of data used in Chapter 11

Correlations between line interview data

See Appendix E 2. Two variables were of particular interest:

49. Desired minus actual general influence of staff departments, scored on the Control Graph (Appendix A).
51. Communication with staff: total score on the following attitude survey items:
    'The cooperation between the line and the production scheduling department is OK' (name of department chosen after the situation in each plant).
    'The people from the controller's department have a lack of understanding of production problems' – scored negatively.
    'The cooperation between the line and the industrial engineers leaves much to be desired' – scored negatively.

Correlation between these variables $r_{49,51} = 0.08$
Correlations with budget motivation and job satisfaction: see fig. 11-4:

Variances:		Correlations with	
		49 Desired minus actual staff influence	51 Communication with staff
17	Relevance (impression)	−0.06(0.10)	−0.18*(−0.03)
18	Relevance (questions)	−0.07(−0.01)	−0.11(0.10)
19	Attitude (impression)	0.06(0.25*)	0.37***(0.37***)
20	Attitude (questions)	0.01(0.32**)	0.15(0.17)
53	Job Satisfaction	0.02(−0.09)	−0.05(0.01)
54	Absence of pressure	0.10(−0.07)	0.19*(0.04)

Figures between brackets are correlations within subgroups
* significant at 0.05 level, ** significant at 0.005 level, *** significant at 0.0005 level

FIG. 11-4. Correlations of Attitudes towards Staff with Budget Motivation and Job Satisfaction.

The correlations of variable 49 with attitude are significant within subgroups and zero over total data. This indicates that the between-subgroup correlation is negative. Using Spearman's rank correlation test between subgroup averages we find $r_{R49,19} = -0.45$ and $r_{R49,20} = -0.52$.
Variable 51 is positively correlated with absence of pressure over total data: good line-staff communication in a plant and low pressure go together.

The staff factor analysis

The 48 staff interviews were divided as follows:
15 with budget accountants, controllers etc.
22 with efficiency engineers, work study engineers, etc.
 5 with quality control engineers
 6 with people charged with production control and scheduling.
The latter two groups were interviewed because they played a role in the total standards system. In the staff factor analysis I have taken efficiency, quality and production control people together.
46 variables were selected from the total staff interview data for the correlation and factor analysis. They are listed in Appendix E 1. The table of results of the staff factor analysis in fig. 11-1 is laid out in the same way as the line factor analysis results of fig. 7-1. For each of the five factors all variables with loadings over 0.35 are again shown. The division of the table into columns tries again to follow causality from left to right. Some of the variables reach the level of a 0.35 loading on none of the factors: the numbers 3, 13, 18, 25, 26, 27, 29, 35, 45. By extending the number of factors in the rotation these variables could obtain higher loadings, but this would make the picture unduly complicated.

Differences between staff and line

Attitude survey items which were included in both line and staff attitude surveys supplied the scores for a correlation analysis over 138 interviewees; the line-staff difference was treated as a variable (value 1 = line, 2 = staff). Significant correlations with the line-staff difference were found for the attitude survey items (Appendix D 5): 3 (-0.19*), 5(-0.19*), 16(-0.21*), 24(0.27**) and 28(-0.15*).
Item no. 24 is one of the F-scale items (authoritarianism; see the statistical section of chapter 9). The other five measures of (non-) authoritarianism are all positively correlated with the line-staff difference, but item no. 24 is the only one for which the correlation reaches a statistically significant level. The fact that the staff is less authoritarian than the line average is also illustrated by fig. 9-4.

CHAPTER 12

SUPERIOR - SUBORDINATE COMMUNICATION : PRESSURE AND GAME SPIRIT IN PRACTICE

Summary of this Chapter

Of all the forces in an organization working upon a budget system the communication between a budgetee and his boss is the most crucial to the functioning of the system, both for its motivation and for its job satisfaction outputs. Contacts between superiors and subordinates contain an element of communication and one of power; for daily operations the first one is more important than the second. The boss in his turn depends on his superior, so there is a vertical flow of ideas through an organization, but this vertical flow is modified by the 'umbrella function' of middle managers.

The way superior-subordinate communication influences budget motivation and job satisfaction is through:

1. Frequent person-to-person contacts about results
2. The use of results in performance appraisal
3. The use of department meetings
4. The creation of a game spirit.

The first two items refer to contacts with individual employees. They increase motivation but also a feeling of pressure. There is the possibility that they disrupt teamwork and lead to undesirable effects like scapegoating and fighting the system.

The second two items represent group leadership. They have positive effects on motivation and job satisfaction, although department meetings in themselves do not increase budget relevance. The game spirit offers the most favorable mix of motivation and a positive job satisfaction effect. It represents motivation of the budgetee from within, not through outside pressure. The game spirit depends strongly upon the leadership skill of the budgetee's superior and how well he exercises his 'umbrella function'. It is easier to realize in smaller companies and in companies of which the parts are less technologically interdependent. For the larger companies a conscious effort of creating scope for the game spirit is desirable. Statistical techniques like the use of control limits known from quality control are recommended for this purpose.

Leadership and subordinateship

Relationships between superiors and subordinates are of tremendous importance for all hierarchical organizations. There is a widespread belief in business that almost any problem can be solved by changing leaders. Many studies have been devoted to leadership, to discover what really is the secret why some leaders succeed and others fail. Factors like job-centeredness, employee centeredness and technical expertise have been related to productivity and employee job satisfaction.[1] When these studies are done seriously, their results are always somewhat disappointing. There are no simple recipes for leadership. The effect of leadership depends as much upon the subordinates and upon factors like culture and technology as upon the leader.

What makes superior-subordinate relationships in organizations so particular is that they combine an element of communication with an element of power. Power is a fascinating thing; so fascinating, that in business often far too much stress is given to the power element and far too little to the communication element in the superior-subordinate relationship. In normal day-to-day operations it is the communication element which determines the effectiveness of the relationship. When

---

[1] For a general picture of the study of leadership see Lammers, 1965. Some results of quantitative investigations into leadership effects are published in Argyle, Gardner & Cioffi 1957, 1958; Indik, Georgopoulos & Seashore 1961; Patchen 1962; Parker1963; Evans 1965.

the power element begins to function, there is often something already wrong.

From a communications point of view a superior and subordinate are just a small group together (Chapter 3). It would often be much easier if it were just that, but there is also the power element which complicates matters. Power breeds misperception: superiors and subordinates perceive each other's behavior differently from similar behavior by other people.[2] We see examples of it in the present study where superiors and subordinates estimated each other's influence on departmental results and on total influence on plant affairs. Superiors tended to overestimate their subordinates' influence on results and to underestimate their influence on total plant affairs, compared to how the subordinates saw it themselves. The reverse was true for subordinates versus their superiors (see Appendix B, fig. B - 2). Differences in perception like these hamper communication.

In spite of misperceptions created by power differences, communication channels between superiors and subordinates can belong to the most effective in an organization by the sheer frequency of the contacts and the relevance of the messages to both parties. For a researcher interviewing various people within a hierarchy it is surprising to discover how ideas often follow vertical lines. To follow the distribution of ideas an organization should in many cases be divided vertically, although the people in it always believe ideas spread horizontally. They overestimate the barriers between hierarchical levels. The vertical distribution of ideas means that a superior in turn depends strongly upon his superior, and so on. However, each individual also contributes something of himself; otherwise the whole organization would reflect only the ideas of the top man. There are of course large organizations where ideas of a strong top man are reflected throughout, but in general the flow of some ideas is stopped and other ideas are generated and sent downwards by middle managers in a hierarchy. The selective passing on of what comes down to him from above – both information and pressure –, the 'umbrella function', is one of the crucial aspects of leadership in any larger organization. The umbrella function is easier to exercise where there is physical distance between a manager and the next higher one (Blau &

[2] For studies about perception distortion see Zalkind & Costello, 1962; Haire, 1962; Read, 1962.

Scott, 1963, p. 171). The personal input downward of the top man in a geographical location is very important.

Leadership and budgets

In the budget case superior-subordinate communication appears to be a key factor to the effectiveness of the system. The statistical analysis on page 271 shows that just from those inputs into the system which could be expressed quantitatively, the four with the strongest overall correlations with budget motivation in the six plants were:

1. Participation in the setting of the budget
2. Frequency of communication about cost and budget variances with the boss
3. Knowing exactly which costs one is responsible for.
4. Frequency and usefulness of group meetings of the boss with his subordinates.

Of these four, the numbers 2 and 4 are direct inputs by the superior. I have classified participation in budget setting as a matter of company policy (ch. 7), but as I measured participation as perceived by the subordinate participant there is also an impact of the superior's leadership behavior on it. 'Knowing exactly which costs one is responsible for' can also be influenced by the boss, although technology appears to have an impact on this too. So actually in all four measurable inputs which correlated strongest with budget motivation the boss plays an important role. Then there are the aspects of the system influenced by the boss which can not easily be expressed in one single score but which are maybe even more important than the others: for example, the game aspect of budgeting. Taking all this together it is certain that *a budgetee's superior has the key role in his motivation to fulfill the budget.*

The influence of the boss through these inputs stretches both to the 'relevance' and to the 'attitude' part of budget motivation: to the real motivating part as well as to the hygienic side. The influence of the superior is much more important than the influence of the budget and standards department staff, which as we saw in chapter 11 is only 'hygienic'. It is the boss who primarily determines the success of a budget system.

The way in which a boss influences budget motivation is, as we have seen, first of all through creating participation in budget setting and through the frequency of his communication with his subordinates about cost and budget variances. These two aspects are both related to the same factor in the factor analysis of line managers' interview data: factor 4, the 'cost-conscious boss'.

There appear to be three other aspects of leader behavior which affect budget motivation, each related to a different factor in the factor analysis: the role played by budget and standards variances in performance appraisal of subordinates (factor 3); the use of meetings of the superior with his subordinates as a group (factor 1) and finally the atmosphere which is created around budgeting: the boss' skill in creating a game environment (factor 5). This last aspect appears to offer the greatest scope for a positive motivation of subordinates without external pressure and negative job satisfaction effects.

The participation issue has been analyzed at length in chapter 9. The other aspects of leader behavior will be discussed in the remaining part of this chapter.

The frequency of personal superior - subordinate contact about budget figures ; the effect of pressure

What I measured was whether an interviewee thought his boss mentioned budget and budget variances or figures expressing technical efficiency results frequently, seldom, or never (see the statistical section at the end of this chapter). The answers to this question appeared to be strongly correlated with budget motivation: they were significantly positively correlated with both measures of budget relevance and both measures of budget attitude, and second in weight for determining budget motivation to budget participation only. I predicted this relationship after the DYNAMO part of the study and the results for the other four plants strongly confirmed the hypothesis. (The variable representing frequency of personal contact with boss about figures was only measured after the DYNAMO phase).

What we are dealing primarily with here is the communication, not the power element in the superior-subordinate relationship. The boss' concern for costs is transferred to the subordinates (Cooper, 1966). We see it in my data from the fact that those who have frequent budget contacts with their boss also see him as cost-conscious ($r_{46,48} = 0,40$***), although seeing the boss as cost-conscious alone is not sufficient for budget motivation.

'The standards should have an impact, because I discuss results with the foremen and they discuss them with their assistant foremen and workers. None of them is happy when the standards are not met' (second-line-manager).

In the factor analysis (fig. 7-1) we find the variables dealing with the boss' communication loading on factor 4: 'cost-conscious boss'. This factor is strongly influenced by the BUROMAT first-line managers, and this explains why 'high participation in budget-setting' has a loading, although not a high one, on the same factor. Factor 4 shows that although having a 'cost-conscious boss' leads to high budget relevance, it also tends to have some negative effects: high pressure and an indication of a lower job satisfaction. This does not mean that budget attitudes are negative: we have seen in chapter 7 that there is no relationship between job satisfaction or pressure and budget attitude. High pressure, besides being undesirable from the personal point of view of the budgetees, has negative consequences for the organization. One is that it disrupts teamwork. Pressure by the boss will lead to an attitude in subordinates of blaming each other, of passing the buck, of scapegoating (Argyris 1953[b], 1954[a]). I found several example of this:

'When we discuss the results with the plant manager, it's a hard fight between departments. For example, the man who is behind on his schedule says: I had no raw material, the purchasing department didn't purchase it in time' (staff interviewee).

'They take an enormous lot of trouble to get some unimportant expenses transferred to another department' (staff interviewee).

'You'd be surprised how some shifts leave the machines for the next shift just to be able to fulfill their target' (staff interviewee).

Attitudes like described here lead to a 'sub-optimization': departments make their own result look as good as possible but this may not necessarily mean the best overall result for the plant as a whole.[3]

Another negative consequence of high pressure is a wrong allocation of effort by the subordinate.

[3] Compare the quotation in chapter 2, page 30 about the disruptive effect of free internal competition between departments.

'People sometimes spill their attention on the wrong side. They fight the standards instead of putting their shoulders under the job. We have exerted too much pressure' (staff interviewee).

Although pressure can be generated in communication without a power element, when the power element in the superior – subordinate relationship begins to operate this will increase the pressure. When a powerful person makes a remark about a negative result this will easily be felt as punitive and not as corrective. This is the case for the interviewees whose scores led to the 'cost-conscious boss' factor. They were motivated, but motivated from above. We will come back to it in the next section when dealing with appraisals.

The question remains how the positive motivational effects of frequent superior-subordinate communication about budgets can be retained without their negative implications of pressure and low job satisfaction. The data indicate that there is another way: the game approach. We will see more about it in a later section of this chapter.

Performance appraisal in superior - subordinate communication

The power element in superior-subordinate communication is expressed most clearly in the act of performance appraisal. Every superior is appraising his subordinate's performance, if not explicitly then at least implicitly: the superior always has an influence upon the subordinate's salary and/or career. In the last resort this is the most essential characteristic of the managerial role (Brown, 1964).

Performance appraisal is one of the most controversial issues in organization.[4] 'Judge not, that you may not be judged yourselves' (S. Matthew, 7 : 1) is a commandment which has deep significance for the performance appraisal situation. It is difficult to make an appraisal interview a positive experience for both appraiser and appraisee or even for either one of them; as we have seen in chapter 3, page 62, its value for motivation is doubtful. Still some form of appraisal is unavoidable.

Appraisal criteria can fall in the categories of personality, ability, effort or results. Modern students of the subject unanimously condemn the use

---

[4] Some recent papers on performance appraisal are those by Odiorne, 1964 and De Wolff et al., 1965. Experimental studies about appraisal practices are described in Rowe, 1964; Stewart, 1965[a] and Meyer, Kay & French, 1965 (see chapter 3).

of personality and ability (= potential but not yet realized performance) as criteria for performance appraisal, although in business practice they are often used, even on official performance rating forms. The criteria which are theoretically acceptable are only effort and results, of which effort represents the point of view of the employee and results the point of view of the company. The problem is that it is very difficult to measure effort; it is already difficult enough to measure results.

Appraisal on the basis of budget variances

Budget variances offer a measurement of results and if they are available they will unavoidably play a role in performance appraisal. This will be the case even if there is no official, mathematical relationship like there is for workers' piece rates or salesmen's quota, but which did not exist in any of my six plants. To measure the role of budget variance in the performance appraisal of line management interviewees I have used the following procedure: I asked them to rank ten cards with possible performance criteria (Appendix D 3, question F 2), in the sequence in which they thought these would be applied by their boss when he actually appraised their performance.[5] The cards bore titles like 'craftmanship', 'leadership' and 'tactfulness'. One of the cards was called 'department's results' and another 'cost-consciousness'. In fig. 12-1 I have plotted the average rank order of 'department's results' and 'cost-consciousness' for the six plants, and separately for higher level- and first-line-management. I used the term 'department's results' because I wanted a common term for all groups, regardless whether they worked under a system of budgets or under non-financial standards. To verify how the card title was understood I asked every interviewee after the ranking, what kind of department's results he had been thinking of. 84% of answers dealt with efficiency, planning, quality or budget performance measured by standards. The other 16% was divided over 'high employee job satisfaction', 'working efficiently, and 'orderliness'. Anyway the vast majority of

---

[5] I have also asked the interviewee to rank the cards in the sequence he would do it for his own subordinates. These could be compared later on to the sequences as the subordinates thought their boss would choose them. I found both cases of striking agreement and of striking disagreement. This appears to be a fair yardstick for the effectiveness of superior-subordinate communication, which, however, I did not evaluate quantitatively. Compare Maier, Hoffman, Hooven & Read, 1961.

people had understood the meaning of the card as it was intended. The card 'cost-consciousness' was added because it deals with the same issues but in a less absolute way, without suggesting measurement by standards. People understood this as 'trying to save materials and supplies' (40%), time (11%) or production equipment (8%); having ideas for savings (14%), knowing the cost of things (13%) and 'behaving as if the plant were his own' (3%). Altogether 89% did not refer to standards in this case, so they agreed with the way the card was intended. The remaining 11% referred to the budget, but nearly all of these came from one plant: BUROMAT. In BUROMAT, 37% of answers on the meaning of 'cost-consciousness' dealt expressly with acting on budget variances. We see in fig. 12-1 that BUROMAT interviewees have the highest scores for

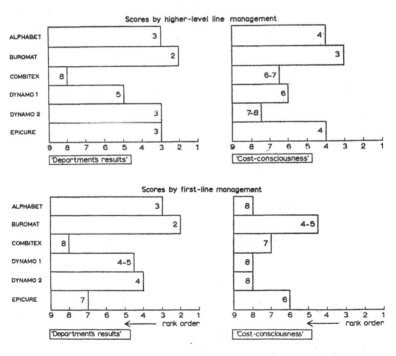

FIG. 12-1. Average Rank Order of Importance of two Appraisal Criteria as Higher Level and First-Line Managers Think their Boss Uses Them.

'cost-consciousness', close to their scores for 'department's results'. To many of them these two cards must have been virtually the same.

Fig. 12-1 shows dramatic differences between plants, especially in the case of 'department's results'. In COMBITEX shortly before the interviews a new performance appraisal form had been introduced. The fact that this form did not mention 'department's results' may explain the extremely low scores of COMBITEX. The rank orders of 'department's results' and of 'cost consciousness' appear to be almost independent of each other ($r = 0.12$).

Through the individual rankings of 'department's results' I am now able to study the effect of a more or less results-oriented appraisal on the budget motivation of my interviewees. The correlation analysis on page 270 shows that an important ranking of 'department's results' increases budget relevance and has a weakly negative impact on budget attitude. ('Cost consciousness' has the same effects but to a lesser extent.) However, the analysis also shows that an important ranking of 'department's results' or 'cost-consciousness' each go together with a feeling that the performance appraisal is *unjust* and that career opportunities are biased. An important ranking of 'department's results' is also correlated with a feeling of high pressure and nervousness. This outcome contains a fair amount of warning against an indiscriminate use of budget results in performance appraisal. It may lead to negative feelings: 'Sometimes I have the feeling that I did everything I could, yet the results are poor. Why do they cling to those rigid figures, can't they see the difficulties?' (first-line-manager).

This quotation shows that to the subordinate it is not the results which count, but the effort spent. Judging by results without taking effort into account is felt as unjust.

The consequences of an overstress on results in appraisal may be serious. It may create in subordinates a tremendous fear of failure with all the adverse consequences of 'management by fear': avoiding to take risks, scapegoating, faking figures so that results 'look right':

'If it is true that my salary increase depends on the figures, it is easy enough to screw up the standards' (third-line-manager).

'The managers have a proletarian attitude towards their budgets. There is little difference between the attitude of a worker towards piece rates and of a plant manager towards his budget' (staff interviewee).

This also means that the chances of success of a financial bonus scheme for managers based on budget results are very small indeed (Bos, 1955, p. 33). The degree of arbitrariness of almost any budget will create evasive activities and negative feelings which will definitely outweigh the increase in budget relevance which the scheme will provide.

The case for appraisal by budget results – however desirable it may seem because of its effect on budget relevance – looks rather weak up to now. Fortunately the factor analysis provides some additional points of view. In the factor analysis (fig. 7-1) the variables dealing with appraisal are grouped together in factor 3: 'upward communication'. As we could expect, the feeling that the appraisal is just goes together with a less important rank order of 'department's results' and 'cost-consciousness' as appraising criteria. Factor 3 is fairly strongly influenced by the COMBITEX and BUROMAT extremes. It shows a number of other things as well, however. An appraisal which is felt as just goes together with a superior-subordinate relationship in which the boss asks his subordinate's ideas. In this same situation, the subordinate feels he has high operational control (influence on results) and a low feeling of pressure. As we have seen in the chapters 10 and 11, this same factor accounts for good understanding of written reports and a good line-staff communication.

The relationship between a lack of upward communication and a feeling of pressure has been found empirically by others (Bass, 1964; Revans, 1964ᵇ). It is very important that upward communication also appears to prevent feelings of injustice in appraisal:

'For appraisal I do not use the figures in an absolute sense, but only in a relative sense. If things go worse I talk with the man and see what the reasons are and if he has taken measures. In this conversation it will appear whether he is fit for his task or not. The mere fact that results become better or worse is an insufficient yardstick' (third-line-manager). The conditon for the use of budgetary results in performance appraisal appears to be a climate of upward communication, so that the results – the company point of view – can be translated back into the efforts – the subordinate point of view.

'It is difficult to appraise realistically. It is easy to base an appraisal on the results of the department, out of proportion to the real difficulties' (third-line-manager).

If appraisal is carried out in proportion to difficulties, department's results will not rank first in the eyes of the subordinate, but they can still retain an important position. As we have seen, the rank order of 'department's results' is related to budget relevance. To keep the budget relevant to the subordinate, results must play a role in appraisal. It is apparent that the dilemma of a manager is to find the right balance between two extremes: an overstress on results in appraisal, leading to feelings of injustice, and too little stress, leading to low relevance of the budget and low motivation. The key to finding this balance lies in upward communication or just simply: listening to the subordinate.

Discussing results in meetings

In chapter 11 we have seen that most line managers dislike meetings. The negative feelings apply mostly to 'line-staff communication' meetings, set up on a routine basis to solve problems, like meetings with efficiency and quality departments. As the line managers see them these meetings are often ineffective, stressful, and a waste of time.

There were few negative comments on what one could call 'department meetings': get-togethers of a superior with the team of subordinates directly reporting to him. These meetings have received a fair amount of attention from social scientists. Guest (1962[a], 1962[b]) reports their use to bring about organizational change. Likert (1961, p. 122 ff.) and Philipsen (1965, p. 117 ff.) relate the use of department meetings among other things to the amount of influence which employees or lower-level managers feel they have on what goes on in the organization. In this study I was able to do the same: I found a positive, but not significant, correlation between successful department meetings and perceived influence on what went on in the plant.[6]

Department meetings have a special function in the case of shift work. Where operations are running in shifts, especially in three shifts, shift supervisors and foremen who use the same equipment and finish each others' job have many problems in common; on the other hand, they never meet as a group unless this is expressly organized. It is very useful

[6] Variables 41 and 45 of Appendix E 2 are correlated with $r = 0.16$. Furthermore, variables 42 and 45 are correlated with $r = -0.30*$, indicating that those who have successful department meetings do not desire more influence on what goes on in the plant.

both from a business and from a human point of view to call them together once a week (Bast, 1960). Three of the plants I studied had three-shift operations, and comments on department meetings were very positive in all cases, although the night shift managers had to make an extra trip to the plant for them:

'The meetings are valuable. At shift relief we have only a short contact. It's good to be able to discuss with the three of us'.

'If I want to stay home I'm allowed to, but the meetings are good for mutual contact'.

'Some of the meetings are useful, some give small benefit, but on the average they are always worthwhile. We can discuss our problems together. It is the only occasion we have for this' (shift foreman).

The use of department meetings for giving attention to budget and standards variances is fairly widespread. Sord and Welsch have made it a special issue in their mail survey of budgeting practices in American Companies. They report (1958, p. 243) that for manufacturing units at plant management level about one half, at supervisor level about one third, and at foreman level about one-fourth of companies use meetings in results feedback. A summary of department meetings' practices within my six plants is shown in fig. 12-2. The role of budget and standards performance feedback in these meetings varies: it may be an occasional issue, it may be a regular agenda item.

	Frequency of department meetings of:		
	plant manager with second-line-managers	second-line with first-line-managers	first-line-managers with employees
ALPHABET	2 weeks	not (once a month with plant mgr.)	not
BUROMAT	1 week	1–4 weeks	2–3 months
COMBITEX	1 week	3 weeks	3–6 months
DYNAMO 1	not	2–6 weeks	not
DYNAMO 2	2 weeks (quality meeting)	1 week	not
EPICURE	1 week	not	not

FIG. 12-2. Frequency of Department Meetings.

Theoretically, meetings are not necessary to discuss budget results where subordinates have their own budget. Problems can be identified with the subordinate affected and the communication is between the superior and the individual subordinate. Meetings are indispensable where subordinates influence budget results collectively, as in the case of shift work mentioned before.

My data show (p. 270) that all in all, meetings have a more positive effect on the *attitude* component of budget motivation than on the *relevance* component. This suggests that they are in many cases not indispensable (at least from the point of view of budget results feedback) but that to the extent that they are seen by the subordinate as valuable, they help create positive attitudes towards the system. Philipsen (1965) has proven that meetings that are *not* seen as valuable are worse than no meetings at all. In my analysis of the effect of department meetings I have consequently treated the use of meetings as an input which can have positive (meetings held and seen as valuable), zero (no meetings held) and negative values (meetings held and seen as a waste of time).

Some quotations from interviews will serve to illustrate how budget and standards variances are used in department meetings and what people think of these meetings in general.

The use of figures:

'We always begin discussing results: reject percentages, which have more meaning to the foremen than money' (second-line-manager).

'In the meeting the department manager explains the results of the department in guilders. Every department is a small-scale plant. We buy from another department and sell again to the next. I think that's good' (first-line-manager).

'The foremen each in turn act as chairmen of the meeting. They must collect all data themselves and interpret them' (second-line-manager).

General usefulness of meetings:

'It is useful that we as managers of different departments learn to speak the same language' (second-line-manager).

'The foremen must believe in the standards to be able to communicate them to the employees. The meetings have a kind of psychological influence on them' (second-line-manager).

'We learn to know each other better. The figures could also be given in another way' (first-line-manager).

'The meetings are useful, even if they are spent on useless subjects' (second-line-manager).
'The stress is on personal contact and giving people a feeling of involvement. The decisions that are taken could also be dictated by me' (third-line-manager).
No meetings:
'In principle my contact with my subordinates is made through walking into their office' (third-line-manager).
'We do not have the foremen together. We meet each other every day' (Second-line-manager).
'I have about a daily contact with my boss and my assistants' (second-line-manager).
Meetings valued negatively:
'The meetings are worthless. I am not so much in favor of this kind of meetings: they often degenerate into nagging. But I see no other way to communicate (third-line-manager).
'No, they are useless. They are a sleepy affair, where always the same people are bickering' (second-line-manager).
'One does not get any support through these meetings, one is just fobbed off with promises if there is a problem' (first-line-manager).

The effects of meetings on attitudes

In the statistical section on page 269 it is shown that interviewees who have an experience of successful meetings with their boss are different in a number of respects from those who miss this experience:

1. They have more frequent contact with their boss about budgetary results and see their boss as more cost-conscious.
2. They participate more in the setting of their budget, they think their department's special problems are sufficiently taken account of in budget setting, and they feel they cannot work without standards.
3. They evaluate their own department s performance more in terms of budget results (see chapter 8, fig. 8-3 and also the DYNAMO case in chapter 8); they think their department is not running efficiently enough, and they expect more improvement in the performance of their department.

4. They have better communications with the budget and standards staff departments and feel less dominated by the staff.
5. Finally, they appear to have a more positive attitude to life in general. They do not believe, for example, that people are nowadays less willing to carry responsibility than they used to be. They are less authoritarian, and feel more free to disagree with the interviewer.

This is confirmed when we study the results of the factor analysis of line management interview data (fig. 7-1). We find 'frequent and useful department meetings' belonging to factor 1 'independence' from which especially the non-authoritarianism which goes with meetings becomes clear. The immediate question is again what is cause and what is effect: do meetings with boss and colleagues make a man less authoritarian, or do non-authoritarians rate meetings as useful and authoritarians as not useful? Looking at the details from my interviews I hold that both explanations are partly true. To some extent at least meetings do make people less authoritarian. The whole idea of two-way communication is non-authoritarian. Besides, higher levels managers are less authoritarian (fig. 9-4) and through meetings they communicate their attitude to their subordinates, using the element of social pressure in any group which meets regularly. Deviant members are pressed to accept the less authoritarian group attitude. Group activities are the most effective way of changing attitudes.

Fig. 12-1 draws also attention to the fact that in BUROMAT and COMBITEX there were periodic department meetings on the employee level. They appeared to function better in BUROMAT, which is not surprising in view of the greater independence of the BUROMAT foremen (compare the BUROMAT case in chapter 9 and the COMBITEX case in chapter 8).

How to make meetings successful

The success of a system of periodic department meetings depends, like any other superior-subordinate interaction, on the ability of the superior (Meuwese 1964), on the attitudes of the subordinates (Zaleznik 1965) and on the situation (Hutte 1959- 60, in particular III, p. 355). This was illustrated with astonishing clarity in the feedback sessions which the researcher conducted with groups of interviewees in the six plants (see chapter 6). The character of the discussions during these meetings varied strongly from plant to plant and even from group to group within each plant, and these differences showed exactly the picture given by interviewees about the department meetings they used to participate in (or not). Groups that were accustomed to have a free exchange of views among themselves had a free exchange of views with the researcher too, even though an unknown observer and sometimes other company officials – up to the president of the company – were present. Groups whose members had complained about frustration in meetings showed a destructive behavior when confronted with the research feedback. Foremen who never participated in department meetings did not communicate in the feedback meetings. It became clear from the feedback sessions that one factor which makes for a successful discussion is an experience of successful discussions in the past. A group has to become a team in order to have good meetings, and this takes time. A department manager who wants to start a program of periodic meetings with his subordinates should realize this and not expect free communication immediately.

It was also clear from the feedback sessions that the ability of second- and third-line-managers to create a permissive atmosphere and to stimulate two-way communication varied widely. There is no substitute for self-awareness and sensitivity of a superior who wants to conduct successful meetings.

The game spirit

Altogether in the factor analysis four factors are positively correlated with both budget relevance and budget attitude (see fig. 272 in the statistical section). They are the factors 1, 4, 5 and 6. Factor 1 ('independence') is related to the use of department meetings. Factor 4 ('cost-conscious boss') is related to frequency of contact between boss and subordinate about budget figures. Both have been analyzed earlier in this chapter. Factor 6 is related to external inputs into the budget system, like the budgetee's age. It will be discussed in chapter 13.

What is left is factor 5 which I called 'cost-conscious self'. It has the highest loading for the 'impression' measure of relevance, but it also has positive loadings for attitude; in its overall effect on motivation it is second only to factor 4, the 'cost-conscious boss'. Then factor 5 is the only factor which has not only positive loadings for budget motivation, but also for job satisfaction and the absence of pressure. Factor 5 appears to represent the situation with the most favorable mix of outputs for the budget system: outputs leading to greater profitability for the enterprise and outputs related to the well-being of its people.

The characteristics of the 'cost-conscious self' situation as they are reflected by the factor analysis table (fig. 7-1) are, in the order of importance shown by the factor loadings:

- the 'cost-conscious self' budgetees know exactly which costs they are responsible for (21)
- there are relatively more of them among the higher-level line management of ALPHABET
- they give the impression of a high budget relevance (17)
- they think trying to attain the standards is a sport (25)
- they consider the feedback information they receive as sufficiently understandable (50)
- they are very satisfied with their job and department (53)
- they are also found among the higher-level line management of EPICURE
- they have produced high scores on the quiz questions about general cost-consciousness, as described in chapter 10 (23).

These people seem to be motivated to fulfill the standards or budgets from within, not through outside forces. They have an interest in cost problems shown by their high quiz scores; they see their own cost responsibility clearly defined. And they see standards attainment as a sport.

'I want to work with standards; then I know where I stand: I think it's a kind of a sport' (second-line-manager).

'If standards are not used to pay people on, then it's a sport. The job must be a sport' (first-line-manager).

'We are stimulated to set high targets, it is a certain sportsmanship: at year-end we have the proud feeling we've made it' (second-line-manager).

'Without standards we would sink away. For me it's a sport to get the people to make it' (first-line-manager).

'To make a budget gain that is as high as possible, that is the sport, but then people should accept a decent challenge in the standards' (staff interviewee).

I think this 'sport' or 'game' aspect is the crucial element which makes the situation of these people different from that of others:
- they show high motivation and involvement
- they feel the standards are challenges for achievement
- they have free scope for acting. They are not pressed from the outside.
- the department's results play a role in their appraisal, but not an extreme role (factor loading 0.24). The interviews give evidence that the department's results are not used in a punitive way by the bosses of those high on the 'cost-conscious self' factor. There is a separation between the 'real-life facts' of appraisal and salary determination and the area of results measured by standards.
- they accept the rules of the budgeting system and the standards when these are set; there are no negative attitudes about any aspect of the budget system loading on factor 5.
- they show a team spirit. In subgroups that have above average loadings on factor 5, there are no signs of 'passing the buck' to another department. The subgroup which is highest on factor 5, the ALPHABET higher-level group, was one of the most interested and constructive groups in the feedback sessions. It was rated favorably on all dimensions of the sessions by both researchers present. There was no need for the group leader to intervene: the discussion just went by itself. The observing researcher described it: 'these people have an easy and playful way of getting along with each other'.

If we compare this list of characteristics of 'cost-conscious self' – budgetees with the list of 'play' characteristics derived from Huizinga in chapter 3 (p. 77), we see they are almost identical, except for the obvious difference that pure play is an activity carried out for its own sake and budget control, we hope, is not. But budget control fits in with the list of elements of human culture which Huizinga shows to have a game character. The interesting fact is now that to the degree that this game character can develop itself the budget system will serve its goals towards both the enterprise and its members better.

How the game spirit is created

The decisive factor in creating the game spirit in budget control is the attitude of the boss. I have met managers in this study who were radiating enthusiasm towards their subordinates: they were the most successful in creating the game spirit. The manager should handle his subordinates as a team, and the use of meetings can be helpful to create the team spirit. The different subordinates are fellow players in the game, not opponents. The opponent is Nature, inefficiency or maybe a competing company. 'The essence of good budgeting is cooperation' (Tovey, 1963). The manager should show interest in his subordinate's results, but in a corrective, not in a punitive way, and he should listen to them before he judges. The most important characteristic for the manager is perhaps trust, which creates the atmosphere of safety in which the team spirit can operate. Finally he should execute his umbrella function and protect his subordinates from any undue pressure or alarming information by higher superiors or staff departments which would spoil the game.

The game spirit will be easier to realize in a small company than in a big one. The need for more coordination in the bigger company will tend to limit the amount of free scope necessary for the game spirit. *There is a danger in the larger corporation that the coordination function of the budget destroys the motivation function of it.* The solution is in deliberately creating the free scope which is psychologically necessary. The use of statistical techniques in budget control analogous to those used in quality control can guarantee that the need for coordination is still satisfied. This was not practised in any company in this study; good applications are still rare. Still I strongly recommend experimentation with the introduction of Control Limits for budgets as described in chapter 4, especially for the larger corporations. They have a promising potential as technical tools to reach an economical and psychological optimum.

It is possible that the technology used in the particular company influences the possibility of creating the game spirit. When for example parts of the organization are technologically independent – this was the case in EPICURE – it is much easier for a manager to know exactly which costs he is responsible for, to feel the challenge and to pass it to his subordinates. The more technologically interdependent a company becomes, the less clear-cut the responsibilities for results, the less clear the challenge of the game. In these situations it will demand more leadership and managerial creativity to maintain the game atmosphere.

The role of the staff departments in bringing about the game spirit is unfortunately again hygienic. By supplying insufficient or unclear information or by exerting undue pressure they can spoil the game, but they cannot create the game spirit on their own. Their wisest policy is probably self-restraint.

Statistical analysis of data used in Chapter 12

Variables used in this Chapter

The variables from the list in Appendix E 2 which are relevant to superior-subordinate communication and have not yet been introduced in previous chapters are:

a. Variables dealing with individual superior-subordinate control and with meetings:

45. Frequency and usefulness of meetings with boss and colleagues. The score was based upon the interviewee's boss' statement about the frequency of these meetings (1 = never to 5 = daily) and the interviewee's judgment about their usefulness (2 = useless, 3 = doubtful, 4 = useful). The score can be read from this table:

frequency:	1	2	3	4	5
usefulness 2	5	4	3	2	1
3	5	5	5	5	5
4	5	6	7	8	9

So if meetings are seen as useless, the higher their frequency, the lower the score; if meetings are seen as useful, the higher their frequency, the higher the score.

46. Frequency of personal superior-subordinate contact about budget figures ('boss discusses budget variances'). This is the combined score on the open question E 6 (Appendix D 3): 'Does your boss ever discuss budget variances or other performance figures of the department with you? and the attitude survey item: 'My boss discusses the department's costs with me'; these two measures are intercorrelated with $r = 0.55***$.

47. Boss asks my ideas; this is the combined score on two attitude survey items: 'My boss rejects my ideas for improvement' (scored negatively). 'My boss asks my opinion about matters concerning my area of work' (scored positively). These two are intercorrelated with $r = 0.34***$.

48. Boss works on cost reduction: this is the score on the attitude survey item: 'My boss is continuously working on cost reduction'. The intercorrelations between these variables are shown in fig. 12-3.

b. Variables dealing with performance appraisal

27. Attitude survey item: 'A foreman's performance can well be appraised on his efforts to meet standards'.

43. Rank order of 'department's results' in boss' appraisal, obtained by ranking of cards (actual rank orders are deducted from 10 so that an important rank is now represented by a high score).

44. Rank order of 'cost-consciousness' in boss' appraisal (scored like 43).

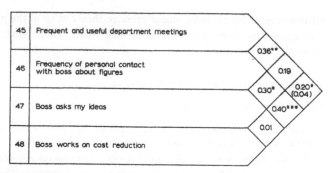

The figure between brackets is the only deviant correlation within subgroups.

   * significant at 0.05 level
  ** significant at 0.005 level
*** significant at 0.0005 level

FIG. 12-3. Intercorrelations of Variables Dealing with Superior-Subordinate Communication

56. My performance is justly appraised and my career depends on myself: this is the combined score on two attitude survey items:
   'I think my performance is justly appraised here'
   'My career opportunities here depend first of all on myself'.
   These two are intercorrelated with $r = 0.35$***.
The intercorrelations between the variables dealing with performance appraisal are shown in fig. 12-4.

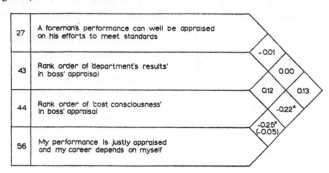

The figure between brackets is the only deviant intercorrelation within subgroups
* significant at 0.05 level

FIG. 12-4. Intercorrelations of Variables Dealing with Performance Appraisal.

c. An important variable is also:

25. Attitude survey item: 'I think trying to attain the standards is a sport'.

Correlations with the output variables

Fig. 12-5 shows the correlation of the 9 variables introduced above with relevance, attitude, job satisfaction and pressure.

We see that *meetings* (45) work predominantly on budget attitude. Other correlations with variable 45: frequent and useful department meetings, besides those in fig. 12-3 and 12-5, are

29. High participation in budget-setting	0.21*
33. Sufficient account of special problems in budget-setting	0.27*
24. Cannot work without standards	0.27*
38. High correlation between own subjective evaluation and budget variance	−0.23*
26. My department not efficient enough	0.25*
36. Expects improvement in performance	0.23*
51. Good communication with staff	0.22*
49. Does not desire less staff influence	−0.24*
58. Positive attitude to life	0.26*
59. Non-authoritarian	0.36**
60. No yes-men	−0.24*

Frequency of contact with boss (46) works on relevance and attitude both, but also on pressure.

Boss asks ideas (47) works on job satisfaction and prevents pressure.

I had expected that 48, the perception that *one's boss works continuously on cost reduction,* would be correlated with relevance: that is, that there would be a correlation between perceived relevance for the boss and relevance for the subordinate. This is not the case. It appears that it is the fact that the boss talks about results figures, not just the fact that he is seen as cost-conscious, which makes for budget relevance in a subordinate.

I had expected that 27, the opinion that *a foreman's performance can well be appraised on his efforts to meet standards,* would be correlated with relevance. This is not the case. The idea of appraising a foreman's performance through his efforts to meet standards is rejected by those with high relevance as much as by those with low relevance.

Rank order of 'department's results' in the boss' appraisal (43) affects relevance and pressure; within subgroups it also affects job satisfaction negatively. That this correlation disappears when we look at total data shows that the amount of 'results' in appraisal accepted as fair must differ from plant to plan or between hierarchical levels.

Rank order of "cost-consciousness" in the boss' appraisal (44) only affects the impression of relevance. Its correlations with the other measure of relevance are negative; all in all, a stress on 'cost-consciousness' without tying it explicitly to the standards does not seem to be very important for motivation . When *performance appraisal is seen as just* (56), this prevents a feeling of pressure.

Seeing attaining the standards as a sport (25) has no direct significant correlations on motivation. It is an intervening variable in factor 5 in the factor analysis and helps to explain this factor.

Variables:		17 Relevance (impression)	18 Relevance (questions)	19 Attitude (impression)	20 Attitude (questions)	53 Job Satisfaction	54 Absence of pressure
45	Frequent and useful department meetings	0.16(0.19)	0.16(0.10)	0.30**(0.14)	0.27*(0.01)	-0.15(0.08)	0.03(0.04)
46	Frequency of personal contact with boss about figures	0.36***(0.22*)	0.23*(-0.01)	0.26*(0.25*)	0.31**(0.26*)	0.00(0.16)	-0.26*(-0.18*)
47	Boss asks my ideas	-0.08(0.04)	0.01(0.14)	0.26*(0.23*)	0.03(0.06)	0.33***(0.47***)	0.25*(0.30*)
48	Boss works on cost reduction	-0.03(-0.10)	0.15(0.20)	-0.01(-0.09)	0.00(-0.08)	0.15(-0.24*)	-0.22*(-0.12)
27	A foreman's performance can well be appraised on his efforts to meet standards	-0.15(0.14)	0.03(-0.08)	-0.08(-0.10)	-0.18(0.09)	0.10(0.02)	0.08(0.03)
43	Rank order of 'departments' results 'in boss' appraisal	0.36***(0.23*)	0.17(-0.00)	-0.15(-0.06)	-0.08(-0.14)	-0.03(-0.25*)	-0.29**(-0.17)
44	Rank order of 'cost consciousness' in boss' appraisal	0.21*(0.04)	-0.12(-0.18*)	0.07(0.07)	0.03(-0.02)	0.02(0.07)	-0.11(-0.08)
56	Performance is justly appraised and my career depends on myself	-0.14(0.06)	0.11(0.24*)	0.08(-0.05)	-0.05(0.05)	0.14(0.05)	0.30**(0.17)
25	I think trying to attain the standards is a sport	0.10(0.18)	0.02(0.08)	-0.13(-0.02)	-0.02(-0.02)	0.21*(0.12)	0.01(0.00)

Variables:	correlations with:			
	17 Relevance (impress.)	18 Relevance (quests.)	19 Attitude (impress.)	20 Attitude (quests.)
29 Budget participation	0.56***	0.34**	0.28**	0.29**
46 Frequency of personal contact with boss about figures	0.36***	0.23*	0.26	0.31**
21 Know exactly for which costs responsible	0.31**	0.28**	0.22*	0.28**
45 Frequent and useful department meetings	0.16	0.16	0.30**	0.27*

* significant at 0.05 level, ** significant at 0.005 level, *** significant at 0.0005 level

FIG. 12-6. Review of Inputs with the Strongest Overall Correlations with Relevance and Attitude.

In fig. 12-6 a review is shown of the four input variables with the strongest overall correlations with relevance and attitude. In the text of this chapter this is used to show the important role of the budgetee's boss in his budget motivation.

Factor loadings for the output variables

Finally fig. 12-7 is a table of factor loadings for the six output variables in the line factor analysis. In the text of this chapter this serves to illustrate the importance of the 'cost-conscious self' factor, which is related to the game spirit and which is the only factor with positive loadings for all six output variables.

←

Figures between brackets are correlations within subgroups

* significant at 0.05 level, ** significant at 0.005 level, *** significant at 0.0005 level

FIG. 12-5. Correlations of Variables dealing with Superior – Subordinate Communication with Relevance, Attitude, Job Satisfaction and Pressure.

Factors:		Factor loadings of:					
		17 Relevance (impress.)	18 Relevance (quests.)	19 Attitude (impress.)	20 Attitude (quests.)	53 Job Satisfaction	54 Absence of pressure
1	Independence	0.16	0.05	0.37	0.42	-0.28	-0.10
2	Budget variance	-0.04	-0.16	0.03	0.08	-0.28	-0.07
3	Upward communication	-0.29	-0.04	0.47	0.21	0.21	0.44
4	Cost-conscious boss	0.20	0.48	0.29	0.28	-0.30	-0.38
5	Cost-conscious self	0.52	0.13	0.14	0.31	0.40	0.15
6	Job rotation	0.34	0.09	0.28	0.02	0.01	-0.02
7	Job involvement	0.01	-0.10	-0.16	-0.13	0.17	-0.10
8	Self-satisfaction	0.06	0.03	-0.06	-0.13	0.34	0.10

FIG. 12-7. Factor Loadings for the Output Measures of the Budget System

Summary of this Chapter

This chapter collects the available conclusions about inputs into the budget system which originate from the kind of people the budgetees are themselves: how old they are, how long they have been in their jobs, what is the influence of their hierarchical and educational level, and which aspects of their personality and their cultural norms play a role in the system. Both youth and being rather new in the job appear to increase the use a budgetee makes of the figures he gets. This indicates that a job rotation policy which limits the period people stay in the same jobs may increase the practical use of budget figures. Hierarchical and educational level in themselves are probably less important as inputs to the system. Hierarchical level goes together with lower authoritarianism, however, which is probably instrumental in creating more favorable budget attitudes. The interview data reveal two other personality factors: job involvement and self-satisfaction. Job involvement is influenced by cultural norms. Although job involvement and self-satisfaction probably affect job motivation and/or job satisfaction in general, they have no direct significance for budget motivation.

Who are the budgetees?

Organizational systems like budget systems are open systems: they

273

interact with the environment. Management alone does not determine how a budget system will function; there are inputs outside management's reach. One group of these 'external' inputs consists of the characteristics of the kind of people the budgetees are: their age and educational background, but also their beliefs and fundamental attitudes which depend on their personalities and also on the cultural influences to which they have been exposed throughout their lives. These inputs to an organization are not wholly external, because management can exert some influence on them through its plant location, hiring, promotion and job rotation policies. If we consider only the budget system we can safely describe them as external inputs however: decisions about plant locations and hiring and promotion of line managers will generally be made on other grounds than their impact on the budget system. This chapter will try to show what the effect of such decisions on a budget system may be. The inputs which will be analyzed in this chapter can be divided into three groups:

1. Age and length of service in the job
2. Hierarchical and educational level
3. Aspects of personality and culture.

Age and job rotation

People's age and the generation they belong to – the two are inseparable of course – influence people's reaction on figures:
'Recently the group of foremen has been somewhat rejuvenated. The younger ones understand figures and want to use them' (staff interviewee). This may be just the way our society develops: modern man has to be more figure-conscious. Groffen (1965), dealing with rationality in business, suggests that younger people will more easily derive satisfactions from working rationally than older people. He relates this to the period in the life of these older people they are in: they question what they have accomplished in life, and not having found it in rationality, they put more weight on feelings and loyalty. This can well make them less easily motivated by figures.

In chapter 8 we have seen both in my data and in the results of Stedry and Kay's experiment that age is a possible determinant of how a budgetee reacts on a budget system. For example, whether he is challenged or discouraged by very tight standards, or whether he expects improvements or not. In the statistical section of this chapter (fig. 13-4) we see that within plants the older people tend to report more pressure. Age is strongly correlated with another aspect: the length of time in the present function. In the factor analysis a short time in the present job and lower age turn up as the decisive variables for factor no. 6. As 'short time in the present job' has the higher loading of the two on this factor, I have called it 'job rotation'. By a policy of job rotation management can deliberately limit the time people serve in a particular job. The 'job rotation' factor in the factor analysis, which also stands for 'younger people', represents a situation where there is more expectation of improvement, more ready knowledge of figures about performance and standards, and a high correlation between own subjective evaluation of performance and budget variance. This is clearly a situation, therefore, of more interest in and use of figures. In chapter 12, fig. 12-7 we see that the 'job rotation' factor has positive loadings for both relevance and attitude, though not very high ones. It is neutral on job satisfaction and pressure.

Above I have offered an explanation for a relationship between preference for figures and youth. It can also be defended that the main cause for the preference for figures is the job rotation. Klein (1965) in describing the situation in a department of a large international company, concludes that the policy this company followed to keep people moving from job to job acted as a second order control: it controlled the controllers and forced them to use the (first-order) controls built into the system, because they had no time to build up the experience to do their job in a different way. The manager who has to tackle a new job will seize all the control tools offered to him. The manager who has been in the job for twenty years will probably feel that the figures can't tell him much he doesn't already know.

Hierarchical and educational level

It is not surprising that there is a strong correlation between the level in the hierarchy of the interviewed line managers (first-line versus higher) and their educational level. In the Netherlands, foremen are mostly promoted from the ranks and they seldom have more than lower vocational training; second-line and higher-level managers are hired for these positions among people with a secondary school, higher vocational or college education. Only in some trades like the graphic trade to which ALPHABET belongs is there an open career path from bottom to top. In this case the people who are promoted are those who extend formal training by evening courses. In one other plant in my sample the second-level managers had come through the ranks; here the career stop was between second-and third-line management.

Educational and hierarchical level of budgetees is correlated to budget relevance and to budget attitude. It is questionable whether this is a direct causal relationship, because, for example, hierarchical level is strongly correlated with budget participation and this in turn is correlated with relevance and attitude. The way the correlations are sorted out by the factor analysis, higher hierarchical level is only important in factor 1: 'independence' which deals with the issue of frequent and useful department meetings and has a positive attitude as an output.

Although it is impossible to get a conclusive picture of causes and effects from my data, my impression is that higher hierarchical level is not so much a cause but as the system was organized in my six plants there just happened to be more inputs which led to higher budget motivation for those at the higher levels in the hierarchy. One of them is non-authoritarianism which will be analyzed below. Educational level does not play an important role in the factor analysis at all, which suggests its influence on the functioning of the budget system is negligible.

Personality and cultural influences: authoritarianism

There were three fundamental attitudes in the budgetees which appeared to play a role in that part of the budget system which I could measure:
a. Authoritarianism
b. The theory Y-attitude in the terminology of McGregor (1960), expressed in the belief that 'working comes naturally to most people'.
c. A feeling of self-satisfaction.

We have met authoritarianism as a characteristic influencing people's reaction on participation in chapter 9. In the statistical section on page 282 it appears that two other attitudes are closely related to authoritarianism: 'yes-men-ship', that is the tendency of interviewees to demonstrate agreement with the interviewer, and a less positive attitude to life in matters like whether people are less willing nowadays to carry responsibility than they used to be.

We see in fiig. 13-3 in the statistical section that authoritarianism is strongly correlated with the hierarchical level: the lower level is more authoritarian. We already saw this in chapter 9 (fig. 9-4). The correlation is with hierarchical level rather than with educational level, which indicates that it is the fact of being a second-line manager rather than the higher education level which explains the lower authoritarianism. Authoritarianism is also corrected with age and period in the job. Age is the probable cause. The correlation of authoritarianism with age shows the difference between generations. It illustrates what I wrote in chapter 1: there is a tendency towards democratization; social norms are shifting in that absolute dependence is no longer accepted (p. 12).

The degree of authoritarianism in the budgetees has some implications for the budget system. Non-authoritarians have more positive attitudes towards the budget system. This fact has already been mentioned in chapter 9 to explain the influence of non-authoritarianism on the relationships between budget participation and budget motivation (p. 187). In plants were managers are less authoritarian they are more positive to the idea of using standards instead of more arbitrary ways of managing. In chapter 13 we have seen that budgetees who participate in successful department meetings with their boss and colleagues tend to be less authoritarian, more positive to life and that they dare to disagree more with the interviewer. So authoritarianism is perhaps not so much an external input to the system as it looks; management can do something about it by using group methods of leadership.

Theory Y and job involvement

Douglas McGregor in his book 'The Human Side of Enterprise' introduces two fundamental managerial attitudes, which he calls 'Theory Y' and 'Theory X'. In short, theory X assumes that the average human being has an inherent dislike of work and will avoid it if he can; he must therefore be controlled and directed. Theory Y assumes that the expenditure of physical and mental effort is as natural as play or rest; people will exercise self-direction and self-control in the service to objectives to which they are committed (McGregor, 1960, p. 33 and 47). I have tried to measure the position of my budgetees between these extremes by an attitude survey item 'Working comes naturally to most people'. People who agree more with this I suppose to be more 'Y', people who disagree to be more 'X'. We have already seen in chapter 11 that staff people as a group are more 'X' than line people.

Theory X is not the same as authoritarianism. The statistical analysis shows that the two are not correlated. I could already notice this during the interviews; for example when one highly non-authoritarian second-line manager said: 'Man in general is born tired'. Although this looks morelike a sophism than a deep-rooted attitude, his score on the attitude survey was toward the 'X' side.

Theory X or Y is not correlated with budget motivation. The factor analysis reveals that theory X or Y is related to a factor which has very few other relationships: no. 7. There is a high loading on this factor for the feeling 'this plant demands my utmost', which is also an attitude survey item. The theory Y attitude ('working comes naturally to most people') and the feeling that 'this plant demands my utmost' are strongly intercorrelated. The 'utmost' feeling is stronger for first-line managers and for 'yes-men' and it is also correlated with pressure. There is one subgroup in the survey which loads much stronger on factor 7 ('theory Y' and 'the utmost') than all the others: this is the first-line-managers group in DYNAMO 2 which we already met in the DYNAMO case study in chapter 8. What is the characteristic of these people? They all originate from the region where the plant is located, and culturally they are not much different from the workers there. About these workers one of the higher-line managers said: "Our labor turnover here is highly dependent on the department's results. If the department does not run well, many people quit. These people are highly interested in their work. An observation upon their work they feel strongly as an observation upon their person. I never noticed anything like this in the other plant (DYNAMO 1). There, people have more the industrial mentality, they are more careless, they just want to earn money".

This is the reason why I called factor 7 'job involvement'. It is the factor of people who think that 'working comes naturally to most people' because it comes very naturally to themselves, and who think that 'this plant demands my utmost' because they like a plant which demands their utmost. 'Job involvement' is both a personality and a cultural factor.

In DYNAMO 2 it is influenced by the particular cultural climate in a rural area somewhere in the northern part of the Netherlands, but the 'job involved' people exist in lesser numbers in other plants as well. Lodahl (1964) and Lodahl & Kejner (1964) have found in the U.S.A. a factor 'job involvement' in the job attitudes of factory workers, nurses, engineers and students which is very similar to the factor described above. Job involvement is described by them as 'a general value-orientation dealing with why people prefer work to idleness' (Lodahl, 1964, p. 513). Lodahl and Kejner see it as operationalizing the 'Protestant Ethic', a cultural norm which operates in people.

The 'job involvement' factor, though probably important for job motivation in general, is fairly neutral on budget motivation, job satisfaction and pressure (fig. 12-7). It is not a crucial input in the budget system. We saw in chapter 8 that job involved people tend to see their standards as tight without having any negative attitudes about this. Job involvement is probably one of the factors which positively influence people's tolerance for tight standards.

Self-satisfaction

The factor analysis revealed one other factor which is rather neutral on budget motivation and pressure, and which only appears to bear some relationship to job satisfaction. I called this factor 'self-satisfaction'. It is the only factor which is distributed equally over all subgroups: all hierarchical groups in all plants have some 'self-satisfaction' people. They are the ones who evaluate their own department's performance highly, but who do not follow the budget variances in their judgment; their ability is rated highly by their boss and the personnel manager. They feel their influence on what goes on in the plant is low and should be higher; nevertheless, they are the ones who participate most in the setting of technical standards and they are more often consulted by their boss than others. These people seem to be the self-confident, clever managers. Their cleverness, however, has no meaning as an input to the budget system.

The impact on budget systems of Dutch, European or Western culture

This entire study was carried out in the specific cultural setting of industry in the Netherlands – a country of 12 million people, 0.4% of the world's population. To what extent are the conclusions drawn valid for budget systems in industry outside the Netherlands?

We can consider various degrees of extension of the scope of our conclusions:

1. From the Netherlands to Western Europe
2. From Western Europe to the 'Western World', including U.S.A. and other non-European 'Western' countries.
3. From the Western World to a world-wide scale.

Although of course every country in Western Europe has its specific cultural idiosyncrasies – which can be much of a problem – there is sufficient similarity in industrial practice and cultural values to assume that a research project like this carried out in another West-European country would not have yielded very different results, provided that the same type of well-organized participating companies were chosen.

The possible influence of the difference between the industrial climates in Europe and U.S.A. must be considered more sharply. It is a problem which intrigues both Americans (Harbison & Burgess, 1954; Kast, 1964) and Europeans (Nowotny, 1964). There are some aspects of the difference which may be relevant to the functioning of budget systems on either side of the Atlantic. For example, American managers are supposed to be more dollar-cost conscious (I would like, however, to see this proven). There is probably more pressure in the U.S. way of managing, and more job rotation, if only because managers are more easily fired. In the European situation there prevails, as we saw in chapter 2, often a more theoretical and less practical attitude of budget accountants, which makes it more difficult for European managers to get the informational services they need to use the budget system as a management tool. Acknowledging these differences I still believe that my conclusions about the functioning of budget systems are meaningful for the American situation too, as so many details in my findings agree with what researchers in the U.S. have found.

I doubt very much if my conclusions are valid outside the industrialized countries and even for non-Western industrialized countries like Japan. Although Likert (1963) sees a trend towards a world-wide theory of management, I believe the influence of Western cultural values like achievement (McClelland, 1961) in the system is so strong that in non-

Western countries systems like these will work quite differently. The game of budget control as I described it is a Western game.

Statistical analysis of data used in Chapter 13

Variables used in this Chapter

a. Demographic variables
1. Hierarchical level
14. Age group (9 classes)
15. Classification number of years in present job (same *level*, not necessary same department; 4 classes)
16. Classification educational level (5 classes).

b. Personality variables
55. Attitude survey item: 'This plant demands my utmost' (scored negatively).
57. Attitude survey item: 'Working comes naturally to most people'.
58. Positive attitude to life. This is the combined score on two attitude survey items, both scored negatively:
    'People nowadays are less willing to carry responsibility than they used to be', and
    'If the labor market gets less tight, personnel management will get tougher again here'.
    These two are intercorrelated with $r = 0.35$***.
59. Non-authoritarianism and 60. Yes-men-index: see the statistical section of chapter 9. Yes-men-index is simply the number of 'always' or 'mostly' answers on attitude survey items.
    The intercorrelations between the demographic variables are shown in fig. 13-1. The variables split into two pairs: age + period in present job, and hierarchical + educational level, each strongly intercorrelated.

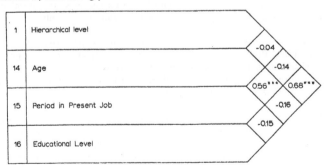

*** significant at 0.0005 level

FIG. 13-1. Intercorrelations Between Demographic Varibales.

The intercorrelations between the personality variables are shown in fig. 13-2. Here we have two groups: 55 + 57 (Theory Y, etc.) and 58-59-60 (non-authoritarianism, etc.).

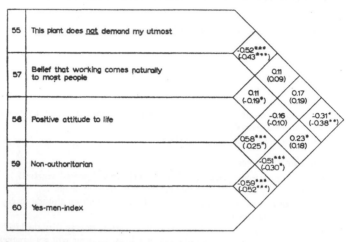

Figures between brackets are correlations within subgroups

* significant at 0.05 level, ** significant at 0.005 level, *** significant at 0.0005 level

FIG. 13-2. Intercorrelations Between Personality Variables

Variable 55 and 57 are also correlated with no. 60 'yes-men-index'. As 55 is scored negatively, this indicates that those who answer more positively to attitude survey questions in general (the yes-men), also score more positively on no. 55 and 57. It points to some bias in the fact that the items 'this plant demands my utmost' and 'working comes naturally to most people' were positively formulated only.

In fig. 13-3 the correlations between demographic and personality variables are shown. The feeling that the plant demands the utmost is weaker for the higher hierarchical level and for those who are more recent in their job.

The three variables of the 'non-authoritarianism' group are stronger correlated with hierarchical level than with educational level and stronger with age than with period in the job.

Finally fig. 13-4 shows the correlations of the demographic and personality variables with the six outputs. There are strong differences between the correlations with the 'impression' and the 'questions' measure of relevance. As we have seen, the interviewer in rating his impression about relevance was rating motivation from within rather than through pressure from outside. This motivation from within is correlated with educational level and with the absence of yes-menship. None of the variables in fig. 13-4 has correlations with budget relevance measured by questions.

282

		correlations with:		
Variables:	I hierarchical level	14 age	15 period in present job	16 educational level
55 this plant does not demand my utmost	0.21*	−0.06(−0.13)	−0.12(−0.20*)	0.08(0.07)
57 belief that working comes naturally to most people	−0.13	0.05(0.12)	0.10(0.05)	−0.02(0.09)
58 positive attitude to life	0.37***	−0.23*(−0.23*)	−0.26*(−0.19*)	0.27*(0.09)
59 non-authoritarian	0.42**	−0.27*(−0.33***)	−0.26*(−0.22*)	0.29*(0.19)
60 yes-men-index	−0.48***	0.25*(0.31*)	0.25*(0.06)	−0.35**(−0.19)

Figures between brackets are correlations within subgroups

* significant at 0.05 level, ** significant at 0.005 level, *** significant at 0.0005 level

FIG. 13-3. Correlations between Demographic and Personality Variables

	correlations with:					
Variables:	17 Relevance (impression)	18 Relevance (questions)	19 Attitude (impression)	20 Attitude (questions)	53 Job Satisfaction	54 Absence of Pressure
1 hierarchical level	0.32**	0.03	0.17	0.30**	-0.12	-0.03
14 age	-0.16(-0.13)	-0.15(-0.15)	-0.09(-0.01)	-0.08(-0.01)	0.12(-0.03)	0.03(-0.21*)
15 period in present job	-0.15(-0.15)	-0.05(-0.02)	0.16(-0.26*)	0.07(0.04)	0.17*(0.11)	0.09(0.09)
16 educational level	0.43***(0.21*)	0.09(0.06)	-0.02(-0.13)	0.21*(0.04)	-0.04(0.13)	-0.14(0.07)
55 this plant does not demand my utmost	0.06(0.16)	-0.13(-0.02)	0.12(0.18*)	0.04(0.00)	-0.09(-0.05)	0.28**(0.24*)
57 belief that working comes naturally to most people	0.11(0.18*)	-0.07(-0.02)	-0.12(-0.09)	0.00(0.02)	0.18*(0.25*)	0.01(0.11)
58 positive attitude to life	0.23*(0.27**)	-0.02(-0.24*)	0.14(0.01)	0.15(-0.02)	-0.18*(0.05)	-0.06(0.10)
59 non-authoritarian	0.19(0.17)	0.06(-0.17)	0.38***(0.18)	0.23*(-0.00)	-0.13(-0.03)	-0.04(0.03)
60 yes-men-index	-0.36**(-0.37**)	-0.11(-0.05)	-0.15(-0.11)	-0.18(-0.06)	0.23*(0.25*)	0.16(0.18)

Figures between brackets are correlations with subgroups

* significant at 0.05 level, ** significant at 0.005 level, *** significant at 0.0005 level

FIG. 13-4. Correlations of Demographic and Personality Variables with Motivation and Job Satisfaction

The correlation between attitude and non-authoritarianism is due to between-plant diffe-ences, it does not hold true within plants. There are level differences in non-authoritarianism, as fig. 9-4 has shown.

The correlation of 'job satisfaction' with 'yes-men-index' points again to the bias of formulating attitude surveys items only positively: both items in the 'job satisfaction' score were formulated this way. The correlation between job satisfaction and the belief that working comes natural to most people may be due to the same cause (both are based on positive attitude survey items).

CHAPTER 14
TECHNOLOGY AND MARKET

Summary of this Chapter

Technological and market influences have an important impact on how budget systems function. Explanations of differences in budget relevance level between plants can be found in three areas:
1. *Differences in the product cost structure between plants, leading to a difference in plant management's possible contribution to profits.*
2. *The difference between a dynamic and a static product cost which is immediately related to the type of product and the technology of its manufacture.*
3. *Differences in the managerial climate which is dominated by the specific interests of the people in top management, who in their turn are influenced by their market.*
These external explanations of what was found in this study serve to complete the picture of influences upon budget systems in an interdisciplinary way.

How technology and market can influence a budget system

In this chapter we will analyze the impact upon a budget system of another group of inputs which are outside management's reach: the particular technology of the plant and forces on the market. In this case there is no doubt about their being fully external to the system (fig. 4-2).

286

The five companies belong to five different trades with different technologies and different markets. The way the budget systems in the five companies can be influenced by these external inputs is for example through:

1. The scope left to plant management in contributing to the profitability of the company.
2. The amount of external pressure for cost reduction and the internal technological possibilities to realize it.
3. The kind of people who are found in the top positions of the organization who are themselves influenced by their market and whose main interest will pervade the organization, as well as the caliber of the people at lower levels in the organization. I will now show how these different kinds of influences worked in the five companies of this study.

Plant management's contribution to profits

A useful economic distinction for our case can be made along the lines of *cost structure* (Mellerowicz, 1958, p. 44). Fig. 14-1 shows the split-up of

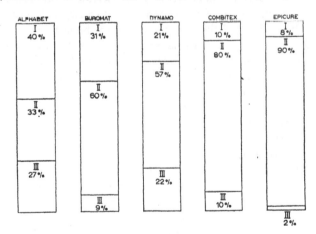

I LABOR COST
II MATERIALS COST
III CAPITAL COST

FIG. 14-1. The Structure of Product Cost in the Five Companies

total product cost in the five companies in three parts: I. wages, salaries and social security cost, that is total cost for direct and indirect labor; II. materials and work done by subcontractors, including 'services', energy and the like; III depreciation and other costs: the cost of capital investments.

We see that only ALPHABET is labor-intensive (labor costs form the largest part of costs); all other companies are materials-intensive. Now in general the scope for cost control by lower-level management is decreasing in the order I-II-III. Management at the lower levels can more often do more percentwise about labor cost than about materials cost and more about materials cost than about capital cost. There are exceptions to this rule, and traditionally in many industries the attention given to labor cost control has perhaps been exaggerated and materials cost control has been neglected, but the rule remains true. Therefore, by ranking the five companies in order of labor cost percentage like in fig. 14-1, we also rank them as well as possible in order of scope for cost control by lower-level-management: this scope is greatest in ALPHABET, smallest in EPICURE. In the food industry where EPICURE operates, 10% of labor savings can be offset by 1% increase of raw materials price, and price fluctuations of raw material are often larger than that.

I have classified the five companies by budget relevance, taking the average score over both higher-level and first-line management and over the 'impression' and the 'questions' measure for budget relevance. The companies rank on this average budget relevance score as follows:

BUROMAT	8.0
ALPHABET	7.3
DYNAMO 1 + 2	7.0
EPICURE	6.9
COMBITEX	6.8

We see that BUROMAT and ALPHABET have the highest relevance, EPICURE and COMBITEX the lowest. The agreement of this sequence with the sequence of labor cost percentage in fig. 14-1 is not accidental, although it does not reach statistical significance. The contribution that good budget control can make to company profits is much greater in BUROMAT and ALPHABET than in EPICURE and COMBITEX.

Of course I have found in the chapter 8 through 12 many internal reasons in management behavior in the plants why ALPHABET and BUROMAT should have higher budget relevance and EPICURE and COMBITEX lower. It looks contradictory that I now relate these differences in relevance to an external cause, but it is not. We may remember from chapter 5 that all five companies were well managed; they belonged to the best organized in their trade. If then management in EPICURE and COMBITEX pays less attention to budget control and therefore the budget relevance in those plants is lower, it is because there is less in it for them: it is not as urgent as it is for BUROMAT and ALPHABET. A good company receives the organization which the circumstances demand. The same phenomena in a system can often be explained externally as well as internally, but the external causes are more fundamental.

The contribution to profits by an individual plant manager is also limited by the degree of technological interdependence between his plant and other parts of the organization such as research and development. On the level of department management, the same is true for technological interdependence between departments and between staff and line. We met this issue earlier: in chapter 10 when dealing with decentralization of account structures and in chapter 12 when dealing with realizing the game spirit. When cost responsibility can be seen only as joint responsibility rather than as individual responsibility, this influences the system. Realizing a high budget relevance in this case will demand greater skills of the budgetee's superiors. A budgetee's scope in contributing to profits is a quantification of his *operational control* as defined in chapter 1. I have tried to measure 'operational control' by subjective ratings (Appendix B). Although these ratings give interesting information about how different levels in the hierarchy see each other, they appear to be too subjective to offer any clues for a comparison between technologies. They contain more information about the interviewee than about his circumstances.

Cost dynamics and cost reduction pressure

The speed of technological development was quite different in the five companies. BUROMAT and DYNAMO were the plants with a highly engineered technical product; their production methods were subject to continuous improvement. In all five plants I have studied the development of the actual production cost of one typical product in the past two years. Taking the slow inflation (about 3% per year) in the Netherlands in this period into account I found for both BUROMAT and EPICURE a cost reduction of around 15% per year. This is based upon one product, and of course the total lifetime of technical products is limited so that new products keep coming in at high cost levels and old product lines are stopped at low cost levels; total departmental cost does not sink 15% a year. Still cost development is clearly dynamic in BUROMAT and DYNAMO. In the other three plants types of products as well as manufacturing development were more static: yearly changes were only a few percents. The difference between dynamic and static cost development is an important input into the budget system. In BUROMAT and DYNAMO a regular adaptation of standards is normal. Everybody knows and expects that next year's standards will be lower than this year's. This attitude guarantees that standards will not easily 'freeze', even for less dynamic parts of the production process. In the other three plants the historical element in standards and budgets is much stronger. As costs tend to be static, budgeting has the character of watching the status quo and seeing that things do not get out of hand rather than of planning cost reduction. It is more difficult to maintain continuous cost-reduction consciousness in this situation, and cost reduction drives (chapter 2, p. 34) every few years may be necessary.

Companies go through periods in which cost reduction pressure from the market is high and periods in which it is lower. In periods of high external cost reduction pressure this will penetrate into the budget system through the management hierarchy.

'It is important for the psychologist to realize . . . that economic pressure is often as important in determining the outlook and conditions within a firm as anything which can readily be changed within the factory itself '(J. A. C. Brown, 1954, p. 118).

The research project did not coincide in any of the plants with a period of exceptionally high budget pressure. Besides I studied each plant at one point in time, so that I have no data for studying how the functioning of the budget system in a particular plant would change through time because of fluctuating outside economic pressure. I assume that it will, however, and the effects of increased pressure through the managerial hierarchy can be concluded from chapter 12.

Technology, market, and managerial climate

In a well-known study about the organization of a bank, Argyris (1954) describes how this type of business automatically selects a certain breed of employees which he calls 'the right type': polite, tactful, security-oriented, non-dynamic. All types of business have to some extent their 'right type' which is found first of all in the top positions. The Dutch sociologist Horringa uses the term 'managerial climate', which he defines as: "the typical atmosphere in a certain type of business, characterized by the kind of people in top management who in their turn are strongly influenced by the market problems they have to cope with; this atmosphere is also partly determined by the technology of the manufacturing process, the educational level of lower management and finally by the kind of workers which are attracted to this type of business" (Horringa, 1965, p. 57, my translation). Horringa gives a typology of managerial climates based on who is the key man in top management: the purchaser's climate, the fashion climate, the engineer's climate and the service climate. Applying Horringa's typology to my five companies I must put ALPHABET in the service climate. ALPHABET, like most graphic companies (Ruckstuhl, 1960) sells services rather than products. Throughout its organization people are impressed with the necessity of following the customer's whims. Emergency orders can change preset plans on very short notice. Strict organizational systems are difficult to realize in such a situation and this will be reflected upon the functioning of budgets and standards. The way these systems actually worked in ALPHABET meant a remarkable managerial achievement.

BUROMAT, COMBITEX and DYNAMO in Horringa's typology belong to the engineer's climate. This one is the most prone to rationality and in this case the functioning of the budget system will meet the least difficulties. EPICURE has an outspoken purchaser's climate. Economically, manufacturing is of secondary importance to EPICURE, which is reflected by the fact that the top manufacturing manager ranks below the top purchasing manager. The key people in such an organization do not have a natural interest in manufacturing cost control. We saw in chapter 11 that the manufacturing standards system in EPICURE was run as an internal affair of the manufacturing function, not integrated in the total company budget control. This is typical for the purchaser's climate.

The interdisciplinary approach

In this chapter we have seen three ways to explain the impact of technology and market on the functioning of budget systems. The three approaches supplement and give greater depth to the micro-analysis of budget systems in the chapters 8 through 13. This chapter has tried to make the analysis of budget systems truly interdisciplinary by adding to the socio-psychological point of view of the previous chapters a number of considerations based on economic, technological and sociological distinctions.

Part IV - The Research Implications

CHAPTER 15
PRACTICAL RECOMMENDATIONS

Summary of this Chapter

In this chapter the results of this study have been translated into practical advice to those in business who have to work – and live – wth budgets and budgetary standards. This advice is based upon the situation of the manufacturing company. There are separate recommendations for:

1. *Company top management*
2. *The top and middle management of the plant*
3. *The plant foremen or first-line-managers*
4. *The company and/or plant controller*
5. *The budget accountant*
6. *The work study engineer*
7. *The personnel manager*

Recommendations to company top management

These recommendations are aimed at top management of a manufacturing company, which for its manufacturing operations either uses budget control and wants to improve its functioning, or does not use budget control and wants to introduce it. The recommendations in this chapter go to some extent beyond the immediate conclusions of this study. This is unavoidable, as any researcher will realize when he steps

293

into a consultant role. My recommendations to company top management are:

Realize that the budget control system is *your* tool to manage your company. Its functioning depends primarily on you, not on your controller (chapter 12).

When setting budgets, have the decisions which must be taken at your level, like the choice of product lines and production volume, taken first and then communicated to your subordinates. Then ask your subordinates to prepare the draft budgets at the lowest possible level of management and have them consolidated at each next higher level. If they cannot be accepted and have to be revised, take the time to discuss this with your subordinates and to explain the reasons. Make sure they do the same with their subordinates. Realize that budgets have a coordinating and a motivating function and that especially in the larger corporations the way the coordination is felt at the lower levels can easily destroy motivation. It is therefore necessary to explain much more than you think you should (chapter 9).

Realize that budgets only motivate when they are tight enough to be a challenge, and that they only offer a challenge if there is a risk that they will not be fully met. If some budgets are not met this is only a sign that the system is healthy and it does not mean that somebody is at fault. If you take the habit of interpreting it in this latter way, budgets will all soon be met, but they will not motivate (chapter 8).

Realize that the fact that motivating budgets are not always met means that the same budget cannot be used both for coordinating and motivating. It will be necessary to reserve a risk percentage for average underattainment of budgets to arrive at actually expected figures which can be used for coordination (ch. 2).

Decide beforehand which percentage variance from the various budgets you can leave to the discretion of your subordinates before you will intervene and let them know this. In other words, set their control limits (chapter 4).

Be sensitive to the reactions of your subordinates to the budgets set for them and keep open grievance channels for those who see their standards as impossibly tight. Be ready to change budgets if this is the case; if you do not do it, actual results will be worse than if you do (chapter 8).

Eliminate the taboo on communicating financial information about budget results to the lowest levels of management, including plant foremen (chapter 10).

Discuss the functioning of the budget system with your controller and make sure he sees his role neither as an auditor nor as a data processor but as a systems architect and educator (chapter 11).

Recommendations to the top and middle management of the plant

Realize that the budget control system is *your* tool to manage your plant. Its functioning within the plant depends primarily on you, not on the controller or his department (chapter 12).

If possible, see to it that budgets and standards are set separately for the responsibility area of each of your foremen, but at least for each second-line manager. Then have your foremen participate in the setting of their technical standards and make their own draft expense budget. Let them have the assistance from the budget accountant they need, but let them do the actual figuring themselves (chapter 9).

If draft budgets are changed afterwards or cut, discuss this with your subordinates and explain the reasons (chapter 9).

If you are running a shift operation so that more foremen are responsible for the same department, the budgeting effort should be done by the lowest level which covers all shifts, but only after consultation with the foremen in meetings. If results can be split by shifts, then again the individual foremen can be the budgetees (chapter 12).

Decide beforehand which percentage variance from the various budgets and technical standards you will leave to the discretion of your subordinates before you will intervene and let them know this. These percentages are their control limits (chapter 4).

Be sensitive to the reactions of your subordinates on the budgets and standards set for them and keep open grievance channels for those who see their standards as impossibly tight. Be ready to change the standard if this is the case (chapter 8).

Take account of the age and personality structure of each of your subordinates in setting targets and standards for them: what will mean a challenge for a young man can mean a discouragingly tight objective for an older man (chapter 13).

Show interest in your subordinates' budget results also when they do not transgress their control limits, but be sure this is seen as interest, not as intervention (chapter 12).

If you have to intervene, get the full story from your subordinate first. Center the conversation around what should be done to correct the situation, not on who is at fault (chapter 12).

Show your subordinates that you consider meeting standards as part of their performance but be careful not to appraise by budget or standards results alone. Realize that while from your point of view results may be the only important factor, in the eyes of your subordinate it is his efforts which determine his merit (chapter 12).

If you are under pressure from your superiors, consider whether it is wise to send this pressure down to your subordinates. Protect your subordinates against influences from above which will in their situation only discourage and demotivate them. Perform your umbrella function (chapter 12).

When budgeting is first started in your plant, do not expect results immediately. Give your subordinates the time to learn to use this tool and learn to use it yourself: this may take a few years. See to it that the budget accounting staff interprets its role not as auditing or policing but as supporting and educating the line in the use of accounting information (chapter 11).

Discuss with your subordinates and with the budget and standards staff which feedback information is desirable from a line management point of view and which is available from a data processing point of view. Try to unite the two. Resist attempts of the line to ask, or of the staff to supply, more information than a normal human being can digest. Review periodically the information received and stop whichever part of it you do not use. Realize, however, that there are key points in your production process about which you should be informed, even if they are never off-standard. They may be off-standard tomorrow (chapter 11).

Realize that the essence of good budget control is cooperation and that you must meet the budget challenge with your subordinates as a team. Realize that the performance of your plant depends on their motivation. Try to develop a game spirit among your team. Show your enthusiasm and respect the responsibilities of your subordinates. Mistrust and undue pressure will destroy the game spirit (chapter 12).

Be sensitive to any signs of passing the buck, scapegoating, fighting the system, or other wasteful activities among your subordinates. If these things happen it is a sign that *you* have failed in leading the game the right way. Try again (chapter 12).

Make sensible use of group meetings with your subordinates. Do not handle problems here which can better be handled on a man-to-man basis, such as budget performances of individual departments. Use them for informal contact and team-building. Use them to supply general information about cost. Let your subordinates use the meetings to help each other in giving meaning to the standards and using them as management tools towards their own subordinates. Meetings can be powerful tools to influence your subordinate's attitudes. However, if you feel your meetings are not useful, it is better not to have them; they will do more harm than good (chapter 12).

Discuss the reorganizations in your management structure with your controller before they are carried out, so that the responsibility and account structures can remain mutually adapted (chapter 10).

Recommendations to the foremen or first-line-managers

Technical performance standards and budgets are a management tool for you to use. They are your guides in the management process and important yardsticks for your managerial achievement (chapter 8).

More and more the first-line-manager will need the kind of information which is supplied by standards and budget systems. In many cases he will be able to do a better job if he gets insight into the financial results of his department as well as the technical results (chapter 10).

Although participation in the setting of an expense budget and sometimes other financial standards takes time and effort, this effort pays off in better budgets and a better understanding of how the business is run (chapter 9).

The foreman who is better informed himself will be able to do a better job at communicating results to the workers. There are many possibilities of involving the workers in the results feedback. The use of periodic meetings is one of them. This study has not included the cost-consciousness and standards fulfilment motivation of workers. From other studies it is clear that one important question is whether or not piece-rates or similar systems are used. Apart from this, the foreman is the key person in determining the cost-consciousness of his workers (chapter 12).

Recommendations to the company and/or plant controller

The success of a budget system does not primarily depend upon the controller, but upon the top line executive. The controller's role is hygienic: he has to satisfy certain minimal requirements but has more scope in making the system fail than succeed. If he considers not only the accounting part but also the human part of the system as his specialty however, he can become the systems architect, catalyst and educator (chapter 11).

The same budget cannot be used for coordinating and for motivating managers. Coordinating budgets should represent actually expected performance; but budgets can be shown to have a motivating effect only when they involve a risk of not being attained. Budgets that are really motivating should be increased with an average risk percentage to arrive at actual expected performance (chapters 2-8).

Consider the use of statistical techniques in cost control and budgeting. From a point of view of motivation it is desirable that, for each budget, control limits are set which guarantee a certain free scope for managers at various levels before their superiors intervene. From a technical point of view this can be solved by statistical techniques like those used in quality control. Controllers should familiarize themselves much more with the possibilities of these techniques (chapter 4).

Split the account structure if possible as far as the responsibility of the individual foremen. Let the foreman draft his own expense budget but have him supplied with all the support from the budget accountant he needs. Eliminate the taboo on financial information in the plant (chapter 9, 10).

Both the system in which individual plant departments are full profit centers buying from and selling to other departments and the system in which they are only expense centers have their drawbacks. In the first case the system is difficult to understand and use for line management and a continuous effort at simplification and instruction is necessary. In the second case expense budgets should be kept flexible enough to adapt to changes in technical performance and line management should have more support in taking economic decisions (chapter 10).

Management information reports should be separated from accounting consolidation reports. In management information there should be a periodic weeding out of over-information, and periodic consultations with management of various levels down to the foreman level about the understandability of information and the desirability of other information (chapter 10).

Establish a close cooperation between work study engineers and budget accountants, although it is not essential that the work study engineers report to the controller (chapter 11).

Man budget accounting departments in such a way that about 25% of total time is available for personal discussions with and support to line management (chapter 11).

When appraising budget accountants and other staff people for salary increases and promotion, ask the line managers with whom they cooperate for their impressions. This has a beneficial effect upon staff behavior and line-staff-cooperation (chapter 11).

The best service to the line is given by budget accountants and other staff people who are competent in their speciality and also tactful (chapter 11).

Develop a career planning for your people (chapter 11).

Recommendations to the budget accountant

When budgets have to be set, let the line managers make the drafts. Assist them with all the information they need. Develop special information sources for this purpose; but let the actual figuring be done by line managers themselves (chapter 9).

Design the management information system yourself after thorough discussion about what line managers at various levels, down to the foreman level, need to know and what you can supply. Do not use reports that serve for accounting consolidation simultaneously for management information. Give more detailed information to lower management levels and more general information to higher management levels (chapter 2-10).

Have periodic consultations with line managers of the different levels about the management information system: desires for new information, improvement of understandability, weeding out of unnecessary information. Beware of overinformation. Managers do not want to know everything; if they miss some information which they need, they will come and ask for it (chapter 10).

Make the management information reports yourself or if they are made by purely clerical people at least check them thoroughly before they are distributed. Managers will use figures only if they feel confident they are right. Frequent mistakes will spoil any information system (chapter 10).

Focus the information on efficiency variances. Omit variances that are caused by pure accounting causes (chapter 10).

Be informed about changes in the responsibility structure of the organization in due time so that you can adapt the account structure accordingly. Budgets should always follow management responsibility (chapter 10).

Be critical as to the raw data you receive. Realize that if people feel they are measured by these data they will tend to make them look right. Data connected with a piece-rate system or which in another way directly influence pay are basically unfit for efficiency information. Always try to anchor the data you receive to actual cash movements, for instance wages paid, which cannot be faked (chapter 10).

Reserve about 25% of your time for personal contacts with the people who receive your management information. Take time to explain figures. Test whether they have understood the information. If they do not it does not mean that they are silly: it means that you have failed in speaking or writing a language they can understand. Try again (chapter 10-11).

Realize that the success of a budget and management information system is not in your hands: it is in the hands of line management. They will not be able to make it successful without your support, however. The success of *your job* depends on the quality of this support: upon your competence and the tactfulness with which you build up your contacts with line management (chapter 11).

Maintain good professional contacts with those responsible for the system of technical standards, such as work study engineers. Keep them informed about the financial side of efficiency results and always base your financial standards on their technical ones (chapter 11).

Recommendations to the work study engineer

Set your standards always in close contact with line management. If line managers see you know your job and you behave tactfully, they will accept you. When they ask your support, always be ready to give it. A staff man should be happy when he is pulled and unhappy when he is pushing (chapter 9-11).

Base standards on external reference information wherever possible, but be careful about how you select these external reference points. If line management does not see them as legitimate and valid for their situation, they will do more harm than good. Take the time to discuss external data with the line managers and let them participate in finding valid reference points (chapter 9).

Realize that the success of your job depends to a large extent on how line people see you (chapter 11).

Maintain good professional contacts with the budget accountants and exchange information with them (chapter 11).

Recommendations to the personnel manager

Keep line management informed about any signs of discouragement of managers through standards that are seen as impossible, as well as about signs of interdepartmental conflict which may be adverse effects of the way the standards and budget system is used for management (chapter 8-12).

A system of job rotation between functions in line management or between line and staff can have its implications not only for the development of the people but also for the development of the control system (chapter 13).

Pay special attention to the development and career planning of staff people like budget accountants and work study engineers. For good line-staff-cooperation is not essential that staff people have line experience; it is more important that they are competent in their speciality and behave tactfully. Include staff people in management development courses and in training in interpersonal relations (chapter 11).

Design the performance appraisal system for staff people for salary increases in such a way that their line counterparts are asked for their impression about the support they get from them and that this impression contributes to the appraisal of the staff man (chapter 11).

CHAPTER 16
THE FUTURE OF BUDGETS AND BUDGET RESEARCH

Summary of this Chapter

This chapter states a number of expectations about the demands which will be put to the manager of tomorrow and about the budget system he will work in. They key question is what balance between control and individual autonomy will be found.
Further research in the field of budget control systems is highly desirable; some possibilities are indicated.

The manager of tomorrow

In Chapter 13 of this book we saw indications of differences in attitude between managers of different generations. The rapid changes in our society are reflected in the demands upon a manager's job and this again influences the people in those jobs. Where are we moving from here?

Some people expect that management will continously become less of an art and more of a science (Leavitt, 1963). The studies about the game aspect in managing through budgets about which this book reports, have convinced me that management will continue to be an art, although it will definitely become more of a science too. By its remaining an art I mean that the personal enthusiasm, sensitivity and creative talent of the manager will still be of key importance. I do not mean that managers are born as such; talents are an asset, but they need to be developed. The growth of the scientific side of management means first of all a more experimental attitude of the manager towards the organizational system in which he works. Preconceived ideas about 'principles of management' will be dropped unless they stand the test of the controlled experiment. We have already seen the gradual fading away of the difference between 'line' and 'staff' (Chapter 11). Probably all managers in the future will need more of the 'spectator' attitude to what goes on in the business which I found in the staff. Terms like 'line' and 'staff' will be replaced by new and easily understandable concepts for describing organizational systems. All management will become systems management. The study of management systems will do away with the borderlines between technology, economics, operations research or social science. Although managers and scientists will probably have their problems of mutual understanding for ever and ever, there will be better cooperation between the two. Researchers will have less difficulties in penetrating into a business (Chapter 5).

The budget system of tomorrow

There is no doubt that the business of tomorrow will need financial planning and goal-setting. There will be more of it than there is today, including companies which could afford to do without it until now. The most significant development in business affecting the budget system is the application of Electronic Data Processing. Budget and management information systems will be more and more computerized and more and more integrated. They will probably be extended to non-accounting data (Leavitt 1965, Gross 1965, Firmin 1966), maybe even to data about employee attitudes and perceptions.

The challenge to business in this development is whether this will lead to increased pressure on the individual or not (Smiddy 1962). The conflict between control and autonomy (Chapter 1) will be fought out in the process of computerization. The outcome of this battle has deep significance for both the individual and the business. What is the value of the Free Enterprise System if freedom exists only at the top? The modern free enterprise corporation is internally a highly guided economy. Will it do any thing better for the people in it than the State Capitalism it rejects?

This study suggests that it should be possible to deliberately plan a certain amount of scope for the individual, even within a system that is computer-controlled. The 'calculated inefficiency' called for in Chapter 1 can save the humanity within the system.

What is the future for the individual within the organization? Let me quote the optimistic point of view:

'If our research leads are correct, the more significant improvements in the human side of enterprise are going to come through changes in the way organizations are controlled, and particularly through changes in the size of the 'influence pie' (Tannenbaum, 1962, p. 255-256).

Suggestions for further research

There is a vast field for further research in management control systems. This study was necessarily still too exploratory. It is desirable to test the hypotheses developed on new data; in particular, to devote further studies to the game aspect of budgeting. Hopefully in psychology the gap caused by the non-existence of a psychology of adult play (Chapter 3) will soon be filled.

The study of budget control systems should be continued with better systems output measures than I was able to find; it should be extended to longitudinal studies (following the same system through time) and to field experiments, like the promising experiment of Stedry and Kay (Chapter 8). It should be extended outside manufacturing units to other functions of the business. How many studies have been devoted to quota setting processes for salesmen? It should be extended from the top management to the non-managerial employee level and to non-business organizations as well. With full acknowledgement of the work that has already been done by several eminent researchers, we have only just started.

Appendices

APPENDIX A
THE CONTROL GRAPH

Description of the technique

The Control Graph technique was developed by staff-members of the Institute for Social Research of the University of Michigan, U.S.A. It is described in, for example, Likert, 1961; Smith and Tannenbaum, 1963; Bowers, 1964.

The technique consists of asking respondents to score 'How much say or influence' they feel several hierarchical levels have on 'what goes on in' their department. These scores are made on five-point scales: little or no influence; some influence; quite a bit of influence; a great deal of influence; a very great deal of influence. So each respondent makes a score for each hierarchical level he is asked about. Subsequently, the scoring is repeated, but now for the *ideal* amount of influence: this is done by asking for the amount of influence that the various levels 'should have' according to the respondents. Positive differences between ideal and actual influence indicate feelings of illegitimacy of the influence actually perceived.

Use of the Control Graph technique in this project

The main purpose of using the Control Graph in the present project was to measure perceptions about the legitimacy of staff influence (chapter 11). Besides, it also proved useful for analyzing perception differences between first-line and higher-level line managers (chapter 12).

The decision to use the Control Graph was only made after the pilot phase of the study in the DYNAMO plants, so that Control Graph scores are only available for the other four plants. The pertinent questions are no. E 15, 16 and 17 in the staff interviews (Appendix D 2) and no. E 25, 26, and 27 in the line interviews (Appendix D 3). Instead of asking for influence in 'your department', I asked for influence in 'this plant', because this is the level at which total line perceptions can be compared to total staff perceptions (unlike in most of chapter 11, staff is defined here so as to include all possible staff departments, not just the budget and standards people).

A qualitative analysis of the kind of influence people said they had been thinking of while scoring on the Control Graph is shown in chapter 1.

In the correlation and factor analysis calculations for the line interviews I used as variables derived from the Control Graph scores (see Appendix E 2):

41. Own estimate of general influence of own level.
42. Desired minus actual influence of own level.
49. Desired minus actual influence of staff departments.

From the staff interviews I derived the following variables (see Appendix E 1):

13. Own estimate of general influence of staff
14. Desired minus actual staff influence
15. Desired minus actual line influence (average over all management levels within the plant).

Control Graph patterns found

The patterns of Control Graphs obtained are shown in fig. A-1. The graphs of fig. A-1 are based on average scores for the combined data from all four plants where the technique was used. Some differences between plants will be analyzed below. The use of line graphs is methodologically debatable in this case as the horizontal axis does not represent a continuum, but I follow the practice used in other studies for reasons of comparison.

General descriptions of Control Graph patterns summarized from many studies in the U.S.A. can be found in Smith and Tannenbaum, 1963. A comparison between their data for business and industrial organizations and mine leads to a number of conclusions:

1. Both in Smith and Tannenbaum's data and in mine all Control Graphs for the line part of the organization have a negative slope (higher control for higher hierarchical levels). This holds true both for the actual and for the desired control.
2. Smith and Tannenbaum state that ideal slopes tend to be more positive (less steep) than actuals. This holds true for my line management data, if we consider just the scores for the level that made the score and the level immediately above. This is also shown by the fact that the differences between desired and actual influence in the line management scores are greatest: for higher-level (mostly second-line) management at the second line, and for first-line management at the first line: so each level sees the difference between desired and actual influence greatest for itself. The staff interviewees, being outside the line hierarchy themselves, perceive the greatest discrepancy between desired and actual influence at the first line of management.
3. Smith and Tannenbaum state that ideal (desired) total control is generally higher than actual. This is clearly the case for my data too; the only case where desired control is below actual is for staff influence as perceived by higher level line management (see chapter 11). If we analyze the situation plant for plant, we find that each subgroup within a plant desires more influence for itself than it feels it has. The only exception is the staff of COMBITEX, which feels it has too much influence (see Chapter 11).
4. Smith and Tannenbaum state a tendency for non-supervisory employees to produce a more positive slope (less steep) than supervisors, at least for desirable influence. I

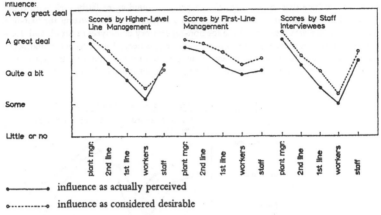

Influence:
A very great deal

| Scores by Higher-Level Line Management | Scores by First-Line Management | Scores by Staff Interviewees |

A great deal

Quite a bit

Some

Little or no

plant mgr. | 2nd line | 1st line | workers | staff | plant mgr. | 2nd line | 1st line | workers | staff | plant mgr. | 2nd line | 1st line | workers | staff

•————• influence as actually perceived

o----------o influence as considered desirable

FIG. A-1. Control Graph Patterns (Averages over Data taken from Four Plants)

have no scores made by non-supervisory employees. However, from my data a clear tendency is visible for first-line managers to produce more positive (less steep) slopes than higher-level line managers, both for actual and desirable influence. My first-line managers are closer to Smith and Tannenbaum's non-supervisory workers than their superiors; they show to some extent a 'worker's attitude' here. There is one exception to this statement. Fig. A-2 B. shows that in the BUROMAT plant the first-line managers produce the same steep slopes as does the higher-level line management elsewhere. In the BUROMAT case study in chapter 9 it is shown that also in other respects (low degree of authoritarianism, budget participation) BUROMAT first-line management is a-typical. The staff tends to produce the same kind of slopes as higher-level line management. In chapter 11, this is interpreted in that the staff identifies itself with the higher line levels.

5. Smith and Tannenbaum state that non-supervisory employees tend to estimate total line control (all levels) lower than supervisors, at least in the case of actual influence. In my data, there is *no* tendency for first-line management to score lower total control than higher-level line management. On the contrary, first-line management tends to score higher. This remains true when we exclude the data for the EPICURE plant, where higher-level line scores are exceptionally low (see fig. A-2 A. and the EPICURE case study in chapter 11). In my data, it can be seen that the estimates for the *own level* are almost equal for higher-level line management and for first-line management. The differences are in the perceptions of the other levels.

6. Smith and Tannenbaum finally state that non-supervisory employees tend to see desired Control Graphs as more positive (less steep) than actual and as above actual to a larger extent than supervisors. In my data, there is no difference between higher-level and first-line management as to the trends in the discrepancies between desired and actual influence.

307

We can conclude that the Control Graph patterns found agree fairly well with those described in the summary study of Smith and Tannenbaum. The patterns for first-line managers in my data resemble those for non-supervisory employees in Smith and Tannenbaum's data, in that they show a more positive (less steep) slope, except for BUROMAT; but they resemble those for higher-level management in the amount of influence scored for the own level and in the differences between desired and actual influence.

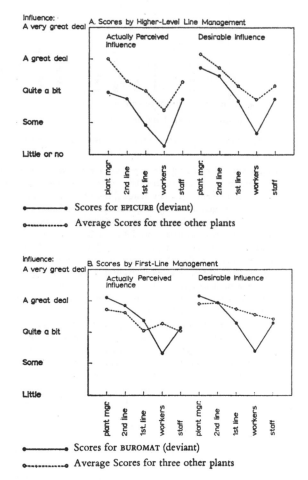

FIG. A-2. Deviating Control Graph Patterns

How much staff influence is desirable?

In fig. A-3 I have collected the Control Graph scores for staff influence, both as actually perceived and as considered desirable.

9 = a very great deal 7 = a great deal 5 = quite a bit 3 = some 1 = little or no	according to first-line-managers		according to higher-level-managers		according to staff interviewees	
	actually perceived	considered desirable	actually perceived	considered desirable	actually perceived	considered desirable
ALPHABET	4.4	5.4	6.0	5.0	5.6	6.0
BUROMAT	5.2	5.7	5.1	5.0	5.2	6.3
EPICURE	5.1	6.3	4.5	4.5	6.1	6.4
TOTAL OF THESE THREE PLANTS	4.9	5.8[2]	5.3	4.9	5.6	6.3[2]
COMBITEX	5.7	5.8	5.8	6.0	7.0[1]	6.5

[1] Difference between COMBITEX and other plants, tested with Wilcoxon's test (two-tailed), significant at 0.05 level, all other differences between plants not significant.
[2] Difference between desirable and actual, tested with Wilcoxon's test (one-tailed) significant at 0.05 level; other differences between columns not significant.

FIG. A-3. Average Control Graph Scores for Staff Influence.

For first line managers and staff the 'desirable' staff influence scores are significantly higher than the actually perceived scores (excluding COMBITEX). For higher-level line managers in ALPHABET and BUROMAT and for staff in COMBITEX desirable scores are lower than actually perceived ones. See chapter 11. Furthermore, most staff scores for actual influence and all staff scores for desired influence are higher than the line scores. The staff sees its own influence greater than the line sees it, and thinks this should be so. There is a fair amount of agreement between staff interviewees in different plants as to which staff influence level is desirable.
Another issue which can be investigated are perception differences between various hierarchical levels as to degrees of influence. This will be done in Appendix B (fig. B-2) for Control Graph scores and Operational Control scores together.

APPENDIX B
ESTIMATES OF OPERATIONAL CONTROL

Available data

The concept of 'Operational Control' is introduced in chapter 1. Chapter 14 has mentioned that the operational control ratings I obtained were not sufficiently objective to use them as a basis for comparing technological situations, but that they convey interesting information about the raters and their perceptions. This will be explored in this Appendix.

'Operational Control' was measured by having interviewees score on a number of scales, separately for each relevant measurable dimension. See Appendix D 3, question D 2, 3, 4. Questions D 2 and 3 served to introduce the scaling:

'How can you yourself influence . . . (the measurable dimension, for example direct labor efficiency or reject percentages) . . . ?

'What kind of factors outside your reach also influence . . . (the measurable dimension) . . . in your department?'

The scoring was done on the following scales:

	my boss	myself	my subordinates	the workers
Results depend 100% on me/him	9 8	9 8	9 8	9 8
	7 6	7 6	7 6	7 6
Results depend 50/50 on me/him and on outside factors	5 4	5 4	5 4	5 4
	3 2	3 2	3 2	3 2
Results depend 100% on outside factors	1	1	1	1

I used a standardized example as an introduction to the first scoring by the interviewee. This example deals with the efficiency of the use of packaging materials in a hypothetical hand-packaging department. Standard scores are for hierarchical levels from the top downwards: 2-6-7-5-7.

Of course, what is obtained by these ratings is a perception by the interviewee of his – and other people's – operational control, not an objective measurement. It is very doubtful if such a thing as operational control can ever be measured objectively. For its effect on budget motivation this question is unimportant: it is precisely *the perception* of operational control that could have a relationship to budget motivation.

Each line interviewee scored the scales for himself, his boss, his immediate subordinates and, possibly, the rank-and-file workers (if these were not the same as his immediate subordinates). Each staff interviewee scored for the various levels in the line. All of these estimates were done for each relevant Measurable Dimension (see chapter 6) separately. In the factor analysis I used only the scores made by line interviewees (not staff) for their own Operational Control (not the Operational Control of their bosses or subordinates) and averaged over the three highest estimated measurable dimensions (Appendix E 2, variable 40). These appeared to be related to factor 3: upward communication.

Those who feel they have a boss who listens to their ideas also tend to feel they have more operational control. Except from this, operational control is not related to any important extent to any aspect of the budget system. It is correlated with the 'yes-men index', var. 60 ($r = 0.38^{**}$), which indicates the possible influence of suggestion by the researcher in the scoring.

Below, the available data will be analyzed in two other ways:

1. For differences between measurable dimensions
2. For differences between somebody's own perception of his Operational Control and the perceptions of his Operational Control by others (superiors, subordinates, staff).

Finally, the line interviews also yielded descriptions by interviewees of the ways in which they could exercise Operational Control (Appendix D 3, question D 2). and of factors that limited their Operational Control (same, question D 3). An analysis and classification of these descriptions will also be given in this Appendix.

Differences between measurable dimensions

Fig. B-2 shows graphs for Operational Control, averaged over all estimates by line interviewees (own level plus other levels) for the plants where data were available. The only measurable dimension not shown is machine hour efficiency (no. 3), because the number of estimates was very small in this case. From fig. B-1 it can be seen that: 1. direct labor, 4. direct materials use, 5. indirect materials and 6. rejection and rework all follow about the same pattern; high scores for workers and first-line management, low scores for higher-level management. No. 2: indirect labor, follows a different pattern: more control for the higher levels, less for the workers. For comparison, I have also shown the Operational Control lines for the two non-cost measurable dimensions mentioned in chapter 6: meeting production schedules and meeting quality level requirements. The graph for 'meeting production schedules' looks somewhat like the one for 'indirect labor'. The Graph for 'meeting quality level requirements' looks like the one for 'direct labor' etcetera, except that the scores for the higher management levels are higher. *Total Operational Control over all levels of management is estimated highest for the quality dimension.*

It is interesting to compare the graphs for Operational Control with the graphs for total control in Appendix A, fig. A-2. They are exactly opposite. Although the lower organizational levels are perceived to have a lot of Operational Control this contributes little to their perceived total control. If we compare only first-line and higher-level line managers, we find that first-line managers estimate their own Operational Control higher than higher-level managers do, but that their estimate of the own level's total control is equal to or lower than those of higher-level managers. Other types of control compensate for the lower Operational Control at the higher management levels. The perceived high Operational Control for first-line management should lead to a careful consideration of their role in standard-setting (chapter 9) and in receiving information (chapter 10). The same holds true for the workers (non-supervisory employees), although it must be stressed that the data mentioned above were only obtained by interviewing managers. I do not have workers' own perceptions.

From the point of view of method, it should be investigated to what extent the shape of the graphs in fig. B-2 could have been influenced by the standard example used to explain the Operational Control scales to interviewees. This example was introduced after the pilot phase of the study, to overcome the difficulty some interviewees had in understanding the rather abstract scales.

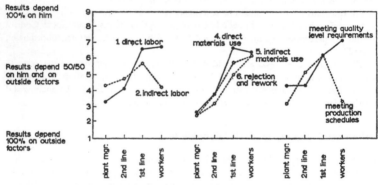

FIG. B-1. Operational Control Estimate Patterns for Various Measurable Dimensions (Averages over data taken from 2-4 plants, not DYNAMO)

It was designed to explain to interviewees what I have named here 'Operational Control': playing one's role in the organizational process, performing, producing, working up to standards, avoiding mistakes. The scores in the example can have influenced the shape of the fig. B-1 graphs to some extent, but they can not explain why for example the scores for department managers (2nd-line management) are far below the example score. Anyhow, as the example was used for all levels and for line and staff equally, it cannot account for any perception differences between levels or between line and staff: nor can it account for differences between measurable dimensions.

Perception differences between individuals, between hierarchical levels and between line and staff

Perception differences between individuals: perception of Operational Control (Appendix E 2, variable 40) is positively correlated with perception of own level's total control on the Control Graph (variable 41): $r_{40,41} = 0.24^{\star}$ (significant at 0.05 level).

This means that those individuals who tend to score high in the one case, also tend to score high in the other.

Perception differences between levels: in the DYNAMO pilot study, it looked as if there were consistent perception differences between hierarchical levels: superiors (people from the next higher levels) tended to score for all levels higher Operational Control. Subordinates (people from the next lower levels) tended to score for all levels lower Operational Control. Staff interviewees tended to score like superiors, that is higher. On the basis of this, I have predicted that the same perception differences would be found in the other four plants. Fig. B-2 is based on the data from the other four plants. For Operational Control, I have only considered here the measurable dimensions 1, 4, 5 and 6 which show about a similar pattern for the Operational Control graphs each (see fig. B-1). From Fig. B-2 we see that my prediction has come true for the estimates by the next lower level (subordinates do estimate lower) and for the staff (staff interviewees do estimate higher). These differences have been tested with the sign test for all available pairs of data (comparing the scores by 2 interviewees, averaged over all measurable dimensions, not only those in fig. B-2). The differences between estimates made by a level and the next lower level are significant at 0.005**; the differences between staff and line at 0.05*. Fig. B-2 shows that for the estimates by the next

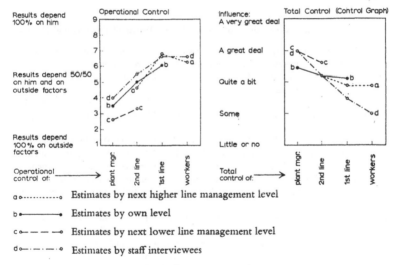

a o ···········o Estimates by next higher line management level

b •————• Estimates by own level

c o— — —o Estimates by next lower line management level

d o—·—·—·o Estimates by staff interviewees

All data are taken over four plants (all except DYNAMO)

Operational control data are taken over four measurable dimensions: direct labor, direct materials use, indirect materials use, rejection and rework

FIG. B-2. Differences in Perception of Operational Control and Total Control for Various Levels of Line Management and for Staff Interviewees

higher level my prediction has come true only for the estimates of Operational Control of first-line managers, not for the estimates of Operational Control of second line managers. The superiors of second-line managers are, of course, the plant managers, and they are only a small group. They score lower than I predicted. They tend to score low also on workers' Operational Control: 5,3 against second-line managers 7.1. The lack of confirmation of my prediction may be due to the smallness of the sample. It is interesting that the staff estimates on the same level as the superiors. I have noted before that the staff tends to identify with the higher levels of line management (see chapter 11).

With regard to the line, the confirmation of my prediction means that the lower management level – having high operational control itself – tends to estimate everybody's operational control lower. In Fig. B-21 I have also shown how perception differences work in the case of Total Control (the Control Graph, Appendix A). We see that the situation is about opposite here: subordinates tend to estimate higher, superiors equal or lower. Now the lower management level – having low total control itself – tends to estimate everybody's total control higher. This could be interpreted in such a way that there is a tendency on both control scales for the own level's estimate to be drawn towards the middle of the scale, and to take the estimates for all other levels along with it.

Analysis of verbal descriptions of elements and limits of Operational Control

Questions D 2 and D 3 in the line interviews (Appendix D 3) served as an introduction to the scoring on the Operational Control scales. The questions were:

D 2: How can you yourself influence . . . (the measurable dimension this part of the interview was dealing with)?

D 3: What kind of factors outside your reach also influence . . . in your department? Analysis of the answers in D 2 revealed that they could be split into four groups ('elements of Operational Control')

1. *Non-routine changes in the production process* (12% of the answers). This is a borderline group between Operational Control and Legislative Decision-Making (see chapter 1). It contains activities like mechanization; technical improvements; improvements in working methods and working conditions; improving the quality of personnel by non-routine training; setting of technical specifications and quality standards; setting of cost standards.

2. *Direct routine intervention into the production process* (not via subordinates or other persons; 31% of the answers). This group contains: distribution of materials, supplies and tools; inspection of incoming goods; work distribution over people and machines; overtime scheduling; studying technical specifications and feedback information; setting production machines and checking machine settings; trouble shooting; record keeping.

3. *Routine intervention via subordinates* (48% of the answers). This group contains: Job instruction and training; supervision on starting and stopping work in time; supervision on working speed and avoidance of stops; supervision on meeting budgets and cost standards; supervision on quality performance and on meeting technical

specifications; discipline, tidiness, safety, consulting subordinates; stimulating communication between subordinates; subordinate appraisal; social leadership, atmosphere, teamwork, personal contact.

4. *Routine intervention via other persons* (9% of the answers). This group contains: informing one's boss, informing one's colleagues, especially giving feedback to managers of earlier stages in the production process, informing staff departments

The answers on question D 3 could be split into four groups as well ('limits of Operational Control'):

1. *Fully external factors* (8% of the answers). These were: the weather; epidemics among the personnel; power supply breakdowns.
2. *Technological constraints* (42% of the answers). These were the technical demands of the production process; quality specifications of the products; age and condition of production machines; quality of materials and supplies; the technological minimum for the number of personnel, taking account of sickness, absence and labor turnover.
3. *Market constraints* (12% of the data). These were sales volume, the production mix, prices of materials and supplies, wage levels, availability of qualified personnel.
4. *Influences of other parts of the organization* (38% of the data). These were the influence of superiors; timely supply of materials; quality performance of earlier stages in the production process; support of staff departments; the influence of subordinates.

The elements of Operational Control were not equally often mentioned by all hierarchical levels. This is illustrated by the table in fig. B-3. Plant managers mainly exercise Operational Control through non-routine changes; first-line managers through routine intervention via subordinates. First-line managers intervene more often directly in the process; plant managers intervene more often through other persons, non-subordinates. Different hierarchical levels are shown in fig. B-3 to have different organizational roles. Each level performs a different function within the organization (Salveson, 1958, p. 212). The lower part of fig. B-3 shows that for the limits of Operational Control there are no such differences between hierarchical levels: they apply fairly equally to all levels.

Obviously, the elements and limits of Operational Control depend on the measurable dimension which is controlled. For example, non-routine changes in the production process (element no. 1) are most frequently mentioned for controlling direct labor cost. Direct routine intervention (element no. 2) is most frequently mentioned for controlling indirect labor cost and indirect materials use. Routine intervention via subordinates (element no. 3) is most frequently mentioned for controlling rejection and rework and direct materials use. Routine intervention via other persons (element no. 4) is most frequently mentioned for controlling machine hour efficiency. As limits of Operational Control, technological constraints (limit no. 2) occur most frequently for the use of direct and indirect materials; market constraints (limit no. 3) for indirect labor cost and machine hours efficiency; the influence of other parts of the organization (limit no. 4) is strongest for direct labor cost, rejection and rework, and meeting quality level requirements.

Finally, the types of elements and limits of Operational Control can be compared from

315

plant to plant. Taking into consideration the vast differences in technology, the distribution of types of elements and limits of Operational Control (taking all measurable dimensions together) is surprisingly equal from plant to plant. Also, the pattern shown in fig. B-3 for the distribution over hierarchical levels is well maintained from plant to plant. The only important differences concern element no. 2: direct routine intervention in the production process. In BUROMAT, DYNAMO and EPICURE, direct intervention is mentioned by first-line managers about twice as frequently as by higher-level managers. In COMBITEX it is mentioned with equal frequency by first-line and higher-level, and in ALPHABET about one-and-a-half times as frequently by higher-level managers. The role differences between first-line managers and higher-level management are least outspoken in COMBITEX and ALPHABET. It is interesting in this respect that in these two plants, contrary to the others, second-line managers are recruited by promotion of first-line managers. In the other plants, second-line managers are attracted from outside; they have a higher level of theoretical education.

% of answers to questions D2–D3 by → dealing with ↓	Plant Managers	2nd-line Managers	1st-line Managers	Total-line Managemt.
D2. Elements of Operational Control:				
1. Non-routine changes in the production process	49	18	5	12
2. Direct routine intervention in the production process	5	30	34	31
3. Routine intervention via subordinates	30	41	54	48
4. Routine intervention via other persons	16	11	7	9
D3. Limits of Operational Control:				
1. Fully external factors	3	8	8	8
2. Technological constraints	47	43	41	42
3. Market constraints	18	12	11	12
4. Influences of other parts of the organization	32	37	40	38

FIG. B3. Distribution of Elements and Limits of Operational Control over Hierarchical Levels.

APPENDIX C
DOCUMENTS FOR THE PREPARATORY PHASE

C 1. Introductory information to top line manager

1. General information about the project (See Appendix D 1).
2. Researcher will be available half-time.
3. Forecast of expected duration of the various phases of the investigation in his plant.
4. Proposal for feedback session.
5. Double confidentiality:
   – no company information to outsiders without management's approval
   – no identification of personal opinions communicated in interviews.
6. First formal line interview will be held with you.
7. Please arrange for introduction to middle management in a short meeting.
8. Please arrange for introductory interviews with plant personnel manager and top functional managers of the departments responsible for maintaining the budget and cost standard system.
9. Please make available a quiet room to conduct the interviews in.
10. Any questions?

C 2. Notes for introductory talk to middle management meeting

1. General information about the project (see Appendix D 1)
2. Stress the difference between budgeting theory – available in accounting textbooks – and the systematic analysis of practice.
3. Forecast expected duration of the various phases of the investigation in this plant.
4. Explain that a sample will be taken: every manager, foreman and staff employee may not be interviewed.
5. Announce that appointments for interviews will be made by the researcher with each manager individually.
6. Any questions?

C 3. Questionnaire for introductory interview with plant personnel manager

1. Could you supply me with an organization chart for this plant, with the names of all managers, foremen and budget/standards staff employees?
2. Is there a system of job classification for the people on this chart? How does it work? What are the job classes of the various people mentioned?
3. Could you prepare a list of all first- and second-line managers, and rate each of them:
   a = promotable
   b = just right at present level
   c = already above his optimal level

4. Could you also rate the same people 1-5 on the basis of their type of leadership:

    1 = authoritarian (prefers clear orders)
    2, 3, 4 = in – between ratings
    5 = democratic (prefers consultation)

5. In what period of the year are management appraisals made and what is the procedure used?
6. What kind of management development activities exist? Who is responsible for these? What subjects are treated in them?
7. Which of the positions in the organization chart have had personnel changes in the past 2 years?
8. Which people on the list have shown signs of overwork, gastric ulcers, and similar psychosomatic complaints?
9. Who represents middle and lower management and staff departments in the Works Council? How does it function?
10. How wholesome are the line-staff relationships?
11. Could you prepare a list of all staff employees and staff managers and rate each of them:

    1 = condemning attitude towards the line
    2, 3, 4 = in – between – ratings
    5 = service attitude towards the line

12. Which line managers are seen as most efficiency-minded?
13. Do you ever perceive any reactions of line managers on budgeting and cost standards? How would you characterize these reactions?
14. If line and staff management meet informally, who sits with whom?
15. If there is an introduction folder for new personnel, could I have a copy?
16. Which personnel newspapers exist? Do they deal with efficiency problems? If so, could I see some examples?
17. Do you have any other information that could be relevant in this context, or any questions?

C 4. Questionnaire for introductory interview with manager(s) of budget and/or efficiency standards department

1. Could you tell me something about the history of this plant?
2. What are the main products and markets?
3. How does this plant fit into the total company structure? (any other desirable information about the company in general).
4. Could you supply me with an organization chart for this plant?
5. Which functions in this chart are responsible for a budget? Are these responsibilities stated in any official document? Could I see it?
6. When did the budget/standards system start in this plant; What is the history of the system?
7. Which staff departments have a role in the system?
8. What is the budget period?

9. What types of budgets are included in the system? Does it lead to a planned income statement?
10. Is the budget system based on engineered direct labor standards, quality standards, planning standards, etc.? Is it integrated with the costing system?
11. Is the budget fixed or variable? What types of budget variances are distinguished?
12. What cost centers and what cost types are distinguished?
13. How is the new budget developed? In what period? Who proposes budget levels? Who is consulted? Who decides? Who signs?
14. Can operating budgets be adjusted during the budget period?
15. To what extent is the budget procedure prescribed by the head office?
16. How are budget variances reported? How frequently? In what form? To whom?
17. Could you make available to me all budgets and variance information covering the past 2 years?
18. What other management information reports are made which show departmental performance? Could you make available to me all information of this type covering the past 2 years?
19. How are the budget and standards staff departments organized? Please give all names.
20. What education and experience level do these people have? Which of them have direct contact with the line?
21. What parts of the budget/cost standards system function best? What parts function least well?
22. What was the total manufacturing cost in this plant in the most recent full year? How was this distributed over departments? How was it distributed over direct materials, direct labor, other expenses? What was total labor cost (direct + indirect wages + salaries + social benefits)?
23. Could you get me a cost calculation of an average product as it is now and as it was (the same product) one year ago and two years ago?
24. Could we draw together a flow chart of the total volume of money flowing yearly through this plant?
25. In a few weeks I will approach you for another interview (formal main staff interview). Do you have any information that could still be relevant to our subject now? Do you have any questions?

APPENDIX D
MAIN INTERVIEW DOCUMENTS

D 1. Scheme for introductory talk to each interviewee

Mr. X, let me explain again briefly the purpose of our interview. I am here for the C.O.P. (follows an explanation why the C.O.P., the Dutch Productivity Committee, was founded, who are represented in it – employers, trade unions and government –, where the money comes from and what kind of research the C.O.P. is sponsoring). The research project I am working for is only a small project: a one-man setup. It was started for the following reason: after World War II we have seen the introduction of modern organization tools in our plants: for instance budgeting, planning, and management information systems. All these tools use *standards* that are set beforehand, to which actual performance is subsequently compared. Now in practice these tools are not so simple to use as in theory and many companies have problems here. Therefore, the C.O.P. has asked five well-organized companies to make their practical experience with these tools available. Your company is the y th of these five that I have come to. I work this way:

First I study the systems that are used in the particular company. Then, I have interviews with various people about their practical experience. They are the 'staff', the people who keep the system going, and the 'line', the foremen and managers of the manufacturing departments. In your company I am interviewing ... (description of the interviewee sample in company terminology). In interviewing I am using a questionnaire, in order to make sure I ask the same questions of everybody, so that I can compare the answers. What I am most interested in is not so much the opinion of any single person, but group opinions. What you tell me is confidential; I will not reveal to anybody what anybody else has said during the interviews. In reporting about the interview results, I will only use your opinion in conjunction with the opinions of others to form a total picture.

When all five companies have been investigated, the results will be published in a report. Such a report looks like this one (a copy of a similar report is shown). These reports are sold like ordinary books to anybody and they are not expensive. The report of our project will try to summarize the general conclusions of the investigation in the five companies. Unfortunately, writing and publishing the report will take quite some time. To avoid keeping you waiting too long, I have promised to your management to give a feedback session in a few months. Then you will hear what I did with all that you and your colleagues told me. Have you any questions? Shall I start asking then?

D 2. Questionnaire for staff interviews (abridged)

A. *General information* (to be filled out beforehand)

1.   Plant number (1 through 6)

2. Date, hour and place of interview
3. Name and initials of interviewee
4. Function of interviewee (type and level)
5. Age at interview date
6. Number of years with the company.

B. *General questions about the job*

1. What is the official title of your present job?
2. How many years have you been in this particular job?
3. To whom are you reporting?
4. And who are the people immediately reporting to you? What jobs do they have?
5. Can you explain to me in a few words what your job consists of?
6. Which part of your job do you consider the most important?
7. Why?
8. Please try to make an estimate of the division of your total working week in the following 3 parts:
   a. Working at your desk without being interrupted.
   b. Talking and listening to others on company premises, including telephoning.
   c. All other activities (observing, travelling etc.).
9. What are your c-type activities?
10. Could you now try to estimate how much of your b-type time (talking and listening) is:
    d. Talking and listening to line managers and workers or mixed line-staff groups.
    c. Talking and listening to other staff people only.
11. What level of line people do you generally have contacts with?
12. What other staff people do you have most contacts with?

C. *Standard-setting*

1. Will you please check on this list, which *standards* and *variances* you have something to do with (checklist of all types of standards in the plant, in which interviewee can check: 'involved in setting standards' and/or 'involved in calculating and publishing variances').
2. Will you please explain your checkmarks?
3. Can you make an estimate of your department's role and the role of the various line managers and other staff departments in the standard-setting processes, on the following scale? (participation scale, see Appendix D 3, question D 12, scored for each type of standard separately).
4. Do you think everyone in this company has the right role in the standard-setting processes? If not, what should be different?
5. Do you think the various standards are tight or loose? Will you please tick one for each type of standard? (loose-tight scale, see Appendix D 3. question D 11).
6. For which areas are good standards lacking still?
7. What is your general opinion about the way standards are set here?

D. Operational control and management information

1. Will you now give an evaluation of the various line departments in terms of their performance on the different points that you think you can judge (evaluation scale, see Appendix D 3., question F 8., to be repeated for each line department).

2. What are the most important improvements that could presently be made in this plant?

3. What conditions must be fulfilled for these improvements to be realized?

4. Will you now estimate the influence of various levels of the line organization on various types of results, on the following scale? (operational control scale, see Appendix D 3., question D 4., to be repeated for each measurable dimension as far as within the scope of the interviewee).

5. For those cases in which you calculate and publish variances to standards, how frequently is this done and who get the reports?

6. What is your general opinion of this type of management information?

7. Are the reports distributed to the right people? Is lower-level management sufficiently informed?

8. Do there exist periodic management information reports that you think could be eliminated?

9. Are there useful figures that should be, but are not reported to management?

10. Are reports timely? Which ones are not?

11. What measures would you propose to increase the impact of the management information system?

12. To what extent are the details of the management information reports prescribed by the head office? What do you think of this?

E. General questions about the control system

1. Do you ever attend meetings of line management where budget or standards variances are discussed? How do these meetings go?

2. Does line management ever come to you, to get explanations about figures? Or do you go to them? Who, in general, takes the initiative for these contacts? Which line managers are involved in this kind of contacts?

3. How frequent are these contacts?

4. When you get the figures and you see a serious underattainment of a standard, what do you do?

5. Which part of the reports is generally best read? Are the reports understood?

6. Could you now estimate the amount of interest various levels of line management show for various types of management information, on the following scale:

He is continuously working with the figures   ⌐ 5
He pays a lot of attention to the figures   ⌐ 4
It is one of the things he pays attention to   ⌐ 3
Occasionaly he pays attention to the figures   ⌐ 2
He is not interested   ∟ 1

(to be repeated for each level of line management for each type of information the interviewee is concerned with).

7. Do the standards that are set influence productivity in this plant?
8. Inasfar as there is a positive influence, in which departments and for which standards is this strongest?
9. Are the line managers stimulated to a better performance by the standards?
10. Do you personally prefer loose or tight standards? Why?
11. What do you consider to be the objective of standard-setting and budgeting?
12. It is sometimes said that budgeting leads to departmental interest prevailing above the general interest. Do you ever feel this holds true for this plant too?
13. How wholesome is the relationship between your department and line management?
14. How wholesome is the relationship between your department and other staff departments?
15. In general, how much say or influence do you feel each of the following persons has on what goes on in this plant? (Control Graph scale, see Appendix D 3., question E 25).
16. Will you please also indicate on the scales what influence you think each person or group *should* have?
17. What kind of influence were you thinking of while asnswering the previous questions?

F. *Appraisals*

1. Who is appraising your performance?
2. Will you have a look at these 10 cards:
   A. Professional knowledge
   B. Understanding production problems
   C. Working hard
   D. Tactfulness towards line people and colleagues
   E. Inventiveness, creativity
   F. Zeal: being an 'eager beaver' for the company
   G. Insight: observing mistakes and using your brains
   H. Leadership: getting things done through subordinates
   I. Personal sympathy of the appraiser
   J. Ability to organize your own work
   Which of these does, in practice, weigh heaviest in the appraisal of your personal performance? Will you please rank all cards in order of actual weight?
3. And how would you rank the cards for your appraisals of your subordinates?
4. Which rating would you give to your own section's present performance?

so-so	satis-factory	fairly good	good	ex-cellent
5	6	7	8	9
☐	☐	☐	☐	☐

Why did you choose this figure and not, for instance, a 9?
5. Will you now rate each of your direct subordinates on the same scale, for his total job performance?

6. Could you illustrate your ratings with a short characterization of the working method of each of your direct subordinates?
7. Do you think the educational level of your people too high, just right, or too low for their present job?

G. *General questions*

1. Will you please try to fill out this attitude survey form (see Appendix D 4-5)
2. If you could choose another job within this company, what type of job would it be?
3. What functions have you had in this company?
4. What types of jobs have you had before?
5. What schools did you attend?
6. Which part of your job do you enjoy most? (Why?)
7. And which part of your job do you dislike most? (Why?)
8. My questions are finished; do you have any more questions?
9. Thank you very much for your participation; please do not discuss the content of the questions with anybody else in the plant within the next two weeks because you might influence another participant.

H. *Interviewer's impressions*

1. General impression:

   Rating of interviews:
2. Openness   low |⎿⎿⎿⎿⎿⎿⎿⎿⎿| high
3. Understanding   low |⎿⎿⎿⎿⎿⎿⎿⎿⎿| high
4. General cost-consciousness   low |⎿⎿⎿⎿⎿⎿⎿⎿⎿| high
5. Relevance of budget/standards   low |⎿⎿⎿⎿⎿⎿⎿⎿⎿| high
6. Attitude towards the line   condemnation |⎿⎿⎿⎿⎿⎿⎿⎿⎿| service

                                             1 2 3 4 5 6 7 8 9

7. Duration of the interview:

D 3. Questionnaire for line interviews (abridged)

'Quiz questions' are marked with★

A. *General information* (to be filled out beforehand)

1. Plant number (1 through 6)
2. Date, hour and place of interview
3. Name and initials of interviewee
4. Function of interviewee
5. Age at interview date
6. Number of years with the company

B. *General questions about the job*

1. What is the official title of your present job?

2. How many years have you been in this particular job?
3. For which department or departments are you responsible?
4. To whom are you reporting?
5. And who are the people immediately reporting to you? What jobs do they have?
6. Will you now have a look at these five cards:
   A. Leading the personnel
   B. Fulfilling production schedules
   C. Maintaining quality
   D. Keeping costs down
   E. Developing new products and processes.
   Probably, all these five subjects demand some of your attention. Will you now please put the one which demands *most* of your attention on top, and the others below in the sequence in which they demand your attention?
7. What kind of special plans do you have for your department in the coming half year?

C. *Checking the relevant measurable dimensions*

1. What sorts of costs must be incurred to keep your department going?
2. Will you now have a look at these 8 cards:
   A. Direct materials cost
   B. Reject cost
   C. Direct labor cost
   D. Indirect labor cost
   E. Maintenance cost of machines and buildings.
   F. Cost of indirect materials, small tools and other supplies
   G. Depreciation of machines and buildings
   H. Energy cost
   (exact descriptions adapted to company situation and terminology).
   Will you now please divide these cards in three groups:
   Costs that cannot be influenced in your department; costs that can somewhat be influenced, and costs that can strongly be influenced in your department. Will you please rank the cards in the third group as to the degree of influence your department has on them?
3. Are there any other costs I should include?
4. (possible probing for explanations of rankings that are not obvious).

D. *Information about each measurable dimension*

(This section is repeated for each relevant measurable dimension. The example is for direct labor. Terminology is again adapted to the company).
1. Let us first discuss direct labor. Which labor in your department is considered as direct?
2. How can you yourself influence direct labor efficiency?
3. What kind of factors outside your reach also influence labor efficiency in your department?

325

4. Will you now estimate the influences of various people on direct labor efficiency on the following scale:

	my boss	my-self	my sub-ordinates	the workers
Results depend 100% on me/him	9 8 7 6	9 8 7 6	9 8 7 6	9 8 7 6
Results depend 50/50 on me/him and on outside factors	5 4 3 2	5 4 3 2	5 5 3 2	5 4 3 2
Results depend 100% on outside factors	1	1	1	1

(Scale is illustrated by a standard example first – this example deals with packaging materials efficiency in a hypothetical hand packaging department – scores are for hierarchical levels from top downwards: 2-6-7-5-7)

5.* How much was the direct labor efficiency in your department over the past period?
6. How frequently do you get information about direct labor efficiencies?
7. From what source do you get this information?
8. What is your general impression of the management information system for direct labor efficiency?
9. In what way are the workers informed about direct labor standards?
10.* At what level of direct labor efficiency is your budgetary standard set?
11. Do you think direct labor standards are tight or loose here? Will you please tick one on this list:

too loose	5	☐
fairly loose	4	☐
just right	3	☐
tight, but attainable	2	☐
too tight	1	☐

12. How are direct labor standards set here? (If interviewee himself plays a role in the standard-setting process): will you please estimate your role in the direct labor standard-setting process and the role of the staff on the following scale (a–b in fig. 9-2)
13. And which roles do you think you and the staff ought to have had in the direct labor standard-setting process (same scale, c–d)
14. Do you expect the direct labor efficiency in your department to improve in the coming year? (Why?)

E. General questions about the control system

1. Do you have regular meetings with your boss and colleagues? (How often, when, who participates, which topics are discussed?)
2. Do you think these meetings are useful? (Why?)
3. Do you have similar meetings with your subordinates?
4. Do you think *these* meetings are useful?
5. Apart from these meetings, how often do you meet with your boss? What topics do you discuss with him then?
6. Does your boss ever discuss budget variances or other performance figures of your department with you? Which figures in particular?
7. Do you receive budget variance reports? What type of reports? How frequently? From whom? What figures in them do you study in particular? What use do you make of these figures?
8. Do you think the budget variance reports are understandable?
9. What is your general impression of the financial information system?
10. With whom in the controller's department do you have contacts? How often, and about what subjects?
11. How wholesome is your relationship with these people?
12. With what other staff departments do you have contacts? How often, about which subjects, and how is your relationship with them?
13. What are the most important improvements that could presently be made in your department?
14.* How many guilders' worth of products passes through your department in a year?
15.* What value is added to one unit of product passing through your department?
16.* What value of materials enters your department to make one unit of product?
17.* How many guilders a year would you save by not hiring one full man?
18.* What is the total investment in machinery within your department?
19. What do you think of the piece-rate system as it is used here? (or any other system used to set workers' wages).
20. Do the standards that are set influence productivity in this plant? Why, and which standards in particular?
21. Would you prefer personally to work with or without standards, or do you have no preference? Why?
22. Do the standards stimulate you yourself to a better performance? Why or why not?
23. If no standards were set, but your instruction would just be to work as efficiently as possible, would this make your job heavier or lighter than it is now? Why?
24. Does your boss, in appraising your personal performance, take into account your department's variances to standards?
25. In general, how much say or influence do you feel each of the following persons or groups has on what goes on in this plant? (interviewee scores on scales);

	little or no influence	some infl.	quite a bit of infl.	a great deal of infl.	a very great deal of infl.
top management	L_____|_____|_____|_____J				
plant manager	L_____|_____|_____|_____J				
line department managers	L_____|_____|_____|_____J				
line foremen	L_____|_____|_____|_____J				
workers	L_____|_____|_____|_____J				
staff-departments	L_____|_____|_____|_____J				
	1	3	5	7	9

26. Will you please also indicate on the scales what influence you think each person or group *should* have?
27. What kind of influence were you thinking of while answering the previous questions?

F. *Appraisal*

1. Who appraises your performance?
2. Will you now have a look at these 10 cards:
   A. Craftmanship and professional knowledge
   B. Department's results
   C. Working hard
   D. Tactfulness towards colleagues and others
   E. Cost consciousness
   F. Zeal; being an 'eager beaver' for the company
   G. Insight: observing mistakes and using your brains
   H. Leadership: getting things done through subordinates
   I. Personal sympathy of the appraiser
   J. Quality consciousness.
   Which of these does, in practice, weigh heaviest in the appraisal of your personal performance? Will you please rank all cards in order of actual weight?
3. And how would you rank the cards for your appraisals of your subordinates?
4. What kind of 'department's results' were you thinking of?
5. How do you judge a person's cost consciousness?
6. How do you judge a person's quality consciousness?
7. Do the workers have sufficient cost and quality consciousness? What, in your opinion, can be done to improve this?
8. Will you now please give an evaluation of how your own department is performing at present on the following points (tick one for each line)

	so-so	satis-factory	fairly good	good	ex-cellent
	5	6	7	8	9
A. Efficiency of materials use	☐	☐	☐	☐	☐
B. Reject rate	☐	☐	☐	☐	☐
C. Efficiency of direct labor	☐	☐	☐	☐	☐
D. Efficiency of indirect labor	☐	☐	☐	☐	☐
E. Efficiency of the use of indirect materials etc.	☐	☐	☐	☐	☐
F. Meeting produc-tion schedules	☐	☐	☐	☐	☐
G. Meeting quality standards	☐	☐	☐	☐	☐

(A through G adapted to plant situation)

9. Will you now rate each of your direct subordinates on the following scale, for his total job performance?

so-so	satis-factory	fairly good	good	ex-cellent
5	6	7	8	9
☐	☐	☐	☐	☐

10. Could you illustrate your ratings with a short characterization of the working method of each of your direct subordinates?

11. How do you rate their leadership towards their subordinates: authoritarian, democratic or in between? Please rate the leadership of each of your direct subordinates on the following scale:

democratic				authoritarian
5	4	3	2	1
☐	☐	☐	☐	☐

G. *General questions*

1. Will you please try to fill out this attitude survey form? (See Appendix D 5).
2. What functions have you had in this company?
3. What types of jobs have you had before?
4. What schools did you attend?

5. Did you ever attend a management development course? What was this course about? Did it deal with budgeting and standard costing?
6. Which part of your job do you enjoy most? (Why?)
7. And which part of your job do you dislike most? (Why?)
8. My questions are finished; do you have any more questions?
9. Thank you very much for your participation; please do not discuss the content of the questions with anybody else in the plant within the next two weeks, because you might influence another participant.

H. *Interviewer's impression*

1. General impression:

Rating of interview:

			1 2 3 4 5 6 7 8 9	
2.	Openness	low	∟_⊥_⊥_⊥_⊥_⊥_⊥_⊥_⊥_⌐	high
3.	Understanding	low	∟_⊥_⊥_⊥_⊥_⊥_⊥_⊥_⊥_⌐	high
4.	General cost-consciousness	low	∟_⊥_⊥_⊥_⊥_⊥_⊥_⊥_⊥_⌐	high
5.	Relevance of budget/standards	low	∟_⊥_⊥_⊥_⊥_⊥_⊥_⊥_⊥_⌐	high
6.	Attitude towards the system	negative	∟_⊥_⊥_⊥_⊥_⊥_⊥_⊥_⊥_⌐	positive

7. Duration of the interview:

D 4. Attitude survey questionnaire - staff

For each sentence, the answer scale was the same:

always   mostly   sometimes   seldom   never

□   □   □   □   □

(It was explained to participants that in cases where this time scale does not apply literally, e.g. "mostly" must be read as "agreement in most cases", etc.).
The sentences used only in the staff survey were the following (there were 40 sentences in total; the numbers not mentioned here are the same as those in the line survey, see Appendix D 5.):
4. The line-managers are ignorant about the job done by my department.
6. Staff departments should leave more to the line.
8. The directives from head-office are limited to a necessary minimum.
9. The line managers are insufficiently cost-conscious.
10. The first task of my department is service to management.
12. The cooperation between staff departments is smooth.
18. A main task of budget variance reports is to show superiors where their subordinates have failed.
19. In my department too, efficiency can be improved.
20. Line-management is sufficiently conscious of the need for reliable clerical data.
22. Line-management is well convinced of the importance of meeting quality standards.

330

26. The cooperation between my department and the line leaves much to be desired.
29. My department is insufficiently consulted in plant problems.
30. My department is undermanned.
32. I would prefer another job in this company.
36. The line managers do not spend enough effort to meet production schedules.
38. Line-management follows our advice.

D 5. Attitude survey questionnaire – line

For each sentence, the answer scale was the same:

always	mostly	sometimes	seldom	never
☐	☐	☐	☐	☐

(It was explained to participants that in cases where this scale does not apply literally, e.g. 'mostly' must be read as 'agreement in most cases'; etc.).
The sentences used were:
1. I like the department I work in.
2. Budgeting is first of all an accounting tool.
3. Working comes naturally to most people.
4. My boss rejects my ideas for improvement.
5. In this plant my private interests are taken account of as much as possible.
6. The management information reports I get are sufficiently understandable.
7. My job makes me agitated and nervous.
8. Budgets are set here without taking sufficient account of my department's special problems.
9. I could work as well without standards.
10. If I am absent for a week, my department still keeps running well.
11. I enjoy my job.
12. The cooperation between the line and the production scheduling department is OK.
13. I think my performance is justly appraised here.
14. Obedience and respect for authority are the most important virtues children should learn.
15. People nowadays are less willing to carry responsibility than they used to be.
16. This plant is well managed.
17. My boss asks my opinion about matters concerning my area of work.
18. I think trying to attain the standards is a sport.
19. My boss is continuously working on cost reduction.
20. The people from the controller's department have a lack of understanding of production problems.
21. A clear order is better than consultation.
22. My boss discusses my department's costs with me.
23. This plant demands my utmost.
24. Young people sometimes get rebellious ideas, but as they grow up they ought to get over them and settle down.
25. It would be possible to work much better and at less cost in this plant.

26. The cooperation between the line and the industrial engineers leaves much to be desired.
27. I feel under pressure in my job.
28. My career opportunities here depend first of all on myself.
29. Taking everything into account, my department runs efficiently enough.
30. A foreman can well be appraised on his efforts to meet standards.
31. Subordinates ought to accept their boss' decisions without reserve.
32. I know exactly which costs I am responsible for.
33. I prefer . . . (ALPHABET etc.) as a place to work above others.
34. People can be divided into two distinct classes: the weak and the strong.
35. There is too much paperwork in this company.
36. Introducing budgeting (standards) has improved efficiency.
37. If the labor market gets less tight, personnel management will get tougher again here.
38. My boss discusses the quality performance of my department with me.
39. If people would talk less and work more, everybody would be better off.
40. I enjoyed participating in this C.O.P. Research Project.

APPENDIX E
LISTS OF FACTORS FOR THE FACTOR ANALYSIS

E 1. Staff factor analysis

Number of cases: 48
Number of variables: 46
The letters + numbers between brackets refer to the questions in the questionnaire of Appendix D 2. Numbers without letters refer to the attitude survey questionnaire of Appendix D 4-D 5.

Variable no:

1. Type of staff function (1 = budget accounting, 0 = other)
2-7 Plant identification for plant 1 — 6 (1 = belongs to plant, 0 = does not belong).
8. Age group.
9. Classification number of years in present job.
10. Classification educational level.
11. Line experience (1 = yes, 0 = no).
12. Interviewer's impression of attitude towards line (H 6).
13. Own estimate of general influence of staff (E 15).
14. Desired minus actual general staff influence (E 16-E 15).
15. Desired minus actual general line influence (average over all management levels within the plant; E 16-E 15).
16 .'Budgeting is first of all an accounting tool' – negative (2).
17. 'Staff departments should leave more to the line' – positive (6).
18 'The first task of my department is service to management' – positive (10).
19. 'A main task of budget variance reports is to show to superiors where their subordinates have failed' – negative (18).
20. Estimated percentage of time spent communicating with the line (B 10 d).
21. 'The line managers are ignorant about the job done by my department' – negative (4).
22. 'The line managers are insufficiently cost-conscious' – negative (9).
23. 'Line management is sufficiently conscious of the need for reliable clerical data – positive (20).
24. 'Line mangement is well convinced of the importance of meeting quality standards' – positive (22).
25. 'The cooperation between my department and the line leaves much to be desired' – negative (26).
26. 'My department is insufficiently consulted in plant problems' – negative (29).
27. 'The line managers do not spend enough effort to meet production schedules'. – negative (36).
28. 'Line management follows our advice' – positive (38).
29. 'The cooperation between staff departments is smooth' – positive (12).

30. 'In my department efficiency can be improved' – negative (19).
31. 'My department is undermanned' – negative (30).
32. 'There is too much paperwork in this company' – negative (35).
33. Average judgment about looseness of standards (C 5, average over all relevant measurable dimensions).
34. Maximum role of own department in the standard-setting process (C 3, maximum score for any relevant measurable dimension).
35. Rank order of 'tactfulness' in boss' appraisal (F 2 D).
36. Rank order of 'understanding production problems' in boss' appraisal (E 2 B).
37. Boss' appraisal of total job performance (F 5 in interview with boss).
38. 'I would prefer another job in this company' – negative (32).
39. 'I like the department I work in' – positive (1). ⎫ total score
    'I enjoy my job' – positive (11). ⎭
40. 'My job makes me agitated and nervous' – negative (7). ⎫ total score
    'I feel under pressure in my job' – negative (27). ⎭
41. 'This plant demands my utmost' – negative (23).
42. 'I think my performance is justly appraised here' – positive (13). ⎫ total
    'My career opportunities here depend first of all on myself' – positive (28). ⎭ score
43. 'Working comes naturally to most people' – positive (3).
44. 'People nowadays are less willing to carry responsibility than they used to ⎫
    be – negative (15). ⎪ total
    'If the labor market gets less tight, personnel management will get tougher⎬ score
    again here' – negative (37). ⎭
45. 'A clear order is better than consultation' – negative (21). ⎫
    'Young people sometimes get rebellious ideas, but as they grow older they ⎪
    ought to get over them and settle down' – negative (24). ⎪ total
    'Subordinates ought to accept their boss' decisions without reserve' – ⎬ score
    negative (31). ⎪
    'People can be divided into two distinct classes, the weak and the strong' – ⎪
    negative (34). ⎭
46. Total number of 'always' or 'mostly' answers in attitude survey (Apendix D 4-D 5).

E 2. Line factor analysis

Number of cases: 90
Number of variables: 60
The letters and numbers between brackets refer to the questions in the questionnaire of Appendix D 3. Numbers without letter refer to the attitude survey questionnaire of Appendix D 5.

Variable no:

1. Hierarchical level (1 = first-line, 2 = higher).
2-13. Plant and level identification for plant 1-6 and first-line, or higher levels (1 = belongs to subgroup, 0 = does not belong).
14. Age group.

15. Classification number of years in present job.
16. Classification educational level.
17. Interviewer's impression of relevance of budget/standards (H 5).
18. 'Do the standards that are set, influence productivity in this plant?' (E 20). } total
    'Do the standards stimulate yourself to a better performance?' (E 22). } score
19. Interviewer's impression of attitude towards the system (H 6).
20. 'Would you prefer personally to work with or without standards, or do
    you have no preference?' (E 21). } total score
    'If no standards were set, but your instruction would just be to work as } score
    efficiently as possible, would this make your job heavier or lighter than it is
    now?' (E 23).
21. 'I know exactly which costs I am responsible for' – positive (32).
22. Total score on quiz questions about actual performance information and about
    standards (D 5 and D 10, summarized over the 3 best known measurable dimen-
    sions).
23. Total score on general cost-consciousness quiz questions (E 14, 15, 16, 17, 18).
24. 'I could work as well without standards' – negative (9).
25. 'I think trying to attain the standards is a sport' – positive (18).
26. 'Taking everything into account, my department runs efficiently enough' – negative
    (29).
27. 'A foreman's performance can well be appraised on his efforts to meet standards'
    – positive (30).
28. Overall budget variance for the department in the past 3 months – derived from
    official figures, and classified:
    1 = very unfavorable (loss more than 5% of total added value)
    2 = unfavorable (loss 1-5% of total added value)
    3 = even (favorable or unfavorable variance not more than 1% of total added
        value)
    4 = favorable (gain 1-5% of total added value)
    5 = very favorable (gain more than 5% of total added value)
    Added value = all costs within department minus direct materials.
29. Own estimate of maximum role in budget setting process (or interviewer's estimate
    if role is so slight that no own estimate was made) (D 12).
30. Discrepancy between desired and actual role in budget setting process (D 13-D 12;
    1 = positive discrepancy, 0 = no discrepancy or negative discrepancy).
31. Own estimate of maximum role in non-financial (technical) standards setting
    process (or interviewer's estimate if role is so slight that no own estimate was
    made) (D 12).
32. Discrepancy between desired and actual role in technical standard setting process
    (D 13-D 12; 1 = positive discrepancy; 0 = no discrepancy or negative discre-
    pancy).
33. 'Budgets are set here without taking sufficient account of my department's special
    problems' – negative (8).
34. Average judgment about looseness of standards (D 11, average over all relevant
    measurable dimensions).

35. Average judgment about looseness of standards by top plant manager and staff people (from interview with top plant manager and staff interviews).
36. Improvement in performance expected (D 14; total score for 3 most relevant measurable dimensions).
37. Average evaluation of present performance of own department (F 8, average over all lines).
38. Lack of correlation between own subjective evaluation of performance and objective budget variance derived from official figures. (See chapter 8 for exact method of determination).
39. Rating of ability, composed of boss' rating of total job performance (F 9 in interview with boss) and promotability rating by personnel manager (question 4 in Appendix C 3).
40. Average estimate of own operational control (D 4, average for the three highest estimated measurable dimensions).
41. Own estimate of general influence of own level (E 25).
42. Desired minus actual general influence of own level (E 26-E 25).
43. Rank order of 'department's results' in boss' appraisal (F 2 B).
44. Rank order of 'cost consciousness' in boss' appraisal (F 2 E).
45. Frequency + usefulness of meetings with boss and colleagues (index on the basis of E 1 and E 2 – see chapter 12).
46. 'Does your boss ever discuss budget variances or other performance figures of your department with you?' (E 6) 'My boss discusses the department's costs with me' – positive (22). } total score
47. 'My boss rejects my ideas for improvement' – negative (4) 'My boss asks my opinion about matters concerning my area of work' – positive (17). } total score
48. 'My boss is continuously working on cost reduction' – positive (19).
49. Desired minus actual general influence of *staff* departments (E 26-E 25).
50. 'The management information reports I get are sufficiently understandable' – positive (6).
51. 'The cooperation between the line and the production scheduling department is O.K.' – positive (12). 'The people from the controller's department have a lack of understanding of production problems' – negative (20). 'The cooperation between the line and the industrial engineers leaves much to be desired' – negative (26). } total score
52. 'There is too much paperwork in this company' – negative (35).
53. 'I like the department I work in' – positive (1). 'I enjoy my job' – positive (11). } total score
54. 'My job makes me agitated and nervous' – negative (7). 'I feel under pressure in my job' – negative (27). } total score
55. 'This plant demands my utmost' – negative (23).
56. 'I think my performance is justly appraised here' – positive (13). 'My career opportunities here depend first of all on myself' – positive (28). } total score
57. 'Working comes naturally to most people' – positive (3).

58. 'People nowadays are less willing to carry responsibility than they used to be
     – negative (15).
     'If the labor market gets less tight, personnel management will get tougher
     again here' – negative (37). } total score

59. 'A clear order is better than consultation' – negative (21).
     'Young people sometimes get rebellious ideas, but as they grow older they
     ought to get over them and settle down' – negative (24).
     'Subordinates ought to accept their boss' decisions without reserve' –
     negative (31).
     'People can be divided into two distinct classes, the weak and the strong' –
     negative (34). } total score

60. Total number of 'always' or 'mostly' answers in attitude survey (Appendix D 5).

Alphabet 102 cases	Budget variance				
	− −	−	o	+	+ +
Evaluation mark 9	0	2	5	2	3
8	0	13	15	9	6
7	0	6	11	7	5
6	0	6	3	1	0
5	0	6	2	0	0

Dynamo 1 60 cases	Budget variance				
	− −	−	o	+	+ +
Evaluation mark 9	1	2	1	2	3
8	4	6	6	10	17
7	3	0	1	0	3
6	1	0	0	0	0
5	0	0	0	0	0

Buromat 87 cases	Budget variance				
	− −	−	o	+	+ +
Evaluation mark 9	0	2	2	1	0
8	3	10	18	0	1
7	2	10	15	1	0
6	5	5	3	2	1
5	3	2	0	1	0

Dynamo 2 60 cases	Budget variance				
	− −	−	o	+	+ +
Evaluation mark 9	0	1	0	1	1
8	1	0	8	10	5
7	1	2	6	4	4
6	1	0	4	3	0
5	3	2	2	0	1

Combitex 83 cases	Budget variance				
	− −	−	o	+	+ +
Evaluation mark 9	0	1	1	1	0
8	4	4	14	4	0
7	3	8	2	2	0
6	5	9	2	1	0
5	8	10	4	0	0

Epicure 74 cases	Budget variance				
	− −	−	o	+	+ +
Evaluation mark 9	1	1	0	2	0
8	7	6	6	11	3
7	3	8	2	9	1
6	5	0	0	7	0
5	0	2	0	0	0

ACKER, H. B., Organisationsanalyse; Verfahren und Techniken Praktischer Organisationsarbeit. *Baden-Baden, Verlag für Unternehmensführung, 1963.*

ADORNO, T. W., E. FRENKEL-BRUNSWIK, D. J. LEVINSON and R. N. SANFORD, The Authoritarian Personality, *New York, Harper & Brothers, 1950.*

AMICUCCI, D. J., Budget Variance Trend Reports, *N. A. A. Bulletin-Management Accounting, New York 1965,* 1st section 11, 9-14.

ANTHONY, R. N., Management Accounting, Text and Cases, *Homewood (Ill.), Irwin, 1956.*

ANTHONY, R. N., Planning and Control Systems – A Framework for Analysis, *Boston, Div. of Research, Graduate School of Business Administration, Harvard University, 1965.*

ARGYLE, M., G. GARDNER and F. CIOFFI, The Measurement of Supervisory Methods, *Human Relations, London, 1957,* 4, 295-312.

ARGYLE, M., G. GARDNER and F. CIOFFI, Supervisory Methods Related to Productivity, Absenteeism, and Labour Turnover, *Human Relations, London, 1958,* 1, 23-40.

ARGYRIS, C., The Impact of Budgets on People, *Ithaca, School of Business and Public Administration, Cornell University, 1952.*

ARGYRIS, C., Diagnosing Defenses Against the Outsider, *Journal of Social Issues, 1952,* 3, 24-34.

ARGYRIS, C., Human Problems with Budgets, *Harvard Business Review, 1953,* 1, 97-110.

ARGYRIS, C., Executive Leadership: An Appraisal of a Manager in Action, *New York, Harper & Brothers, 1953.*

ARGYRIS, C., Leadership Pattern in the Plant, *Harvard Business Review, 1954,* 1, 53-76.

ARGYRIS, C., Organization of a Bank, A Study of the Nature of Organization and the Fusion Process, *New Haven (Conn.), Labor and Management Center, Yale University, 1954.*

ARGYRIS, C., Personality and Organization, The Conflict between System and the Individual, *New York, Harper & Brothers, 1957.*

ARGYRIS, C., Creating Effective Research Relationships in Organizations, *Human Organization, 1957,* 1, 34-40.

ARGYRIS, C., The Organization: What Makes It Healthy? *Harvard Business Review, 1958,* 6, 107-106.

ARGYRIS, C., Organizational Effectiveness Under Stress, *Harvard Business Review, 1960,* 3, 137-136.

ARGYRIS, C., Interpersonal Competence and Organizational Effectiveness, *Homewood, Ill., Irwin Dorsey series in behavioral science in business, 1962.*

ARGYRIS, C., Integrating the Individual and the Organization, *New York, John Wiley & Sons, 1964.*

339

BAKKE, E. W., Bonds of Organization – An Appraisal of Corporate Human Relations, *New York, Harper & Brothers*, 1950.

BARR, R. D., The Real Problem of Controllership – Administration, *Financial Executive, Brattleboro (Vt.)*, 1964, 4, 32-36.

BASS, B. M., Some Experimental Approaches to the Study of Organizational Psychology, *Management International., Wiesbaden*, 1963, 3/4, 90-97.

BASS, B. M., and H. J. LEAVITT, Some Experiments in Planning and Operating, *Management Science, Baltimore*, 1963, 4, 574-585.

BAST, G. H., Ploegenarbeid in de Industrie, Verslag van het Sociologische Deel van een Onderzoek, *Arnhem, Van Loghum Slaterus*, 1960.

BECKER, S. W., and D. GREEN, JR., Budgeting and Employee Behavior, *Journal of Business, Chicago*, 1962, 4, 392-402.

BECKER, S. W., and D. GREEN, JR., Budgeting and Employee Behavior: A Rejoinder to a "Reply", *Journal of Business, Chicago*, 1964, 2, 195-197.

BEINUM, H. J. J. VAN, Een Organisatie in Beweging, *Leiden, Stenfert Kroese*, 1963.

BELDEN, T. G. and M. R. BELDEN, The Lengthening Shadow: The Life of Thomas J. Watson, *Boston, Toronto, Little, Brown & Co.*, 1962.

BENARD, C., Mesure des Responsabilités par la Comptabilité de Gestion, *Travail et Methodes, Paris*, 1963, 184, 38-42.

BENNIS, W. G., Revisionist Theory of Leadership, *Harvard Business Review*, 1961, 1, 26-34.

BERNE, E., Games People Play: The Psychology of Human Relationships, *London, André Deutsch*, 1966.

BLAU, P. M. and W. R. SCOTT, Formal Organizations, *London, Routledge & Kegan Paul*, 1963.

BLOK-VAN DER VOORT, E. M., Kwantificering in de Sociologie, *Statistica Neerlandica*, 1964, 3, 341-346.

BLOM, F. W. C., Organisatie voor Directe Kostenbeheersing, *Tijdschrift voor Efficiëntie en Documentatie, Den Haag*, 1964, 6, 312-316.

BLOM, F. W. C., De Controller, *De Naamloze Vennootschap, Roermond*, 1965, 9, 141-143.

BOERS, E. P. J. A., De Delegatie van Verantwoordelijkheid, Psychologisch Beschouwd, *Mededelingen Bureau Personeelsbeheer en Organisatie van de Vereniging van Nederlandse Gemeenten, Den Haag*, 1962, 3, 13-41.

BOLLE DE BAL, M., Sociologisch Onderzoek en Industriele Praktijk, *Synopsis, Brussel*, 1965, 89, 1-22.

BONHAM-CARTER, A. D., Centralisation and Decentralisation in Unilever, *Appendix VII in Edwards and Townsend, Business Enterprise, Its Growth and Organisation, London, Macmillan & Co.*, 1958.

BONINI, C. P., Simulating Organizational Behavior, *Chapter 15 in Cooper et al., New Perspectives in Organization Research, New York/London, John Wiley & Sons*, 1964.

BONINI, C. P., Simulation of Organizational Behavior, *in Bonini et al., Management Controls, New York/London, McGraw Hill*, 1964.

BOS, A. H., Sociologische en Psychologische Aspecten van Bedrijfssignalering, *Bedrijfssignalering, verslag Efficiencydagen 1955, Publicatie no. 350 van het N.I.V.E. Den Haag*, 1955, 15-38.

BOSBOOM, P. H., Te Stellen Hogere Eisen aan de Samenhang in de Organisatie en Mogelijke Organisatorische Oplossingen, *Gemeenschappelijk Informatie- en Documentatie-*

bureau voor Organisatiewerk in de Rijksdienst, Publicatie no. 65, Den Haag, 1962.

BOWERS, D. G., Organizational Control in an Insurance Company, *Sociometry* 1964, 2, 230-244.

BRADSHAW, T. F. and C. C. HULL (eds.), Controllership in Modern Management, *Chicago, Irwin, 1950.*

BROWN, J. A. C., The Social Psychology of Industry, *Harmondsworth, Pelican Book, 1954.*

BROWN, W. B. D., Exploration in Management, *London, Heinemann, 1960.*

BROWN, W. B. D., Organisation and Science, *Work Study and Management, London, 1964, 5, 208-215.*

BUCHANAN, P. C., The Leader Looks at Individual Motivation, *Looking into Leadership Monograph, Washington, Leadership resources Inc., 1961.*

BUITER, J. H., Production Standards, Financial Incentives and the Reactions of Workers, *Work Study and Management, London, 1964, 8, 354-362.*

BURKENS, J. C. J., Het Moderne Ziekenhuis: Prestatie en Probleem, *Wending, Den Haag, 1956/57, 10/11, 609-625.*

BUZZARD, R. B., People in Industry – Statistical Indices and Records, *Personnel Management, London, 1962, 361, 157-170.*

CARZO, R., JR., Some Effects of Organization Structure on Group Effectiveness, *Administrative Science Quarterly, Ithaca, 1963, 4, 393-424.*

CASSEE, E. TH., Leidinggeven in Ziekenhuizen: een nadere beschouwing, *Mens en Onderneming, Leiden, 1965, 3, 197-207.*

CAUSSIN, R., Les Bases Psychologiques du Controle Budgétaire, *Organisation Scientifique, Bruxelles, 1947, 11, 254-258.*

C.B.S. (Centraal Bureau voor de Statistiek), Statistisch Zakboek 1965, *Hilversum, W. de Haan N.V., 1965.*

CHARNES, A. and A. C. STEDRY, Further Explorations in the Theory of Multiple Budgeted Goals, *Research Paper no. 12, Organization Research Program, School of Industrial Management, M.I.T., Cambridge (Mass.), 1963.*

CHARNES, A., and A. C. STEDRY, Investigations in the Theory of Multiple Budgeted Goals, in Bonini et al., *Management Controls, New York/London, Mc Graw Hill, 1964.*

CHARNES A. and A. C. STEDRY, Exploratory Models in the Theory of Budget Control, *Chapter 13 in Cooper et al., New Perspectives in Organization Research, New York/London, John Wiley & Sons, 1964.*

CHARNES, A. and A. C. STEDRY, The Attainment of Organization Goals Through Appropriate Selection of Sub-Unit Goals, *Publication no. 86, Research Program on the Organization and Management of R. and D., Sloan School of Management, M.I.T., Cambridge (Mass.), 1964.*

CHILD, I. L. and J. W. M. WHITING, Determinants of Level of Aspiration: Evidence from Everyday Life, *in Brand (ed.) The Study of Personality, New York/London, John Wiley & Sons, 1954.*

CHURCHILL, N. C. and W. W. COOPER, Effect of Auditing Records: Individual Task Accomplishment and Organization Objectives, *Chapter 14 in Cooper et al., New Perspectives in Organization Research, New York/London, John Wiley and Sons, 1964.*

CHURCHMAN, C. W., and A. H. SCHAINBLATT, The Researcher and the Manager: A Dialectic of Implementation, *Management Science, Baltimore, 1965, 4, B-69-87.*

CHURCHMAN, C. W. and others, Commentaries on "The Researcher and the Manager: A Dialectic of Implementation", *Management Science, Baltimore*, 1965, 2, B-1-55.

COCH, L. and J. R. P. FRENCH, JR., Overcoming Resistance to Change, *Human Relations, London*, 1948, 4, 512-534 *(also in Cartwright & Zander, Group Dynamics, New York, Row, Peterson & Comp*, 1953, 237).

COFER, C. N. and M. H. APPLEY, Motivation: Theory and Research, *New York/London, John Wiley & Sons*, 1963.

COHEN, J., P. COOPER and P. THORNE, A Note On Communication in a Factory, *Occupational Psychology, London*, 1965, 1, 25-30.

COLEMAN, C. J., Avoiding the Pitfalls in Results-Oriented Appraisals, *Personnel*, 1965, 24-34.

COOPER, R., Leader's Task Relevance and Subordinate Behaviour in Industrial Work Groups, *Human Relations, London*, 1966, 1, 57-84.

CROZIER, M., Le Contexte Sociologique des Relations Hiérarchiques, *Organisation Scientifique, Bruxelles*, 1964, 2, 29-36.

CYERT, R. M. and J. G. MARCH, The Behavioral Theory of the Firm; A Behavioral Science – Economics Amalgam, *Chapter 16 in Cooper et al., New Perspectives in Organization Research, New York/London, John Wiley and Sons*, 1964.

DALE, E., Functions of the Manager of Tomorrow, *Training Directors Journal*, 1963, 9, 25-36.

DALZIEL, S. and L. KLEIN, The Human Implications of Work Study, The Case of Pakitt Ltd., *Stevenage (Herts.) Human Sciences Unit, Warren Spring Laboratory*, 1960.

DAVIS, K., The Case for Participative Management, *Business Horizons, Bloomington (Ind.)*, 1963, 3, 55-60.

DOORN, J. A. A. VAN, et al., Produktiebeheersing m.b.v. Normstelling in Dienstverlenende Afdelingen, *De Ingenieur, Den Haag*, 1964, 50/51, A 761-782.

DREVER, J., A Dictionary of Psychology, *London, Penguin Reference Book*, 1952.

DRUCKER, P. F., The Practice of Management, *London, Heinemann*, 1961.

DRUCKER, P. F., Control, Controls and Management, *in Bonini et al., Management Controls, New York/London, Mc Graw Hill*, 1964.

DUNNINGTON, R. A., D. SIROTA and S. M. KLEIN, Research for Organization Theory and Management Action, *Industrial Relations Research Association*, 1963.

EGLIN, R., Management Accounting in Practice, *Business (The Management Journal), London*, 1965, 11, 76-80.

EILON, S., Control Systems with Several Controllers, *The Journal of Management Studies, Oxford*, 1965, 3, 259-268.

EILON, S., A Classification of Administrative Control Systems, *The Journal of Management Studies, Oxford*, 1966, 1, 36-48.

ERP, TH. M. VAN, Variabele Budgettering en Kostenbeheersing, *Tijdschrift voor Efficiëntie en Documentatie, Den Haag*, 1965, 13, 978-982.

ESHBACH, A. R. and L. A. SHENE, Selling a Cost Control Program to the Foreman, *Cost and Management, Hamilton*, 1964, 1, 11-17.

EVAN, W. M., Organization Man and Due Process of Law, *American Sociological Review*, 1961, 4, 540-547.

EVAN, W. M., Les Conditions Fonctionnelles d'Existence d'Organisations Industrielles Volontaires, *Sociologie du Travail, Paris*, 1963, 237-247.

EVAN, W. M., Indices of the Hierarchical Structure of Industrial Organization, *Management Science*, Baltimore, 1963, 3, 468-478.

EVANS. M. G., Supervisors' Attitudes and Departmental Performance, *The Journal of Management Studies*, Oxford, 1965, 2, 174-190.

FESTINGER, L., A Theory of Social Comparison Processes, *Human Relations*, London, 1954, 2, 117-140.

FESTINGER, L., A Theory of Cognitive Dissonance, *Evanston, Row, Peterson & Company*, 1957.

FESTINGER, L. and D. KATZ, (eds.), Research Methods in the Behavioral Sciences, New York, The Dryden Press, 1953.

FIRMIN, P. A., The Potential of Accounting as a Management Information System, *Management International*, Wiesbaden, 1966, 2, 35-55.

FORRESTER, J. W., Industrial Dynamics, New York, The M.I.T. Press & John Wiley & Sons, 1961.

FRASER, J. M., Human Relations in a Fully Employed Democracy, London, Sir Isaac Pitman and Sons Ltd., 1960.

FRENCH, J. R. P. JR., J. ISRAEL and D. AAS, An Experiment on Participation in a Norwegian Factory: Interpersonal Dimensions of Decision Making, *Human Relations*, London, 1960, 1, 3-20.

FRENCH, J. R. P. JR., E. KAY and H. H. MEYER, Participation and the Appraisal System, *Human Relations*, London, 1966, 1, 3-20.

FUYUUME, J., Working with Operating Management, *N.A.A. bulletin – Management Accounting*, 1965, 1st section, 1, 51-57.

GAYNOR, E. W., Use of Control Charts in Cost Control, *N.A.C.A. Bulletin*, 1954, 1st section, 10, 1300-1308.

GELLERMAN, S. W., Motivation and Productivity, New York, American Management Association, 1963.

GIBBS, C. B. and I. D. BROWN, Increased Production from the Information Incentive in a Repetitive Task, *The Manager*, London, 1956, 374-379.

GORDON, M. J., Toward a Theory of Responsibility Acounting Systems, *N.A.A. Bulletin* 1963, 1st section, 4, 3-10.

GRAAF, M. H. K. VAN DER, Psychologische Aspecten van de Planning, *Maandblad voor Bedrijfsadministratie en -organisatie*, Den Haag, 1965, 814, 9-11.

GROFFEN, W. H., Horizontaal Organiseren, *Alphen a/d Rijn, Samson*, 1963.

GROFFEN, W. H., Gevoelens in een Rationele Bedrijfshuishouding, *Doelmatig Bedrijfsbeheer*, Alphen a/d Rijn, 1965, 9, 386-390.

GROOT, A. M., De Engels-Amerikaanse Methode van Budgettering, *De Naamloze Vennootschap*, Roermond, 1960, 10/11, 211-213.

GROOT, A. D. DE, Methodologie, Grondslagen van Onderzoek en Denken in de Gedragswetenschappen, Den Haag, Mouton & Co. 1961.

GROSS, B. M., What are Your Organization's Objectives? *Human Relations*, London, 1965, 3, 195-216.

GUEST, R. H., Organizational Change: The Effect of Successful Leadership, Homewood, Ill., *Irwin Dorsey series in behavioral sciehce in business*, 1962.

GUEST, R. H., Managerial Succession in Complex Organizations, *The American Journal of Sociology*, Chicago, 1962, 1, 47-57.

343

GURIN, G., Work Satisfactions, in *The Worker in the New Industrial Environment*, Ann Arbor, Mich. *Foundation for Research on Human Behavior*, 1962.

GURIN, G., J. VEROFF and S. FELD, Americans View Their Mental Health, New York, *Basic Books Inc.*, 1960.

HAIRE, M., The Concept of Power and the Concept of Man in *Argyris et al.*, *Social Science Approaches to Business Behavior*, Homewood, Ill., Irwin, 1962.

HAIRE, M., The Social Sciences and Management Practices, *California Management Review*, 1964, 4, 3-10.

HALL, J. G., Human Relations – A Challenge to Accountants, *Cost and Management*, Hamilton, 1963, 11, 512-515.

HALL, J. G., Something Old, Something New: Acounting-Management Relationship, *Cost and Management*, Hamilton, 1964, 4, 155-161.

HALL, M. P., Communication within Organizations, *The Journal of Management Studies*, Oxford, 1965, 1, 54-70.

HARBISON, F. H. and B. W. BURGESS, Modern Management in Western Europe, *The American Journal of Sociology*, Chicago, 1954, 1, 15-23.

HARMAN, H. H., Modern Factor Analysis, *London/Chicago*, *The University of Chicago Press*, 1965.

HECKHAUSEN, H., Leistungsmotivation, *in Handbuch der Psychologie, 2. Band, Allgemeine Psychologie II, Motivation*, Göttingen, *Verlag für Psychologie*, 1965.

HENDERSON, P. W. and B. R. COPELAND, Application of Probability to Cost Control Reports, *Financial Executive*, Brattleboro (Vt.), 1965, 12, 40-44.

HENRICI, S. B., New Views on Standards, *N.A.A. Bulletin-Management Accounting*, 1965, 1st section 11, 3-9.

HERZBERG, F., B. MAUSNER and B. B. SNYDERMAN, The Motivation to Work, New York, *John Wiley and Sons*, 1959.

HESSELING, P. G. M., Sociaal-Psychologische Aspecten van Taakstelling voor Handenarbeid in de Industrie, *Arbeidskundig Tijdschrift*, Den Haag, 1963, 72, 76, 77, 11-23, 206-216, 238-258.

HOFSTEDE, G. H., Normstelling als Gereedschap voor Managers, *Doelmatig Bedrijfsbeheer*, Alphen a/d Rijn, 1964, 6, 7, 8, 9, 214-216, 273-277, 309-310, 340-342.

HOFSTEDE, G. H., Arbeidsmotieven van Volontairs, *Mens en Onderneming*, Leiden, 1964, 373-392.

HOLDEN, P. E., L. S. FISH and H. L. SMITH, Top Management Organization and Control, A Research Study of the Management Policies and Practices of Thirty-one Leading Industrial Corporations, *Calif./London*, *Stanford University Press*, 1941.

HORRINGA, D., Bestuursklimaat in Relatie tot Medezeggenschap, *Chapter III in Marka-Pocket no. 16*, Utrecht/Antwerpen, Marka Boeken, 1965.

HUGHES, C. L., Goal Setting, Key to Individual and Organizational Effectiveness, New York, *American Management Association*, 1965.

HUIZINGA, J., Homo Ludens, Proeve ener Bepaling van het Spel-Element der Cultuur, Haarlem, *H. D. Tjeenk Willink & Zoon*, 1958 (English edition: London, Routledge, 1949).

HUTTE, H. A., Ontwerp voor een Nederlandse Arbeids-Sociatrie, *Mens en Onderneming*, Leiden, 1959/1960, several numbers (8).

344

HUTTE, H. A., Decision-Taking in a Management Game, *Human Relations, Londin,* 1965, 1, 5-20.

HUTTE, H. A., Sociatrie van de Arbeid, *Assen, Van Gorcum,* 1966.

INDIK, B. P., B. S. GEORGOPOULOS and S. E. SEASHORE, Superior-Subordinate Relationships and Performance, *Personnel Psychology, Baltimore,* 1961, 4, 357-375.

IRLE, M., Demokratische Betriebsführung – Ein Weg der Produktivitätssteigerung?, *Rationalisierung, Munchen,* 1963, 7, 160-162.

IRLE, M., Informationen und Entscheidungen in der Linien – Stabsorganisation, *Psychologie und Praxis, Stuttgart,* 1963, 3, 97-104.

I.S.R. (Institute for Social Research of the University of Michigan), Manual for Interviewers, *Survey Research Center, Ann Arbor,* 1960.

I.S.R., Manual for Coders (Content Analysis), *Survey Research Center, Ann Arbor,* 1961.

JASINSKY, F. J., Use and Missue of Efficiency Controls, *Harvard Business Review,* 1956, 4, 105-112.

JOHNSON, R. A., F. E. KAST and J. E. ROSENZWEIG, The Theory and Management of Systems, *New York, McGraw Hill,* 1963.

JONGE, H. DE and G. WIELENGA, Statistische Methoden voor Psychologen en Sociologen, *Groningen, Wolters,* 1963.

KAHN, R. L. and C. F. CANNELL, The Dynamics of Interviewing, *New York, John Wiley & Sons,* 1957.

KAHN, R. L. and N. C. MORSE, The Relationship of Productivity to Morale, *The Journal of Social Issues,* 1951, 3, 8-18.

KAHN, R. L., D. M. WOLFE, R. P. QUINN, J. D. SNOEK and R. A. ROSENTHAL, Organizational Stress: Studies in Role Conflict & Ambiguity, *New York, John Wiley & Sons,* 1964.

KAST, F. E., Management Concepts and Practices – European Style, *Business Horizons, Bloomington (Ind.),* 1964, 4, 25-36.

KLEIN, L., Rationality in Management Control, *The Journal of Management Studies, Oxford,* 1965, 3, 351-361.

KNIGHT, W. D. and E. H. WEINWURM, Managerial Budgeting, A Behavioral Approach to the Successful Adaptation of a Budgeting System from a Managerial Viewpoint, *New York, The Macmillan Co., London, Collier-McMillan Ltd.,* 1964.

KOLAJA, J., A Yugoslav Workers' Council, *Reprint fron Human Organization, by the Center for Productivity Motivation, The University of Wisconsin,* 1960.

KÖNIG, R., Das Interview: Formen, Technik, Auswertung, *Köln/Berlin, Kiepenheuer & Witsch,* 1962.

LAMMERS, C. J., De Sociologische Studie van Leiderschap in Organisaties, *Mens en Onderneming, Leiden,* 1965, 3, 131-152.

LAMMERS, C. J. et al., Medezeggenschap en Overleg in het Bedrijf, *Marka-pocket no. 16, Utrecht/Antwerpen, Marka Boeken,* 1965.

LAWLER, E. E., Ability as a Moderator of the Relationship between Job Attitudes and Job Performance, *Personnel Psychology, Baltimore,* 1966, 2, 153-164.

LAWRENCE, L. C. and P. C. SMITH, Group Decision and Employee Participation, *Journal of Applied Psychology,* 1955, 5, 334-337.

LEAVITT, H. J., Unhuman Organizations, *Harvard Business Review,* 1962, 4, 90-98.

LEAVITT, H. J., The Manager of To-Morrow, *Training Directors Journal,* 1963, 9, 37-45.

LEAVITT, H. J., Applied Organization Change in Industry: Structural, Technical and Human Approaches, in Cooper et al., *New Perspectives in Organization Research*, New York/London, John Wiley & Sons, 1964.

LEAVITT, H. J., A Framework for Thinking About Future Management Information Systems (Informatie technologie en het management van morgen), *Doelmatig Bedrijfsbeheer*, Alphen a/d Rijn, 1965, 5, 209-300.

LEENT, J. A. A. VAN, Sociale Psychologie in Drie Dimensies, *Utrecht/Antwerpen, Aula-boek*, 1963.

LEVINSON, H., C. R. PRICE, K. J. MUNDEN, H. J. MANDL and C. M. SOLLEY, Men, Management and Mental Health, *Cambridge (Mass.), Harvard University Press*, 1964.

LEWIN, K., Field Theory in Social Science, Selected Theoretical Papers, *New York, Harper & Brothers*, 1951.

LEWIN, K., T. DEMBO, L. FESTINGER and P. S. SEARS, Level of Aspiration, in *J. M. Hunt (ed.), Personality and the Behavior Disorders*, New York, The Ronald Press Company, 1944.

LIEBERMAN, S., The Effects of Changes in Roles on the Attitudes of Role Occupants, *Human Relations*, London, 1956, 4, 385-403.

LIKERT, R., Effective Supervision: An Adaptive and Relative Process, *Personnel Psychology*, Baltimore, 1058, 3, 317-332.

LIKERT, R., New Patterns of Management, *New York, Mc Graw Hill*, 1961.

LIKERT, R., New Patterns in Sales Management, *Michigan Business Papers, Ann Arbor*, 1962, 37.

LIKERT, R., Trends Toward A World-Wide Theory of Management, *Institute for Social Research Newsletter, Ann Arbor*, oct., 1963.

LIKERT, R. and R. LIPITT, The Utilization of Social Science, in *Festinger & Katz*, (eds.), *Research Methods in the Behavioral Sciences*, New York. The Dryden Press, 1953.

LIKERT, R. and S. E. SEASHORE, Making Cost Control Work, *Harvard Business Review*, 1963, 6, 96-108.

LIMPERG, TH. JR., Bedrijfseconomie, Deel V, Leer van de Inwendige Organisatie, *Deventer, Kluwer*, 1965.

LODAHL, T. M., Patterns of Job Attitudes in Two Assembly Technologies, *Administrative Science Quarterly*, Ithaca, 1964, 8, 482-520.

LODAHL, T. M. and M. KEJNER, The Definition and Measurement of Job Involvement, *Ithaca, publication of the Graduate School of Business and Public Adinistration, Cornell University*, 1964.

LOGAN, H. H., Line and Staff: An Obsolete Concept?, *Personnel*, New York, 1966, 1, 26-33.

LUPTON, T. and J. H. HORNE, The Work Activities of "Middle" Managers; an Exploratory Study, *Journal of Management Studies*, Oxford, 1965, 1, 14-34.

LUYK, H., Doelmatige Taakvorming, *Doelmatig Bedrijfsbeheer*, Alphen a/d Rijn, 1963, 9, 348-352.

MCCALL, R. J., Invested Self-Expression: A Principle of Human Motivation, *Psychological Review, American Psychological Association*, 1963, 4, 289-303.

MCCLELLAND, D. C., The Achieving Society, *Princeton, N. J., D. Van Nostrand Co. Inc.*, 1961.

MCGRATH, J. E., Toward A "Theory of Method" for Research on Organizations,

Chapter 28 in Cooper et al., *New Perspectives in Organization Research, New York/ London, John Wiley & Sons,* 1964.

MCGREGOR, D., An Uneasy Look at Performance Appraisal, *Harvard Business Review,* 1957, 3, 89–94.

MCGREGOR, D., The Human Side of Enterprise, *New York, McGraw Hill,* 1960.

MCMURRY, R. N., The Case for Benevolent Autocracy, *Harvard Business Review,* 1958, 1, 82–90.

MACNAUGHTON, J. D., A Study of Foreman's Communication, *Personnel Practice Bulletin, Canberra,* 1963, 1, 10–20.

MAIER, N. R. F., Psychology in Industry, A Psychological Approach to Industrial Problems, *London, George G. Harrap & Co. Ltd.,* 1959.

MAIER, N. R. F., Hoe de Beslissingen op het Peil van de Bedrijfsleiding te Verbeteren, *Synopsis, Brussel,* 1964, 71, 39–48.

MAIER, N. R. F., L. R. HOFFMAN, J. J. HOOVEN and W. H. READ, Superior – Subordinate Communication in Management, *New York, American Management Association,* 1961.

MANAGER, The, Who Wants Social Research in Industry?, *The Manager, London,* 1964, 21–23.

MARCH, J. G. and H. A. SIMON, Organizations, *New York, John Wiley & Sons,* 1958.

MARIS, M., Het Masterbudget, *De Naamloze Vennootschap, Roermond,* 1960, 10/11, 207–210.

MARRIOTT, R., Incentive Payment Systems; A Review of Research and Opinion, *London, Staples Press,* 1961.

MASLOW, A. H., Motivation and Personality, *New York/London, Harper & Row,* 1954.

MASON, J. I., Operating Variance Analysis, *The Cost Accountant, London,* 1964, 8, 300–303.

MATTESSICH, R., Accounting And Analytical Methods, *Homewood (Ill.), Irwin,* 1964.

MAYNTZ, R., Zum Gegenwärtigen Stand der Organisationssoziologie, *Betriebswirtschaftliche Mitteilungen, no. 29, Bern, Verlag Paul Haupt,* 1964.

MECHANIC, D., Sources of Power of Lower Participants in Complex Organizations, in *New Perspectives in Organization Research, New York/London, John Wiley & Sons,* 1964.

MELLEROWICZ, K., Betriebswirtschaftslehre der Industie, *Freiburg im Breisgau, Rudolf Haufe Verlag,* 1958.

MERTON, R. K., Social Theory and Social Structure, *Glencoe (Ill.), The Free Press,* 1957.

METCALF, H. C. and L. URWICK (eds.), Dynamic Administration, The Collected Papers of Mary Parker Follett., *New York & London, Harper & Brothers,* 1940.

MEUWESE, W., The Effect of the Leader's Ability and Interpersonal Attitudes on Group Creativity under Varying Conditions of Stress, *Groningen, V.R.B.,* 1964.

MEY, A., Bedrijfsbegroting en Bedrijfsbeleid, *Leiden, Stenfert Kroese N.V.,* 1951.

MEY, J.L., Organisatie, Budgettering en Administratieve Verantwoording, *'s Gravenhage, Delwel,* 1960.

MEYER, H. H., E. KAY and J. R. P. FRENCH, JR., Split Roles in Performance Appraisal, *Harvard Business Review,* 1965, 1, 123–129.

MEYNEN, J., Werknemers-Medezeggenschap en de Oplossing van het Sociale Vraagstuk in de Onderneming, *Amsterdam, H. Sijthoff's Financiële Bladen,* 1961.

MILES, R. E. and VERGIN, R. C., Behavioral Properties of Variance Controls, *California Management Review,* 1966, 3, 57–65.

MILLER, V. V., Human Behavior and Budget Controls, *Advanced Management – Office Executive*, 1962, 12, 30–34.

MONHEMIUS, W., Besliskunde, een Vlag die de Lading Dekt? *Statistica Neerlandica*, 1963, 4, 363–383.

MORRIS, W. T., Management Science in Action, *Homewood Ill., Richard D. Irwin Inc.*, 1963.

MORSE, N. E. and E. REIMER, The Experimental Change of a Major Organizational Variable, *Journal of Abnormal & Social Psychology*, 1956, 1, 120–130.

MORSE, N. C., E. REIMER and A. S. TANNENBAUM, Regulation and Control in Hierarchical Organizations, *The Journal of Social Issues*, 1951, 3, 41–49.

MULDER, M., Machtsmotief, Positieve en Negative Identificatie, in *Mulder et al.*, Mensen, Groepen, Organisaties, Assen, Van Gorcum, 1963.

MULDER, M., Decisie Structuur en Groepsprestatie, in *Mulder et al.*, Mensen, Groepen, Organisaties, Assen, Van Gorcum, 1963.

MULDER, M., R. VAN DIJK, T. STELWAGEN, J. VERHAGEN, S. SOUTENDIJK and J. ZWEZERIJNEN, Illegitimacy of Power and Positivity of Attitudes Toward the Power Person, *Human Relations*, London, 1966, 1, 21–38.

MYERS, M. S., Who Are Your Motivated Workers?, *Harvard Business Review*, 1964, 1, 73–88.

N.A.A. BULLETIN, Departures in Communicating Accounting Data to Foremen; A Summary of Practice, *N.A.A. Bulletin*, 1963, 3rd section, 5, 3–21.

NAUS, P. J., De Effectiviteit van Schriftelijke Mededelingen in een Bedrijf, *Tijdschrift voor Psychologie, Gawein*, Nijmegen, 1963, 3, 199–233.

N.I.C.B. (National Industrial Conference Board) Behavioral Science – What's in it For Management? *Business Management Record*, 1963.

N.I.P.G. (Nederlands Instituut voor Praeventieve Geneeskunde), Hoe Denkt U Over Uw Werk?, *Den Haag, C.O.P.*, 1958.

NOBLE, C. E., Calculating Control Limits for Cost Control Data, *N.A.C.A. Bulletin*, 1954, 1st section, 10, 1310–1317.

NOWOTNY, O. H., American Vs. European Management Philosophy, *Harvard Business Review*, 1964, 2, 101–108.

ODIORNE, G. S., Do the Best Men Get To the Top? *Challenge, The Magazine of Economic Affairs*, New York, 1964.

O.E.E.C. (A. V. DeMarco), Cost Reduction in Industry, an Integrated Approach to the Practical Application of Progressive Management Techniques for the Control and Reduction of Cost, *Paris, OEEC European Productivity Agency*, 1961.

OUBRIDGE, V. W., Management Control, *The Manager*, London, 1960, 513–517.

PARKER, T. C., Relationships Among Measures of Supervisory Behavior, Group Behavior, and Situational Characteristics, *Personnel Psychology*, Baltimore, 1963, 4, 319–334.

PATCHEN, M., Supervisory Methods and Group Performance Norms, *Administrative Science Quarterly*, Ithaca, 1962, 3, 275–294.

PATCHEN, M., Alternative Questionnaire Approaches To The Measurement Of Influence in Organizations, *The American Journal of Sociology*, Chicago, 1963, 1, 41–52.

PATCHEN, M., Participation in Organizational Decision-Making and Member Motivation: What is the Relation?, *Personnel Administration*, 1964, 24–31.

PATCHEN, M., Labor-Management Consultation at TVA, Its Impact on Employees, *Administrative Science Quarterly*, 1965, 2, 149-174.

PELZ, D. C., Leadership Within a Hierarchical Organization, *The Journal of Social Issues*, 1951, 3, 49-56.

PELZ, D. C., Freedom in Research, *International Science and Technology*, New York, 1964. 54-63.

PHILIPSEN, H., Medezeggenschap in de Vorm van Werkoverleg, *in Marka-pocket no. 16*, Utrecht/Antwerpen, Marka Boeken, 1965.

PHILIPSEN, H. and E. TH. CASSEE, Verschillen in de Wijze van Leidinggeven Tussen Drie Typen Organisaties, *Mens en Onderneming*, Leiden, 1965, 3, 172-184.

POTTER, S., The Theory and Practice of Gamesmanship, *Harmondsworth, Penguin Books*, 1962.

PUTTEN, A. VAN, Budgettering en Planning, *De Naamloze Vennootschap*, Leiden, 1960, 10/11, 222-224.

PYM, D., Effective Managerial Performance in Organizational Change, *The Journal of Management Studies*, 1966, 1, 73-84.

RAIA, A. P., Goal Setting and Self-Control, An Empirical Study, *The Journal of Management Studies*, 1965, 1, 34-53.

RATHE, A. W., Management Controls in Business, *in D. G. Malcolm & A. J. Rowe, Management Control Systems*, New York, John Wiley & Sons, 1960.

READ, W. H., Upward Communication in Industrial Hierarchies, *Human Relations*, London, 1962, 1, 3-15.

REINOUD, H., Personnel Management and Business Efficiency, *Personnel Management*, London, 1961/1962, 358/359, 245-251, 33-45.

REINOUD, H., Bedrijfsbegroting en Planning op Lange Termijn, *Tijdschrift voor Efficiëntie en Documentatie*, Den Haag, 1965, 1, 31-32.

REVANS, R. W., Quantitative Methods in Management, *Management International*, Wiesbaden, 1964, 3, 27-36.

REVANS, R. W., Attitudes Toward Operational Change, *Lecture for IBM WTC Executive Development Department, Blaricum (Neth.)*, 1964.

REVANS, R. W., Science and the Manager, London, MacDonald, 1965.

RICE, A. K., The Enterprise and its Environment, a System Theory of Management Organization, *London, Tavistock Publications*, 1963.

RIDGWAY, V. F., Dysfunctional Consequences of Performance Measurements, *Administrative Science Quarterly*, Ithaca, 1956, 2.

RILEY, W. P., Staff and Line Responsibilities for Overhead Cost, Control, *AMA Management Bulletin*, 1961, 14, 9-13.

ROBERTS, E. B., Industrial Dynamics and the Design of Management Control Systems, *in Bonini, et al., Management Controls*, New York, London, McGraw Hill, 1964.

ROTTER, J. B., Social Learning and Clinical Psychology, *Psychology Series*, New York, Prentice Hall Inc., 1954.

ROWE, K. H., An Appraisal of Appraisals, *The Journal of Management Studies*, Oxford, 1964, 1, 1-25.

RUCKSTUHL, P., La Gestion dans l'Imprimerie, Paris, Dunod, 1960.

RÜSSEL, A., Spiel und Arbeit in der Menschlichen Entwicklung, *in Entwicklungspsycho-*

logie, 3. Band vom Handbuch der Psychologie, Göttingen, Verlag für Psychologie, 1958.

RUSSEN GROEN, R. D. VAN, Berichtgeving aan Lager Kader in Twee Fabrieken te Stads-kanaal, *Philips Administration Review, Eindhoven,* 1965, 1, 7-14.

SALVESON, M. E., An Analysis of Decisions, *Management Science, Baltimore,* 1958, 3, 203-217.

SCHAAFSMA, A. H., Produktieplanning, Hulpmiddel bij het Besturen van de Onder-neming, *De Ingenieur, Den Haag,* 1963, 47, A 641-644.

SCHACHTER, S., B. WILLERMAN, L. FESTINGER & R. HYMAN, Emotional Disruption and Industrial Productivity, *Journal of Applied Psychology,* 1961, 4, 201-213.

SCHLEH, E. C., The Fallacy in Measuring Management, *Dun's Review and Modern Industry,* 1963, 49-54.

SCHOLMA, C., Budgettering en Standaardkosten, *Alphen aan de Rijn, Samson,* 1961.

SCHROEFF, H. J. VAN DER, Staforganen en Staffuncties in de Organisatie, *Maandblad voor Accountancy en Bedrijfshuishouding, Purmerend,* 1958, 3, 91-108.

SCHWARTZ, M. M., E. JENUSAITIS and H. STARK, Motivational Factors, Among Supervisors in the Utility Industry, *Personnel Psychology, Baltimore,* 1963, 1, 45-53.

SEASHORE, S. E. and D. G. BOWERS, Communications and Decision Processes as Deter-minants of Organizational Effectiveness, *Survey Research Center ISR, Ann Arbor,* 1962.

SEASHORE, S. E., B. P. INDIK and B. S. GEORGOPOULOS, Relationships Among Criteria of Job Performance, *Journal of Applied Psychology,* 1960, 3, 195-202.

SHILLINGLAW, G., Divisional Performance Review: An Extension of Budgetary Control, *in Bonini et al., Management Controls, New York, Mc Graw Hill,* 1964.

SIMON, H. A., The New Science of Management Decision, *New York, Harper & Bros,* 1960.

SIMON, H. A., On the Concept of Organizational Goal, *Administrative Science Quarterly, Ithaca,* 1964, 1, 1-22.

SIMON, H. A., H. GUETZKOW, G. KOZMETSKY and G. TYNDALL, Centralization Vs. Decen-tralization in Organizing the Controller's Department, *New York, Controllership Foundation Inc.,* 1954.

SLATER, P. E. and W. G. BENNIS, Democracy is Inevitable, *Harvard Business Review,* 1964, 2, 51-59.

SMIDDY, H. F., Notes on the Nature and Function of Professional Managing, *Management International, Wiesbaden,* 1962, 5, 5-18.

SMITH, C. G. and A. S. TANNENBAUM, Organizational Control Structure: A Comparative Analysis, *Human Relations, London,* 1963, 4, 299-316.

SORD, B. H. and G. A. WELSCH, Business Budgeting, A Survey of Management Planning and Control Practices, *New York, Controllership Foundation,* 1962.

SPITZ, J. C., Statistiek voor Psychologen, Pedagogen, Sociologen, *Amsterdam, Noord-Hollandsche Uitgevers Mij.,* 1965.

STARBUCK, W. H., Level of Aspiration, *Psychological Review, American Psychological Association,* 1963, 1, 51-60.

STARREVELD, R. W., Leer van de Administratieve Organisatie, *Alphen a/d Rijn, Samson,* 1962.

STARREVELD, R. W., Bedrijfsleiding en Informatie-Economie, *Maandblad voor Accountancy en Bedrijfshuishoudkunde, Purmerend,* 1965, 9, 322-334.

STEDRY, A. C., Budget Control and Cost Behavior, *Englewood Cliffs N.J., Prentice-Hall, Inc.*, 1960.

STEDRY, A. C., Aspiration Levels, Attitudes, and Performance in a Goal-Oriented Situation, *Industrial Management Review, School of Industrial Management, M.I.T., Cambridge (Mass.)*, 1962, 2, 60-76.

STEDRY, A. C., Budgeting and Employee Behavior: A Reply, *Journal of Business, Chicago*, 1964, 2, 195-202.

STEDRY, A. C., Budgetary Control: A Behavioral Approach, *publication no. 43 of the School of Industrial Management, M.I.T., Cambridge (Mass.)*, 1964.

STEDRY, A. C. and A. CHARNES, Some Models of Organization Response to Budgeted Multiple Goals, *Research publication no. 1 of the School of Industrial Management, M.I.T., Cambridge (Mass.)*, 1964.

STEDRY, A. C. and E. KAY, The Effects of Goal Difficulty on Performance, *Publication BRS-19 by Behavioral Research Service, General Electric Company, Crotonville, N.Y.*, 1964

STEDRY, A. C. and E. KAY, The Effects of Goal Difficulty on Performance: A Field Experiment, *publication of Sloan School of Management, M.I.T., Cambridge (Mass.)*, 1964.

STEWART, R., Reactions to Appraisal Interviews, *The Journal of Management Studies, Oxford*, 1965, 1, 83-100.

STEWART, R., The Use of Diaries to Study Managers' Jobs, *The Journal of Management Studies, Oxford*, 1965, 2, 228-235.

STEWART, R. N., Basic Reports for Management, *Advanced Management – Office Executive*, 1963, 7, 14-17.

STOK, TH. L., De Arbeider en de Zichtbaarmaking van de Kwaliteit, *Leiden, Stenfert Kroese*, 1959.

TANNENBAUM, A. S., Control in Organizations: Individual Adjustment and Organizational Performance, *Administrative Science Quaterly, Ithaca*, 1962, 2, 236-257.

TANNENBAUM, A. S. and S. E. SEASHORE, Some Changing Conceptions and Approaches to the Study of Persons in Organizations, *Survey Research Center, University of Michigan, Ann Arbor*, 1963.

TANNENBAUM, R. and W. H. SCHMIDT, How to Choose A Leadership Pattern, *Harvard Business Review*, 1958, 2, 95-101.

TEULINGS, A. W. M. and C. J. LAMMERS, Medezeggenschap in een Tiental Bedrijven, *Sociologische Gids*, 1965.

THEIL, H. and D. B. JOCHEMS, De Kunst van het Begroten, *De Naamloze Vennootschap, Roermond*, 1960, 10/11, 181-184.

THOMAE, H. (editor), Allgemeine Psychologie II: Motivation, *Göttingen, Verlag für Psychologie*, 1965.

THOMAE, H., Das Problem der Motivarten, *in Handbuch der Psychologie, 2. Band: Allgemeine Psychologie II, Motivation, Göttingen, Verlag für Psychologie*, 1965.

THOMAS, K., Die Betriebliche Situation der Arbeiter, *Stuttgart, Ferdinand Enke Verlag*, 1964.

TOAN, A. B., JR., Power, Influence, Persuasion and Management Reports, *Financial Executive, Brattleboro (Vt.)*, 1965, 8, 11-15.

TORGERSON, W. S., Theory and Methods of Scaling, *New York/London, John Wiley & Sons/ Chapman & Hall*, 1958.

TOVEY, D. E., The Accountant's Role in Budgeting, *Lausanne, unpublished participants paper of IMEDE*, 1963.

TRULL, S. G., Strategies of Effective Interviewing, *Harvard Business Review*, 1964, 1, 89-94.

VAJDA, S., An Introduction to Linear Programming and the Theory of Games, *London/ New York, Methuen & Co./John Wiley & Sons*, 1960.

VROOM, V. H., Some Personality Determinants of the Effects of Participation, *The Journal of Abnormal and Social Psychology*, 1959, 3, 322-327.

VROOM, V. H., Work and Motivation, *New York/London, John Wiley & Sons*, 1964.

VROOM, V. H., Some Psychological Aspects of Organizational Control, *in Cooper et al., New Perspectives in Organization Research, New York/London, John Wiley & Sons*, 1964.

VROOM, W. H. and F. C. MANN, Leader Authoritarianism and Employee Attitudes, *Personnel Psychology, Baltimore*, 1960, 2, 125-140.

WEINWURM, E. H., Budgeting and Operations Research, *Business Budgeting*, 1962, 5, 13-19.

WELSCH, G. A., Budgeting – Profit Planning and Control, *Englewood Cliffs N. J., Prentice Hall Inc.*, 1964.

WENTWORTH, G. O., A. T. MONTGOMERY, J. A. GOWEN and T. W. HARREL, The Accounting Process, A Program for Self-Instruction, *New York, McGraw Hill*, 1963.

WHITE, R. W., Motivation Reconsidered: The Concept of Competence, *Psychological Review, American Psychological Association*, 1959, 5, 297-333.

WHYTE, W. F., Money and Motivation, An Analysis of Incentives in Industry, *New York, Harper & Brothers*, 1955.

WHYTE, W. H. JR., The Organization Man, *New York, Doubleday Anchor Books*, 1956.

WIENER, N., The Human Use of Human Beings, Cybernetics and Society, *New York, Doubleday Anchor Books*, 1954.

WILLEMZE, F. G., Kwaliteitsbeleid en Industriële Organisatie "Morgen", *Statistica Neerlandica*, 1964, 2, 189-200.

WILLIAMS, L. K., The Process of Feedback in Research, *Ithaca, New York State School of Industrial and Labor Relations, Cornell University*, 1963.

WOLFF, CH. J. DE, et al., Toch Moeten we Beoordelen, *Leiden, Stenfert Kroese, Publ. no. 45, Nederlandse Vereniging van Bedrijfspsychologie*, 1965.

YDO, M. G., Prestatie en Beloning in een Nieuw Licht, *Alphen aan de Rijn, Samson*, 1965.

ZALEZNIK, A., The Dynamics of Subordinacy, *Harvard Business Review*, 1965, 3, 119-131.

ZALKIND, S. S. and T. W. COSTELLO, Perception: Some Recent Research and Implications for Administration, *Administrative Science Quarterly, Ithaca*, 1962, 2, 218-235.

ZANNETOS, Z. S., On the Theory of Divisional Structures: Some Aspects of Centralization and Decentralization of Control and Decision-Making, *Management Science, Baltimore*, 1965, 4, B. 49-68.

ZOBRIST, A., Psychologische Aspekte Betriebswirtschaftlicher Kontrollsituationen, *Referat für Betriebswirtschaftliches Doktorandenseminar der Universität Freiburg (Schweiz)* 1965.

ZOBTHOUT, D. A. C., De Technische en Organisatorische Aspecten van Bedrijfssignalering, *Bedrijfssignalering, verslag Efficiencydagen 1955, Publicatie no. 350 van het N.I.V.E., Den Haag*, 1955, 5-14.

NAME INDEX

Aas, D. 14, 71, 72
Acker, H. B. 111
Adorno, T. W. 196
Amicucci, D. J. 98
Anthony, R. N. 10, 11, 31, 35, 36
Appley, M. H. 46, 47, 64, 79
Argyle, M. 248
Argyris, C. 10, 12, 13, 41, 42, 44 ff., 49, 59, 60, 67, 70, 80, 105, 231, 252, 291

Bakke, E. W. 10, 87
Barr, R. D. 243
Bass, B. M. 68, 257
Bast, H. H. 259
Bat'a, T. 23, 30
Bavelas, A. 71
Becker, S. W. 20, 40, 73, 97, 146, 150
Beinum, H. J. J. van 13, 16
Belden, T. G. and M. R. 2nd title page
Benard, C. 30
Bennis, W. G. 12, 81
Berne, E. 52, 77
Bertalanffy, L. von 86
Blau, P. M. 225, 236
Blok, E. M. 111

Blom, F. W. C. 28, 35
Boers, E. P. J. A. 12
Bolle de Bal, M. 14
Bonham-Carter, A. D. 14
Bonini, C. P. 83, 91, 92
Bos, A. H. 32, 34, 72, 210, 257
Bosboom, P. H. 102
Boulding, K. 86
Bowers, D. G. 9, 11, 305
Bradshaw, T. F. 61
Brown, I. D. 64
Brown, J. A. C. 290
Brown, W. B. D. 87, 253
Buchanan, P. C. 51
Buiter, J. H. 12
Burgess, E. W. 280
Burkens, J. C. J. 103
Buzzard, R. B. 111

Carzo, R. Jr. 72
Cannell, C. F. 111
Cassee, E. Th. 176, 186
Caussin, R. 40
Charnes, A. 83, 90, 93, 94, 118, 176, 177
Child, I. L. 65

353

SUBJECT INDEX

Decision Theory 85
delegation 29, 102
democracy 12
developmental research 105
direct costing 28
discipline 10
distance 81
– geographical 58, 249, 250
drives 46
DYNAMO company 109, 132, 134, 135,
  155, 157ff., 161ff., 183, 185, 192, 204,
  209, 211, 224, 225, 228, 230, 232, 233,
  251, 255, 259, 261, 278, 279, 287ff.,
  305, 313, 316

economic influences 97, 286ff., 315, 316
educational background 274ff., 281ff.
education role of staff 244, 295, 296
efficiency variance 31, 206, 300
effort allocation 94, 252
empire-building 220
EPICURE company 109, 132, 133, 134,
  153, 157ff., 183, 186, 209, 228, 230,
  234, 235, 242, 243, 255, 259, 264, 266,
  287ff., 307ff., 316
esteem needs 52, 61, 62, 74
evaluation marks 156ff., 169ff., 261
exception, management by 36, 37, 61,
  94
expectancy 47ff.
expectation of improvement 153, 154,
  168ff., 172, 261
expected actual cost 24
expense center 30, 189, 203ff., 242, 298
expense variance 31, 206
external reference points 95, 176ff.,
  182ff., 195, 301

factor analysis 46, 120, 121, 130ff.
– of line interview data 131ff., 272
– of staff interview data 225ff., 246
failure 64ff., 156, 168
feedback 17, 84, 95ff., 206
feedback sessions 116, 164, 262, 263, 265
field study 41, 42, 46, 104ff.

fighting the system 50, 81, 212ff., 253
  297
financial incentives 15, 44, 257
forecasting 15, 22, 23
freedom 13
free enterprise 303, 304
frequency of superior-subordinate con
  tact about figures 250, 251ff., 261
  267, 268

game 76ff.
– and budgeting 17, 18, 264, 265
– and business 78
– and standard-setting 81, 82, 190, 19;
– definition of 77
gamesmanship 77
game spirit 73ff., 263ff., 296
Game Theory 77
geographical location 58, 249, 250
goals 48
goal difficulty 44
goal discrepancy 65, 154
goal setting 37
graphs 34, 208, 306
group formation 37, 58ff., 262

Hawthorne Experiments 40, 42
hedonism 53
hierarchical authority 10, 11
hierarchical level 159, 185ff., 189, 275
  276, 281ff., 306ff., 312ff.
Homo Ludens 74
Human Relations 40
hygiene 54, 76, 185, 224, 266, 298

ideology 14
incentives 15, 37, 44, 46, 257
independence 13, 70, 72
Independence factor 132, 182, 187, 251
  262, 263, 276
Industrial Dynamics 90, 91
industrial engineer 27, 93, 113, 114, 152
  184, 195, 222, 235, 242, 301
industrial trades 108
influence 9, 304, 305ff., 310ff.